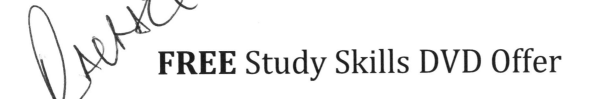

FREE Study Skills DVD Offer

Dear Customer,

Thank you for your purchase from Mometrix! We consider it an honor and a privilege that you have purchased our product and we want to ensure your satisfaction.

As a way of showing our appreciation and to help us better serve you, we have developed a Study Skills DVD that we would like to give you for <u>FREE</u>. This DVD covers our *best practices* for getting ready for your exam, from how to use our study materials to how to best prepare for the day of the test.

All that we ask is that you email us with feedback that would describe your experience so far with our product. Good, bad, or indifferent, we want to know what you think!

To get your FREE Study Skills DVD, email <u>freedvd@mometrix.com</u> with *FREE STUDY SKILLS DVD* in the subject line and the following information in the body of the email:

- The name of the product you purchased.
- Your product rating on a scale of 1-5, with 5 being the highest rating.
- Your feedback. It can be long, short, or anything in between. We just want to know your impressions and experience so far with our product. (Good feedback might include how our study material met your needs and ways we might be able to make it even better. You could highlight features that you found helpful or features that you think we should add.)
- Your full name and shipping address where you would like us to send your free DVD.

If you have any questions or concerns, please don't hesitate to contact me directly.

Thanks again!

Sincerely,

Jay Willis
Vice President
<u>jay.willis@mometrix.com</u>
1-800-673-8175

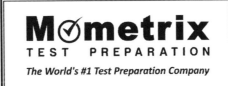

OCN SECRETS

Study Guide
Your Key to Exam Success

OCN Test Review for the
ONCC Oncology Certified Nurse Exam

Published by
Mometrix Test Preparation
Mometrix Nursing Certification Test Team

Written and edited by the Mometrix Nursing Certification Test Team

Printed in the United States of America

This paper meets the requirements of ANSI/NISO Z39.48-1992 (Permanence of Paper).

Mometrix offers volume discount pricing to institutions. For more information or a price quote, please contact our sales department at sales@mometrix.com or 888-248-1219.

Mometrix Media LLC is not affiliated with or endorsed by any official testing organization. All organizational and test names are trademarks of their respective owners.

Paperback
ISBN 13: 978-1-61072-388-6
ISBN 10: 1-61072-388-0

Ebook
ISBN 13: 978-1-62120-440-4
ISBN 10: 1-62120-440-5

Hardback
ISBN 13: 978-1-5167-0551-1
ISBN 10: 1-5167-0551-3

Dear Future Exam Success Story:

First of all, **THANK YOU** for purchasing Mometrix study materials!

Second, congratulations! You are one of the few determined test-takers who are committed to doing whatever it takes to excel on your exam. **You have come to the right place.** We developed these study materials with one goal in mind: to deliver you the information you need in a format that's concise and easy to use.

In addition to optimizing your guide for the content of the test, we've outlined our recommended steps for breaking down the preparation process into small, attainable goals so you can make sure you stay on track.

We've also analyzed the entire test-taking process, identifying the most common pitfalls and showing how you can overcome them and be ready for any curveball the test throws you.

Standardized testing is one of the biggest obstacles on your road to success, which only increases the importance of doing well in the high-pressure, high-stakes environment of test day. Your results on this test could have a significant impact on your future, and this guide provides the information and practical advice to help you achieve your full potential on test day.

Your success is our success

We would love to hear from you! If you would like to share the story of your exam success or if you have any questions or comments in regard to our products, please contact us at **800-673-8175** or **support@mometrix.com**.

Thanks again for your business and we wish you continued success!

Sincerely,
The Mometrix Test Preparation Team

Need more help? Check out our flashcards at: http://MometrixFlashcards.com/ONCC

TABLE OF CONTENTS

Introduction

Thank you for purchasing this resource! You have made the choice to prepare yourself for a test that could have a huge impact on your future, and this guide is designed to help you be fully ready for test day. Obviously, it's important to have a solid understanding of the test material, but you also need to be prepared for the unique environment and stressors of the test, so that you can perform to the best of your abilities.

For this purpose, the first section that appears in this guide is the **Secret Keys**. We've devoted countless hours to meticulously researching what works and what doesn't, and we've boiled down our findings to the five most impactful steps you can take to improve your performance on the test. We start at the beginning with study planning and move through the preparation process, all the way to the testing strategies that will help you get the most out of what you know when you're finally sitting in front of the test.

We recommend that you start preparing for your test as far in advance as possible. However, if you've bought this guide as a last-minute study resource and only have a few days before your test, we recommend that you skip over the first two Secret Keys since they address a long-term study plan.

If you struggle with **test anxiety**, we strongly encourage you to check out our recommendations for how you can overcome it. Test anxiety is a formidable foe, but it can be beaten, and we want to make sure you have the tools you need to defeat it.

Secret Key #1 – Plan Big, Study Small

There's a lot riding on your performance. If you want to ace this test, you're going to need to keep your skills sharp and the material fresh in your mind. You need a plan that lets you review everything you need to know while still fitting in your schedule. We'll break this strategy down into three categories.

Information Organization

Start with the information you already have: the official test outline. From this, you can make a complete list of all the concepts you need to cover before the test. Organize these concepts into groups that can be studied together, and create a list of any related vocabulary you need to learn so you can brush up on any difficult terms. You'll want to keep this vocabulary list handy once you actually start studying since you may need to add to it along the way.

Time Management

Once you have your set of study concepts, decide how to spread them out over the time you have left before the test. Break your study plan into small, clear goals so you have a manageable task for each day and know exactly what you're doing. Then just focus on one small step at a time. When you manage your time this way, you don't need to spend hours at a time studying. Studying a small block of content for a short period each day helps you retain information better and avoid stressing over how much you have left to do. You can relax knowing that you have a plan to cover everything in time. In order for this strategy to be effective though, you have to start studying early and stick to your schedule. Avoid the exhaustion and futility that comes from last-minute cramming!

Study Environment

The environment you study in has a big impact on your learning. Studying in a coffee shop, while probably more enjoyable, is not likely to be as fruitful as studying in a quiet room. It's important to keep distractions to a minimum. You're only planning to study for a short block of time, so make the most of it. Don't pause to check your phone or get up to find a snack. It's also important to **avoid multitasking**. Research has consistently shown that multitasking will make your studying dramatically less effective. Your study area should also be comfortable and well-lit so you don't have the distraction of straining your eyes or sitting on an uncomfortable chair.

The time of day you study is also important. You want to be rested and alert. Don't wait until just before bedtime. Study when you'll be most likely to comprehend and remember. Even better, if you know what time of day your test will be, set that time aside for study. That way your brain will be used to working on that subject at that specific time and you'll have a better chance of recalling information.

Finally, it can be helpful to team up with others who are studying for the same test. Your actual studying should be done in as isolated an environment as possible, but the work of organizing the information and setting up the study plan can be divided up. In between study sessions, you can discuss with your teammates the concepts that you're all studying and quiz each other on the details. Just be sure that your teammates are as serious about the test as you are. If you find that your study time is being replaced with social time, you might need to find a new team.

Secret Key #2 – Make Your Studying Count

You're devoting a lot of time and effort to preparing for this test, so you want to be absolutely certain it will pay off. This means doing more than just reading the content and hoping you can remember it on test day. It's important to make every minute of study count. There are two main areas you can focus on to make your studying count:

Retention

It doesn't matter how much time you study if you can't remember the material. You need to make sure you are retaining the concepts. To check your retention of the information you're learning, try recalling it at later times with minimal prompting. Try carrying around flashcards and glance at one or two from time to time or ask a friend who's also studying for the test to quiz you.

To enhance your retention, look for ways to put the information into practice so that you can apply it rather than simply recalling it. If you're using the information in practical ways, it will be much easier to remember. Similarly, it helps to solidify a concept in your mind if you're not only reading it to yourself but also explaining it to someone else. Ask a friend to let you teach them about a concept you're a little shaky on (or speak aloud to an imaginary audience if necessary). As you try to summarize, define, give examples, and answer your friend's questions, you'll understand the concepts better and they will stay with you longer. Finally, step back for a big picture view and ask yourself how each piece of information fits with the whole subject. When you link the different concepts together and see them working together as a whole, it's easier to remember the individual components.

Finally, practice showing your work on any multi-step problems, even if you're just studying. Writing out each step you take to solve a problem will help solidify the process in your mind, and you'll be more likely to remember it during the test.

Modality

Modality simply refers to the means or method by which you study. Choosing a study modality that fits your own individual learning style is crucial. No two people learn best in exactly the same way, so it's important to know your strengths and use them to your advantage.

For example, if you learn best by visualization, focus on visualizing a concept in your mind and draw an image or a diagram. Try color-coding your notes, illustrating them, or creating symbols that will trigger your mind to recall a learned concept. If you learn best by hearing or discussing information, find a study partner who learns the same way or read aloud to yourself. Think about how to put the information in your own words. Imagine that you are giving a lecture on the topic and record yourself so you can listen to it later.

For any learning style, flashcards can be helpful. Organize the information so you can take advantage of spare moments to review. Underline key words or phrases. Use different colors for different categories. Mnemonic devices (such as creating a short list in which every item starts with the same letter) can also help with retention. Find what works best for you and use it to store the information in your mind most effectively and easily.

Secret Key #3 – Practice the Right Way

Your success on test day depends not only on how many hours you put into preparing, but also on whether you prepared the right way. It's good to check along the way to see if your studying is paying off. One of the most effective ways to do this is by taking practice tests to evaluate your progress. Practice tests are useful because they show exactly where you need to improve. Every time you take a practice test, pay special attention to these three groups of questions:

- The questions you got wrong
- The questions you had to guess on, even if you guessed right
- The questions you found difficult or slow to work through

This will show you exactly what your weak areas are, and where you need to devote more study time. Ask yourself why each of these questions gave you trouble. Was it because you didn't understand the material? Was it because you didn't remember the vocabulary? Do you need more repetitions on this type of question to build speed and confidence? Dig into those questions and figure out how you can strengthen your weak areas as you go back to review the material.

Additionally, many practice tests have a section explaining the answer choices. It can be tempting to read the explanation and think that you now have a good understanding of the concept. However, an explanation likely only covers part of the question's broader context. Even if the explanation makes sense, **go back and investigate** every concept related to the question until you're positive you have a thorough understanding.

As you go along, keep in mind that the practice test is just that: practice. Memorizing these questions and answers will not be very helpful on the actual test because it is unlikely to have any of the same exact questions. If you only know the right answers to the sample questions, you won't be prepared for the real thing. **Study the concepts** until you understand them fully, and then you'll be able to answer any question that shows up on the test.

It's important to wait on the practice tests until you're ready. If you take a test on your first day of study, you may be overwhelmed by the amount of material covered and how much you need to learn. Work up to it gradually.

On test day, you'll need to be prepared for answering questions, managing your time, and using the test-taking strategies you've learned. It's a lot to balance, like a mental marathon that will have a big impact on your future. Like training for a marathon, you'll need to start slowly and work your way up. When test day arrives, you'll be ready.

Start with the strategies you've read in the first two Secret Keys—plan your course and study in the way that works best for you. If you have time, consider using multiple study resources to get different approaches to the same concepts. It can be helpful to see difficult concepts from more than one angle. Then find a good source for practice tests. Many times, the test website will suggest potential study resources or provide sample tests.

Practice Test Strategy

When you're ready to start taking practice tests, follow this strategy:

Untimed and Open-Book Practice

Take the first test with no time constraints and with your notes and study guide handy. Take your time and focus on applying the strategies you've learned.

Timed and Open-Book Practice

Take the second practice test open-book as well, but set a timer and practice pacing yourself to finish in time.

Timed and Closed-Book Practice

Take any other practice tests as if it were test day. Set a timer and put away your study materials. Sit at a table or desk in a quiet room, imagine yourself at the testing center, and answer questions as quickly and accurately as possible.

Keep repeating timed and closed-book tests on a regular basis until you run out of practice tests or it's time for the actual test. Your mind will be ready for the schedule and stress of test day, and you'll be able to focus on recalling the material you've learned.

Secret Key #4 – Pace Yourself

Once you're fully prepared for the material on the test, your biggest challenge on test day will be managing your time. Just knowing that the clock is ticking can make you panic even if you have plenty of time left. Work on pacing yourself so you can build confidence against the time constraints of the exam. Pacing is a difficult skill to master, especially in a high-pressure environment, so **practice is vital**.

Set time expectations for your pace based on how much time is available. For example, if a section has 60 questions and the time limit is 30 minutes, you know you have to average 30 seconds or less per question in order to answer them all. Although 30 seconds is the hard limit, set 25 seconds per question as your goal, so you reserve extra time to spend on harder questions. When you budget extra time for the harder questions, you no longer have any reason to stress when those questions take longer to answer.

Don't let this time expectation distract you from working through the test at a calm, steady pace, but keep it in mind so you don't spend too much time on any one question. Recognize that taking extra time on one question you don't understand may keep you from answering two that you do understand later in the test. If your time limit for a question is up and you're still not sure of the answer, mark it and move on, and come back to it later if the time and the test format allow. If the testing format doesn't allow you to return to earlier questions, just make an educated guess; then put it out of your mind and move on.

On the easier questions, be careful not to rush. It may seem wise to hurry through them so you have more time for the challenging ones, but it's not worth missing one if you know the concept and just didn't take the time to read the question fully. Work efficiently but make sure you understand the question and have looked at all of the answer choices, since more than one may seem right at first.

Even if you're paying attention to the time, you may find yourself a little behind at some point. You should speed up to get back on track, but do so wisely. Don't panic; just take a few seconds less on each question until you're caught up. Don't guess without thinking, but do look through the answer choices and eliminate any you know are wrong. If you can get down to two choices, it is often worthwhile to guess from those. Once you've chosen an answer, move on and don't dwell on any that you skipped or had to hurry through. If a question was taking too long, chances are it was one of the harder ones, so you weren't as likely to get it right anyway.

On the other hand, if you find yourself getting ahead of schedule, it may be beneficial to slow down a little. The more quickly you work, the more likely you are to make a careless mistake that will affect your score. You've budgeted time for each question, so don't be afraid to spend that time. Practice an efficient but careful pace to get the most out of the time you have.

Secret Key #5 – Have a Plan for Guessing

When you're taking the test, you may find yourself stuck on a question. Some of the answer choices seem better than others, but you don't see the one answer choice that is obviously correct. What do you do?

The scenario described above is very common, yet most test takers have not effectively prepared for it. Developing and practicing a plan for guessing may be one of the single most effective uses of your time as you get ready for the exam.

In developing your plan for guessing, there are three questions to address:

- When should you start the guessing process?
- How should you narrow down the choices?
- Which answer should you choose?

When to Start the Guessing Process

Unless your plan for guessing is to select C every time (which, despite its merits, is not what we recommend), you need to leave yourself enough time to apply your answer elimination strategies. Since you have a limited amount of time for each question, that means that if you're going to give yourself the best shot at guessing correctly, you have to decide quickly whether or not you will guess.

Of course, the best-case scenario is that you don't have to guess at all, so first, see if you can answer the question based on your knowledge of the subject and basic reasoning skills. Focus on the key words in the question and try to jog your memory of related topics. Give yourself a chance to bring the knowledge to mind, but once you realize that you don't have (or you can't access) the knowledge you need to answer the question, it's time to start the guessing process.

It's almost always better to start the guessing process too early than too late. It only takes a few seconds to remember something and answer the question from knowledge. Carefully eliminating wrong answer choices takes longer. Plus, going through the process of eliminating answer choices can actually help jog your memory.

Summary: Start the guessing process as soon as you decide that you can't answer the question based on your knowledge.

How to Narrow Down the Choices

The next chapter in this book (**Test-Taking Strategies**) includes a wide range of strategies for how to approach questions and how to look for answer choices to eliminate. You will definitely want to read those carefully, practice them, and figure out which ones work best for you. Here though, we're going to address a mindset rather than a particular strategy.

Your chances of guessing an answer correctly depend on how many options you are choosing from.

How many choices you have	How likely you are to guess correctly
5	20%
4	25%
3	33%
2	50%
1	100%

You can see from this chart just how valuable it is to be able to eliminate incorrect answers and make an educated guess, but there are two things that many test takers do that cause them to miss out on the benefits of guessing:

- Accidentally eliminating the correct answer
- Selecting an answer based on an impression

We'll look at the first one here, and the second one in the next section.

To avoid accidentally eliminating the correct answer, we recommend a thought exercise called **the $5 challenge**. In this challenge, you only eliminate an answer choice from contention if you are willing to bet $5 on it being wrong. Why $5? Five dollars is a small but not insignificant amount of money. It's an amount you could afford to lose but wouldn't want to throw away. And while losing $5 once might not hurt too much, doing it twenty times will set you back $100. In the same way, each small decision you make—eliminating a choice here, guessing on a question there—won't by itself impact your score very much, but when you put them all together, they can make a big difference. By holding each answer choice elimination decision to a higher standard, you can reduce the risk of accidentally eliminating the correct answer.

The $5 challenge can also be applied in a positive sense: If you are willing to bet $5 that an answer choice *is* correct, go ahead and mark it as correct.

Summary: Only eliminate an answer choice if you are willing to bet $5 that it is wrong.

Which Answer to Choose

You're taking the test. You've run into a hard question and decided you'll have to guess. You've eliminated all the answer choices you're willing to bet $5 on. Now you have to pick an answer. Why do we even need to talk about this? Why can't you just pick whichever one you feel like when the time comes?

The answer to these questions is that if you don't come into the test with a plan, you'll rely on your impression to select an answer choice, and if you do that, you risk falling into a trap. The test writers know that everyone who takes their test will be guessing on some of the questions, so they intentionally write wrong answer choices to seem plausible. You still have to pick an answer though, and if the wrong answer choices are designed to look right, how can you ever be sure that you're not falling for their trap? The best solution we've found to this dilemma is to take the decision out of your hands entirely. Here is the process we recommend:

Once you've eliminated any choices that you are confident (willing to bet $5) are wrong, select the first remaining choice as your answer.

Whether you choose to select the first remaining choice, the second, or the last, the important thing is that you use some preselected standard. Using this approach guarantees that you will not be enticed into selecting an answer choice that looks right, because you are not basing your decision on how the answer choices look.

This is not meant to make you question your knowledge. Instead, it is to help you recognize the difference between your knowledge and your impressions. There's a huge difference between thinking an answer is right because of what you know, and thinking an answer is right because it looks or sounds like it should be right.

Summary: To ensure that your selection is appropriately random, make a predetermined selection from among all answer choices you have not eliminated.

Test-Taking Strategies

This section contains a list of test-taking strategies that you may find helpful as you work through the test. By taking what you know and applying logical thought, you can maximize your chances of answering any question correctly!

It is very important to realize that every question is different and every person is different: no single strategy will work on every question, and no single strategy will work for every person. That's why we've included all of them here, so you can try them out and determine which ones work best for different types of questions and which ones work best for you.

Question Strategies

Read Carefully

Read the question and answer choices carefully. Don't miss the question because you misread the terms. You have plenty of time to read each question thoroughly and make sure you understand what is being asked. Yet a happy medium must be attained, so don't waste too much time. You must read carefully, but efficiently.

Contextual Clues

Look for contextual clues. If the question includes a word you are not familiar with, look at the immediate context for some indication of what the word might mean. Contextual clues can often give you all the information you need to decipher the meaning of an unfamiliar word. Even if you can't determine the meaning, you may be able to narrow down the possibilities enough to make a solid guess at the answer to the question.

Prefixes

If you're having trouble with a word in the question or answer choices, try dissecting it. Take advantage of every clue that the word might include. Prefixes and suffixes can be a huge help. Usually they allow you to determine a basic meaning. Pre- means before, post- means after, pro - is positive, de- is negative. From prefixes and suffixes, you can get an idea of the general meaning of the word and try to put it into context.

Hedge Words

Watch out for critical hedge words, such as *likely, may, can, sometimes, often, almost, mostly, usually, generally, rarely*, and *sometimes*. Question writers insert these hedge phrases to cover every possibility. Often an answer choice will be wrong simply because it leaves no room for exception. Be on guard for answer choices that have definitive words such as *exactly* and *always*.

Switchback Words

Stay alert for *switchbacks*. These are the words and phrases frequently used to alert you to shifts in thought. The most common switchback words are *but, although*, and *however*. Others include *nevertheless, on the other hand, even though, while, in spite of, despite, regardless of*. Switchback words are important to catch because they can change the direction of the question or an answer choice.

Face Value

When in doubt, use common sense. Accept the situation in the problem at face value. Don't read too much into it. These problems will not require you to make wild assumptions. If you have to go beyond creativity and warp time or space in order to have an answer choice fit the question, then you should move on and consider the other answer choices. These are normal problems rooted in reality. The applicable relationship or explanation may not be readily apparent, but it is there for you to figure out. Use your common sense to interpret anything that isn't clear.

Answer Choice Strategies

Answer Selection

The most thorough way to pick an answer choice is to identify and eliminate wrong answers until only one is left, then confirm it is the correct answer. Sometimes an answer choice may immediately seem right, but be careful. The test writers will usually put more than one reasonable answer choice on each question, so take a second to read all of them and make sure that the other choices are not equally obvious. As long as you have time left, it is better to read every answer choice than to pick the first one that looks right without checking the others.

Eliminate Answers

Eliminate answer choices as soon as you realize they are wrong, but make sure you consider all possibilities. If you are eliminating answer choices and realize that the last one you are left with is also wrong, don't panic. Start over and consider each choice again. There may be something you missed the first time that you will realize on the second pass.

Avoid Fact Traps

Don't be distracted by an answer choice that is factually true but doesn't answer the question. You are looking for the choice that answers the question. Stay focused on what the question is asking for so you don't accidentally pick an answer that is true but incorrect. Always go back to the question and make sure the answer choice you've selected actually answers the question and is not merely a true statement.

Extreme Statements

In general, you should avoid answers that put forth extreme actions as standard practice or proclaim controversial ideas as established fact. An answer choice that states the "process should be used in certain situations, if…" is much more likely to be correct than one that states the "process should be discontinued completely." The first is a calm rational statement and doesn't even make a definitive, uncompromising stance, using a hedge word *if* to provide wiggle room, whereas the second choice is a radical idea and far more extreme.

Benchmark

As you read through the answer choices and you come across one that seems to answer the question well, mentally select that answer choice. This is not your final answer, but it's the one that will help you evaluate the other answer choices. The one that you selected is your benchmark or standard for judging each of the other answer choices. Every other answer choice must be compared to your benchmark. That choice is correct until proven otherwise by another answer choice beating it. If you find a better answer, then that one becomes your new benchmark. Once you've decided that no other choice answers the question as well as your benchmark, you have your final answer.

Predict the Answer

Before you even start looking at the answer choices, it is often best to try to predict the answer. When you come up with the answer on your own, it is easier to avoid distractions and traps because you will know exactly what to look for. The right answer choice is unlikely to be word-for-word what you came up with, but it should be a close match. Even if you are confident that you have the right answer, you should still take the time to read each option before moving on.

General Strategies

Tough Questions

If you are stumped on a problem or it appears too hard or too difficult, don't waste time. Move on! Remember though, if you can quickly check for obviously incorrect answer choices, your chances of guessing correctly are greatly improved. Before you completely give up, at least try to knock out a couple of possible answers. Eliminate what you can and then guess at the remaining answer choices before moving on.

Check Your Work

Since you will probably not know every term listed and the answer to every question, it is important that you get credit for the ones that you do know. Don't miss any questions through careless mistakes. If at all possible, try to take a second to look back over your answer selection and make sure you've selected the correct answer choice and haven't made a costly careless mistake (such as marking an answer choice that you didn't mean to mark). This quick double check should more than pay for itself in caught mistakes for the time it costs.

Pace Yourself

It's easy to be overwhelmed when you're looking at a page full of questions; your mind is confused and full of random thoughts, and the clock is ticking down faster than you would like. Calm down and maintain the pace that you have set for yourself. Especially as you get down to the last few minutes of the test, don't let the small numbers on the clock make you panic. As long as you are on track by monitoring your pace, you are guaranteed to have time for each question.

Don't Rush

It is very easy to make errors when you are in a hurry. Maintaining a fast pace in answering questions is pointless if it makes you miss questions that you would have gotten right otherwise. Test writers like to include distracting information and wrong answers that seem right. Taking a little extra time to avoid careless mistakes can make all the difference in your test score. Find a pace that allows you to be confident in the answers that you select.

Keep Moving

Panicking will not help you pass the test, so do your best to stay calm and keep moving. Taking deep breaths and going through the answer elimination steps you practiced can help to break through a stress barrier and keep your pace.

Final Notes

The combination of a solid foundation of content knowledge and the confidence that comes from practicing your plan for applying that knowledge is the key to maximizing your performance on test day. As your foundation of content knowledge is built up and strengthened, you'll find that the strategies included in this chapter become more and more effective in helping you quickly sift through the distractions and traps of the test to isolate the correct answer.

Now it's time to move on to the test content chapters of this book, but be sure to keep your goal in mind. As you read, think about how you will be able to apply this information on the test. If you've already seen sample questions for the test and you have an idea of the question format and style, try to come up with questions of your own that you can answer based on what you're reading. This will give you valuable practice applying your knowledge in the same ways you can expect to on test day.

Good luck and good studying!

Care Continuum

Relationship of Health Promotion to Oncology

Cancer is the second leading cause of death in the United States. Although mortality rates have shown improvement over the past few decades, one in four deaths is related to cancer, with over half a million cancer deaths estimated this year. Strategies such as smoking cessation, diet modification and exercise promotion, early detection through cancer screening, and the development of new agents such as cancer vaccines should be promoted as **primary prevention strategies**. **Secondary prevention strategies** are aimed at detecting and treating the cancer early, when it is most likely to be curable.

The vast majority of risk factors that place a person at risk for cancer development are modifiable. Estimates show that up to one-third of cancer deaths can be attributed to tobacco use, poor nutrition, and obesity. One of the US Department of Health and Human Services (HHS) Healthy People 2020 goals is to "reduce the number of new cancer cases, as well as the illness, disability, and death caused by cancer."

Cancer Screening Tests

Cancer screening tests help with early detection of a disease, which enables early treatment. They are also used for maintenance to monitor for recurrence of disease or to determine a patient's risk of developing cancer based on genetic or risk factors. Screening tests can be evaluated based on their sensitivity, specificity, and predictive value:

- *Sensitivity* refers to how sensitive a test is to the outcome for which it is testing. For example, an erythrocyte sedimentation rate (ESR) is very sensitive to inflammation but does not delineate exactly where the inflammation is occurring.
- *Specificity*, on the other hand, refers to how accurate a test will be in testing for one particular item. For example, an ESR is very specific for inflammation.
- The *predictive value* refers to the chance a test will have a false reading. This can be a *false positive* when there is a positive result when it should actually be negative or a *false negative* when there is a negative result when it should actually be positive.

Types of Disease Screening

- **Mass screening** is testing that is done to a large group of people. An *example* of this is state-mandated testing that is performed on newborns after delivery.
- **Selective or prescriptive screening** is testing that is done for a specific disease on patients who are at risk for developing that disease. An *example* of this would be genetic testing for the presence of a tumor marker when there is a family history of a genetic disease, such as cystic fibrosis.
- **Single screening** is done to check for the presence of a specific disease, such as hypercholesterolemia.
- **Multiple screening** is looking for at least two abnormalities at one time. An *example* would be screening for elevated cholesterol and testing a PSA at the same time.
- **Multiphasic screening** is looking at a person over a period of time for the development of any conditions. An *example* of this is assessing children for appropriate development with each well-child visit.

Breast Cancer Screening

Early detection is the most important factor in the management of breast cancer. Survival is directly related to the stage of the disease at the time of diagnosis. The American Cancer Society recommends a combination of regular clinical breast exams and counseling to increase awareness of breast cancer symptoms. Annual mammography is recommended beginning at age 40. In 2007, the American Cancer Society issued additional recommendations regarding adjunct screening with MRI. Screening with MRI is recommended for women with a 20% to 25% or greater lifetime risk of breast cancer. This includes women with a strong family history of breast cancer or ovarian cancer and women who were treated for Hodgkin disease.

The **breast self-examination (BSE)** is a simple examination that women can perform at home. It includes inspection and palpation of the breasts in both the standing and lying positions. By performing breast self-examination, women can learn to know the appearance and feel of their own breasts so that they can identify changes. The majority of palpable breast lumps are discovered through breast self-examination.

<u>Breast Cancer Screening Procedures</u>

- **Breast self-exams** are a woman's first line of screening for breast cancer detection. Unfortunately, most breast cancers are not palpable, but it is important for women to perform these monthly in case a mass does develop that can be felt. These should be performed monthly, but not at the same time the woman has her period. Breast exams should also be performed annually by a healthcare provider.
- **Mammograms** involve firm compression of the breast tissue while an x-ray is taken to detect calcified tissue within the breast. These are usually started at age 40, or earlier if there is a familial history. These are usually repeated annually. Abnormalities on the mammogram are further examined by ultrasound to determine whether the tissue change is solid or cystic in nature.
- Women who are at higher risk can undergo a procedure called **ductal lavage** in which cells are collected from the breast ducts and examined for any changes. Contrast dye can also be injected through the duct system to detect any tissue changes.

Cervical Cancer and Lung Cancer Screening

According to the American Cancer Society, the American Society for Colposcopy and Cervical Pathology (ASCCP), and the American Society for Clinical Pathology (ASCP), **screening for cervical cancer** (using cytology, either conventional or liquid based) for women 21-29 years of age is recommended every 3 years. Screening should begin at age 21, regardless of the age of onset of sexual activity. Recommendations for screening of women who have received the HPV vaccination are the same as those for women who have not received the vaccination.

In 2012, the American Lung Association (ALA) issued an interim guideline of **lung cancer screening recommendations**. The best way to prevent lung cancer associated with tobacco use is to never start smoking or to cease smoking. Low-dose computed tomography (CT) screening should be recommended to people who are current or former smokers 55 to 74 years of age or those who have a smoking history of a least 30 pack-years. People with a history of lung cancer should not be screened using low-dose CT. Chest x-rays are not recommended for lung cancer screening.

Colon and Rectal Cancer Screening

According to the US Preventive Services Task Force (USPSTF) recommendations, **colon cancer screening** should begin at age 50. For patients with a close relative with colorectal polyps or colorectal cancer, patients with inflammatory bowel disease, or patients with a familial adenomatous polyposis (FAP), screening may be recommended at an earlier age. Screening can be performed using high-sensitivity fecal occult blood testing (recommend yearly testing), sigmoidoscopy (recommend every 5 years or, if performed in combination with high-sensitivity fecal occult blood testing, every 3 years) or colonoscopy (recommend every 10 years).

Some additional tests that can be utilized for **colorectal cancer screening** include double contrast barium enema, CT colonography, and stool DNA tests. Double contrast barium enemas, also known as a lower GI series, use barium sulfate and air to outline the colon and rectum to view abnormalities. CT colonography, also known as a virtual colonoscopy, can be used in colon cancer screening by creating 2 and 3 dimensional views of the colon via computed tomography. Lastly, stool DNA tests can identify fragments of the DNA of cancer cells that have shed into the stool. Stool DNA tests are not being used any longer in the United States.

Advance Directives

In accordance to Federal and state laws, individuals have the right to self-determination in health care, including decisions about end of life care through **advance directives** such as living wills and the right to assign a surrogate person to make decisions through a durable power of attorney. Patients should routinely be questioned about an advanced directive as they may present at a healthcare provider without the document. Patients who have indicated they desire a do-not-resuscitate (DNR) order should not receive resuscitative treatments for terminal illness or conditions in which meaningful recovery cannot occur. Patients and families of those with terminal illnesses should be questioned as to whether the patients are Hospice patients. For those with DNR requests or those withdrawing life support, staff should provide the patient palliative rather than curative measures, such as pain control and/or oxygen, and emotional support to the patient and family. Religious traditions and beliefs about death should be treated with respect.

Epidemiology

Cancer Incidence, Prevalence, Mortality, Case-Fatality, and Survival

- **Cancer incidence** refers to the amount of new cases of cancer that are diagnosed each year. This is usually described as a ratio of how many diagnoses of a certain type of cancer are diagnosed out of every 100,000.
- **Cancer prevalence** refers to the total number of people who had a diagnosis of cancer in the past. This statistic can include those who are currently fighting the disease, those in remission, or those who have been cured.
- **Cancer mortality** refers to the number of people who have died from cancer. With cancer being the number two cause of death in this country, this number can be quite high.
- **Case-fatality** refers to mortality from a specific type of cancer, such as colon cancer. This gives information on how deadly a certain type of cancer may be.
- **Cancer survival** refers to the number of patients who were diagnosed with cancer at least five years previously. This includes patients who are in remission, currently battling the disease, or those who have been cured.

Absolute Risk, Relative Risk, Attributable Risk, and Cumulative Risk

- **Absolute risk** refers to the number of cancer diagnoses as far as incidence and cancer death are concerned. This number is actually an average of cancer diagnoses within a group of people, usually out of 100,000.
- **Relative risk** refers to the chance of being diagnosed with cancer because of certain risk factors that are specific to a certain cancer. For example, the relative risk of a person who smokes cigarettes developing lung cancer is much higher than the relative risk of a person who does not smoke.
- **Attributable risk** refers to the number of cancer diagnoses that could be prevented if the patient did not have certain risk factors. An example would be the decrease in the incidence of lung cancer that would result if people no longer smoked.
- **Cumulative risk** is the chance of a person developing cancer throughout their lifetime. It does not take into account specific risk factors that may be present in different individuals.

Ethnic Grouping and Cancer

Culture or ethnic factors that influence cancer are many and varied. The most affected ethnic group overall are *African Americans*, who have the highest rate of cancer from all sources; more than any other ethnic group. The group with the lowest rate of cancer overall is *Native Americans.* Prostate cancer incidence is highest in African American males. The *Japanese* have the highest 5-year survival rate from all types of cancer; whereas the Native Americans have the lowest 5-year survival rate. One factor common to all groups and influencing all groups is the *lower socio-economic class*. This class has the highest incidence of cancer whatever the ethnic group.

Epidemiology of Lung Cancer

Lung cancer causes more deaths in both men and women in this country than any other type of cancer. Approximately 90% of all people who develop lung cancer are *smokers*. There are known risks for lung cancer with second-hand exposure to smoke, but no exact figures are known for incidence of cancer in this population. It is known that when smokers quit smoking, some repair occurs within the lung tissue. This does not immediately decrease the risk of developing lung cancer, but the risk will begin to decrease at least 5 years after quitting smoking.

Other factors that increase the risk of developing lung cancer include ***environmental exposure to carcinogens***, such as asbestos, uranium, and radon.

Overall, lung cancer has a very ***poor prognosis***, though this depends on how far advanced the disease is at the time of diagnosis and whether metastasis develops. The 5-year survival rate for non-small cell lung cancer is approximately 15%, wheras the survival rate for small cell lung cancers is approximately 5%.

Bladder Cancer Risk Factors

Men are three times more likely to develop **bladder cancer** than women. The risk is increased in men over the age of 60, and Caucasians are twice as likely to develop bladder cancer as African Americans. The incidence of bladder cancer has slowly increased over time.

- ***Smoking cigarettes*** has been proven to be the most likely cause in over one-half of all cases of bladder cancers in men. About one-quarter of all bladder cancers in women are linked to cigarette smoking.
- Working with certain ***industrial chemicals*** also places a person more at risk for developing bladder cancer. The industries that show the highest incidence of bladder cancer include paint manufacturing, textiles, and leathers.
- ***Poor dietary habits*** and frequently eating fried or fatty foods increase the risk of developing bladder cancer. The fat-soluble vitamins A and E have shown to help prevent the formation of bladder malignancies as well as the mineral zinc.

Prostate Cancer Risk Factors

The incidence of **prostate cancer** has gradually decreased, which is most likely due to more screening being performed with prostate specific antigen (PSA) testing. Overall, prostate cancer accounts for 1 in 3 cancers in men. The prognosis for patients with prostate cancer has slowly improved in all groups except for African American males.

- Prostate cancer is more common in ***older men*** and it has been found that prostate cancer affects over one-half of men 90-years-old or older.
- Prostate cancer is more likely to occur in ***African American men*** than Caucasian men.
- There is a proven ***genetic link*** to prostate cancer and men whose female relatives had breast cancer may also be at an increased risk for prostate cancer.
- Men who work in the ***farming industry*** or in the ***manufacture of batteries*** are more susceptible to prostate cancer than others. This is due to an increased exposure to the element cadmium.

Head and Neck Cancer Risk Factors

Most cancers that occur in the **head and neck** occur in the mouth. The second most common is laryngeal cancer following by oropharyngeal cancer. Men are more likely than women to develop a head or neck cancer and these are more common in people over the age of 50.

- ***Smoking*** is the number one risk factor that greatly increases the chance of developing head and neck cancer.
- ***Alcoholism*** greatly increases the risk for mouth cancer and cancer of the pharynx.
- ***Chewing tobacco*** can greatly increase the risk for oral cancer.

- Cancers that occur on the outside of the mouth are mostly caused by *UV, or sunlight, exposure.*
- *Carcinogenic inhalants*, such as cigarette smoke, asbestos, or wood dust, can greatly increase the risk for cancers of the nasal passages, nasopharynx, or larynx.
- Cancers of the oropharynx are usually caused by *excessive alcohol consumption* or can even result from *poor oral hygiene.*

Colorectal Cancer Risk Factors

Patients over the age of 50 have a much greater chance of developing **colorectal cancer** than those who are younger.

- Patients who *do not have access to or do not choose* to have regular screening procedures for colon cancer may develop the disease and not know until symptoms become bothersome. This puts them at risk for having more advanced disease if they do develop colon cancer.
- *Chronic inflammatory diseases* that involve the colon, rectum, and anus can increase the chances for developing colon cancer. These include Crohn's disease, ulcerative colitis, or a history of villous adenoma polyps.
- Patients with *diets high in fat and low in fiber* are more likely to develop colon cancer. Those who work in environments in which they are exposed to air particles from wood or metal manufacturing are also at risk.
- A *family history* of colon cancer or familial polyposis also increases the chance for developing colon cancer.

Human Papillomavirus

Some types of the sexually transmitted disease **human papillomavirus (HPV)** cause cancer. Approximately 26,000 cases of cancer diagnosed each year are directly attributable to HPV. The CDC recommends an **HPV vaccine** for females 13-26 years of age and for males 13-21 years of age. There are two vaccines available, Gardasil and Cervarix, and both are indicated for the prevention of human papillomavirus-associated diseases including cervical cancer, genital warts, vulvar neoplasia, and vaginal neoplasia. The vaccines are not 100% reliable in the prevention of cervical cancer and does not protect against all causes of gynecological malignancies or sexually transmitted infections. No pretreatment laboratory tests are required. Patient with an allergy to yeast should not receive this vaccine. The drug is administered as an IM injection and given in three separate doses. The vaccine has been proven to be most effective when all three doses have been given before the patient begins sexual activity. Side effects include headache, nausea/vomiting, fainting, fever, and irritation and pain at the injection site.

Survivorship

Available Resources to Assist Navigating the Healthcare System

Patients with a cancer diagnosis must make many decisions about surgery, radiation, and/or chemotherapy, often with little assistance. Resources available to assist patients and families in **navigating the healthcare system** include:

- *Physicians*: The patient should go to the physician with a written list of questions about any issues of concern. Patients often become intimidated by physicians and forget to ask or are afraid to ask crucial questions.
- *Nurse navigators/Patient advocates*: Some nurses are specially trained to assist patients in understanding their options, making appointments, organizing lab and imaging reports, and finding resources.
- *National Cancer Institute*: The NCI provides extensive information about different types of cancer and current options for treatment.
- *Survivorship/Support groups*: These groups can provide emotional support and practical advice about dealing with cancer and the treatments required.
- *Community agencies/organizations*: Programs may be available to assist with meals, transportation, and lodging.
- *Internet resource:* Cancer.net provides much information about navigating cancer care for children and adults.

Survivor and Secondary Survivors

In the past, a survivor was the friend or family member who lost a loved one to cancer. They were the ones who cared for the patient and took care of them until the patient died and left them behind. Now, these caregivers and family members are called **secondary survivors**. The patient does not have to die from cancer for there to be secondary survivors.

A **survivor** is now considered the cancer patient and he or she is called this from the moment of diagnosis. Surviving cancer is now measured in the amount of time since the person has finished treatment or since they were diagnosed with cancer. Most healthcare workers refer to the survival of the patient in relation to 5 years. Oftentimes, prognosis of a disease is measured in the mortality rate from a certain type of cancer 5 years after diagnosis. A cancer survivor is considered a survivor their whole life, even if they have a recurrence.

Different Stages of Survival

1. The **acute stage** is the initial stage of the disease when a person is first diagnosed with cancer. Nursing interventions at this level are focused on education, which will continue throughout all stages. This includes education on the disease process, treatments available, and community resources available for support and further education, and the importance of compliance with the medical treatment plan.
2. The **extended stage** occurs after selected treatments are completed and includes the stage at which long-term therapy may occur. Nursing interventions at this stage are focused on continued compliance with any long-term therapy that will be started. This includes educating on the importance of continuing screening procedures to monitor for cancer recurrence.

3. The **permanent stage** is that stage in which a patient is considered to be cancer-free. This is frequently monitored by a patient being cancer-free for 5 years. Nursing interventions at this stage are once again focused on education, especially the importance of continued compliance with screening for cancer recurrence.

Physical Effects on Survivors of Cancer

There are multiple long-term **physical effects** that a cancer survivor may experience as a result of the cancer itself or its treatment.

- *Cardiac effects* such as heart failure, heart disease, and cardiomyopathy may occur, especially if a patient has received an anthracycline agent as part of their treatment.
- *Pulmonary toxicity* and inflammation of the lungs can occur as a result of chemotherapy (especially bleomycin), radiation treatment, or steroid use.
- *Endocrine problems* can occur after chemotherapy administration, hormone therapy, or surgery.
- Patients may have long-term effects on *fertility*.
- *Bone and joint pain* as well as *osteoporosis* can occur after administration of chemotherapy, hormone therapy, or radiation.
- *Nerve damage*, including peripheral neuropathy and hearing loss, can occur after chemotherapy.
- Surgery, radiation therapy, and chemotherapy can have long-term effects on *digestion and absorption of nutrients.*
- For patients who have had lymph nodes removed, *lymphedema* may occur, causing swelling and pain from the abnormal buildup of lymph fluid.
- Some cancer survivors may experience long-term learning, memory, and attention difficulties as well.

Recurrence Rates for Common Cancers

Recurrence is a common fear for many cancer survivors. The chance of a cancer recurrence is dependent upon many **factors**, including the stage and grade of the cancer, the type of cancer, the treatment the patient received, and how long of a time period has passed since the treatment was completed.

- In *breast cancer patients*, the highest risk of recurrence is within the first 2 years following treatment. HER2 positive breast cancer is more likely to recur than HER2 negative breast cancer. Triple negative breast cancer is also more likely to recur in comparison with other breast cancers.
- *Colon cancer* is most likely to recur within 3 years of the initial treatment. The liver is the most common site for recurrence. The patient's age, preoperative CEA level, tumor location, size and cell differentiation, and the involvement of lymph nodes all play a large role in the likelihood of recurrence. The 5-year survival rate for stage 1 colon cancer is 74%, while the survival rate for stage IV colon cancer is only 6%.

Types of Rehabilitation Therapy

Rehabilitation encompasses many different aspects of a patient's life and helps them with accomplishing goals that enable them to function independently. The healthcare team works together to provide the resources necessary to assist the patient in achieving these goals.

- **Physical therapy** is used to help patients with movement, relieve pain, and allow them to perform simple activities such as walking, standing, sitting, bending. It also helps to build strength and energy levels after illness.
- **Occupational therapy** helps patients perform ADLs independently, such as dressing, basic hygiene, cooking, and maintaining household needs.
- **Respiratory therapy** helps patients to maintain optimal respiratory health through deep breathing, administering breathing treatments, and building respiratory strength.

There are many other forms of therapy that can be utilized for various medical conditions that are more specific and specialized for a patient and their condition and limitations. Therapy can also be oriented toward psychological needs, such as spiritual, financial, or relationship-oriented therapies.

Goal of Rehabilitation

The **aim of rehabilitation** is the cure of the patient, or as near to that as possible, with the reinsertion of the patient back into his/her original environment; with the same job, duties and interpersonal relationships the patient had before the cancer diagnosis.

Adaptation of the patient as a consequence of treatment, with all limitations acknowledged and overcome to the fullest extent possible without compromising the patient's quality of life that was present before. The goal is to reenter life as before or as near to previous life as possible. There are many organizations that can give support and comfort, and ease the transition back into normal life.

Reintegration

Reintegration describes the process of assisting the patient to return to work through a program with their employers to understand the needs of each other and how to work together to reach the goal of **re-employment**.

Long-Term Follow-Up Guidelines

Survivors of Childhood, Adolescent, and Young Adult Cancers

The Children's Oncology Group (COG) has developed long-term follow-up guidelines for **survivors of childhood, adolescent, and young adult cancers**. The guidelines were developed with the objective of providing **standardization** and **enhancement** of follow-up care provided to survivors of pediatric cancers. The guidelines are evidence based and collectively compiled by a panel of experts with experience in pediatric cancers. The guidelines were most recently updated in 2013 and are available to health care providers who provide ongoing care to childhood cancer survivors. Each guideline is either based on the cancer itself or its treatment (e.g., surgery, chemotherapy, radiation). The therapeutic agent used as part of the cancer treatment is listed, along with the potential late effects the person may experience, risk factors, highest risk factors, the recommended periodic evaluation and health counseling, and further considerations.

Breast Cancer and Colorectal Cancers

The American Society of Clinical Oncology (ASCO) has developed guidelines for the long-term follow-up care of **breast and colorectal cancer survivors**. For **breast cancer patients** who have completed primary therapy with a curative intent, regular history and physical exams and mammography are recommended. During the first 3 years post treatment, it is recommended that physical exams be performed every 3 to 6 months. For years 4 and 5 post treatment, physical exams should be performed every 6 to 12 months and then completed annually (after year 5), post treatment. For patients that have had a breast-conserving surgery, a post treatment mammogram is recommended 1 year after the initial mammogram was completed and at least 6 months after the completion of radiation therapy.

For **colorectal cancer survivors**, ASCO guidelines state that a medical history and physical examination coupled with carcinoembryonic antigen (CEA) testing should be performed every 3 to 6 months for a period of 5 years. Computed tomography scanning of the abdomen and chest should be completed annually for the 3-year period after treatment. Surveillance colonoscopy is recommended 1 year after the initial surgery and then every 5 years after (depending on the clinical findings of the last colonoscopy performed).

Employment Discrimination Laws Protecting Survivors of Cancer

There are several laws that protect cancer survivors from **employment discrimination** related to their cancer.

- The ***Americans with Disabilities Act (ADA)*** and the ***Federal Rehabilitation Act*** are federal laws that prohibit employers from discriminating against their employees based on a disease or disability. The ADA prohibits discrimination based on genetic information related to a disease.
- In addition, the ***Genetic Information Nondiscrimination Act (GINA)*** also provides protection from discrimination of employees based on the results of a genetic test or a family history of a disease or illness. The GINA law covers the same employers that are covered under the ADA law (those with at least 15 employees).
- The ***Family and Medical Leave Act*** requires employers of at least 50 or more employees to provide up to 12 weeks of unpaid leave during any 12-month period to attend to their own serious health condition or that of an immediate family member.

Health Insurance Concerns for Survivors of Cancer

According to the Annual Report to the Nation on the Status of Cancer (1975-2012), 66% of people treated for cancer survive 5 years after diagnosis. Many cancer survivors experience financial hardship as a result of their treatment. Follow-up care continues for cancer survivors and may include expensive testing and treatment to manage long-term side effects and potential disabilities. Some insurance plans will deny coverage for cancer-related illnesses if the condition is deemed "preexisting." Cancer survivors may have difficulty keeping and maintaining coverage. Resources such as prescription drug assistance programs may be of assistance for those who qualify.

- The **Patient Advocate Foundation** is a foundation that assists patients who have a chronic, life-threatening, or debilitating illness and may be experiencing difficulties with access to health care, job retention or discrimination, or a debt crisis related to their illness.
- **COBRA** is a federal law that gives an employee the right to choose to temporarily keep group health insurance benefits that would otherwise be lost due to a decrease in working hours, quitting a job, or loss of a job.

Financial Assistance Resources for Cancer Survivors

Numerous local, state, and national organizations are available to provide cancer patients with **financial assistance**. Organizations include:

- *Patient Advocate Foundation* (http://www.patientadvocate.org): Provide assistance for co-pays and transportation expenses for cancer patients and has aid programs specifically for those with metastatic breast cancer and multiple myeloma.
- *Partnership for Prescription Assistance* (PPA) (https://www.pparx.org): Provides information about free or low cost prescription drugs.
- *PAN Foundation* (https://panfoundation.org/index.php/en/): Offers financial assistance to pay medical costs through 60 disease-specific programs.
- *Healthwell Foundation* (https://www.healthwellfoundation.org/): Provides financial assistance through the Emergency Cancer Relief Fund.
- *CancerCare* (http://www.cancercare.org): Has a financial assistance program that assists with costs of transportation, home care, child care, and co-payments. Breast cancer patients can receive financial assistance for medications, lymphedema supplies, and durable medical supplies.
- *The Samfund* (https://www.healthwellfoundation.org/): Provides twice yearly grants to assist young (21-39) cancer patients with living expenses, tuition, education, medical bills, and various other health-related expenses.

Support Programs for Cancer Survivors

There are many **support programs** specific to survivorship for people who have experienced cancer in their lives. **Cancer Hope Network** is a not-for-profit organization that provides confidential one on one support to cancer survivors at no cost. Cancer Hope Network utilizes volunteer staff that have also experienced cancer in their lifetime, and matches those volunteers with clients who have had a similar cancer experience. In addition to the one on one support they provide, Cancer Hope Network has a social network known as Hope Net that allows cancer survivors to create or join groups specific to their cancer experience.

The American Cancer Society along with the George Washington University Cancer Institute collaborated to form the **National Cancer Survivorship Resource Center**. The program provides survivorship resources and tools to cancer survivors, caregivers, and health care providers.

Support Programs for Family Members of Cancer Survivors

There are several foundations that offer support programs specifically for **family members of cancer survivors**. In addition, individual facilities in which the patient received cancer treatment may offer support groups or programs for family members.

- *The Angel Foundation* offers a variety of different camps, retreats, and support groups for family members of cancer survivors. They offer a free 3-day camp that is designed just for children who have a parent with cancer.
- *The Live Strong Foundation*, founded by cancer survivor Lance Armstrong, offers a multitude of services through its foundation for all cancer survivors, caregivers, family, and friends.

- The Live Strong Foundation has developed **Survivorship Centers** at leading medical institutions throughout the United States. These Survivorship Centers provide direct survivorship services as well as continue to advance in the field of cancer survivorship through research and the sharing of best practices.

Treatment Related Conditions

Delayed-Onset Side Effects Resulting from Chemotherapy Treatment

Fatigue and activity intolerance	Onset usually with a week of having chemotherapy. Activities must be geared to the patient's ability with adequate rest periods, and patients taught to recognize the signs of physical overactivity.
Itching	Dry, itchy skin (pruritus) common after beginning chemotherapy. Changing medications or adding antihistamines may alleviate itching. Topical corticosteroids may also help for limited areas and applying moisturizers to dry skin.
Nausea and vomiting	Many chemotherapy drugs cause nausea and vomiting, especially drugs such as hexamethylmelamine, procarbazine, imatinib, and cyclophosphamide. Cold food, small frequent meals, ginger ale, and anti-emetics may relieve nausea.
Diarrhea	Chemotherapy and immunotherapy may cause diarrhea. Use dietary modification, bulk formers, and antidiarrheals
Hair loss	Drugs that result in hair loss include carboplatin, cisplatin, cyclophosphamide, docetaxel, doxorubicin, epirubicin, 5-FU, paclitaxel, and vincristine. Wigs, other hairpieces, or scarves may be used to cover hair loss
Neutropenia	Patient's blood count must be monitored and patient protected from exposure to infection. Antibiotics may be needed for infection. In some cases, granulocyte transfusions, corticosteroid treatment, or administration of G-CSF, filgrastim may be necessary.

Chronic and/or Permanent Side Effects from Chemotherapy Treatment

Chronic and/or permanent side effects of chemotherapy include:

- *Early menopause/Ovarian failure/Infertility:* Chemotherapy, especially high dose, often results in cessation of menses, which may be permanent in women over age 40. Some chemotherapy may result in male infertility as well as erectile dysfunction
- *Birth defects:* Long-term therapy, such as tamoxifen, may pose a risk of birth defects, so patients are advised to avoid pregnancy.
- *Increased weight:* Gains of up to 15 pounds are common, especially for those who go into early menopause.
- *Chronic fatigue:* Some people develop long-term fatigue unresolved by sleep or rest.
- *Cognitive impairment:* Commonly referred to as having "chemo brain," some patients have difficulty concentrating and suffer memory loss. Cognitive impairment may persist for up to 2 years or longer, especially in older adults.
- *Cardiovascular problems:* Anthracyclines (such as doxorubicin, and epirubicin), targeted therapies (such as bevacizumab and trastuzumab), and mitoxantrone may cause cardiomyopathy, heart failure, dysrhythmias, myocarditis, or endocarditis if not discontinued at the first indication of cardiovascular damage.
- *Osteoporosis:* Hormone (testosterone, estrogen) deprivation resulting from hormone therapy for breast/prostate cancer or steroid therapy may result in bone thinning.
- *Hearing loss:* Some chemotherapy, such as platinum-based chemotherapeutic agents (cisplatin, carboplatin) damage the inner ear.

Delayed-Onset Side Effects Resulting from Radiation Therapy

Delayed-onset side effects of radiotherapy depend on the type of radiation, dosage, and area of the body irradiated. Typical problems include:

- *Skin irritation:* Ranging from mild redness and itching to blistering, peeling, and severe burns and ulcerations. Onset is usually within 7-14 days of beginning radiotherapy. Management includes bathing with warm (not hot) water, patting dry, and avoiding applications of heat or cold to irradiated areas. Patients should wear loose clothing. Topical antibiotics may be needed for infection. Aloe gel, Radiacare Gel®, topical steroids, and Aquaphor may help soothe skin between treatments.
- *Fatigue:* Onset is within a few weeks of beginning radiotherapy. Management includes adequate rest periods and avoiding over-exertion.
- *Head/neck issues:* Dry mouth may lead to dental problems. Dysphagia may result from fibrosis, edema, or narrowing of the throat. Management includes, mouth rinses for dry mouth, avoidance of whitening toothpastes, small soft meals for dysphagia, moisturizer, soft-bristled toothbrushes and avoidance of dental floss.
- *Chest issues*: Problems can include taste changes, pulmonary fibrosis, heart failure, anorexia, and radiation pneumonitis. Management includes sleeping with head of bed elevated to relieve dyspnea, fans to move air, oxygen for severe dyspnea.
- *Abdominal issues:* Problems can include nausea and vomiting, diarrhea, enteritis, indigestion, gas, gastric ulcers, and renal damage. Management includes dietary modification, antiemetics, and antidiarrheals.
- *Pelvic issues:* Problems can include rectal bleeding, incontinence (urine and stool), enteritis, painful urination and defecation, fertility problems, and sexual problems (including erectile dysfunction). Management includes monitoring urinary output, fertility preservation measures, absorbent pads and good skin care for incontinence.
- *Anemia:* May result from radiation to large body areas or pelvic, extremity, or chest bones, especially if chemotherapy is given concurrently. Management may include transfusions, nutritional supplementation.

Chronic and/or Permanent Side Effects from Radiation Therapy

Chronic and/or permanent side effects of radiation therapy vary according to radiation target and include:

- *Breast/chest:* Skin may darken and become dry and thin. Telangiectasias may be evident. Breast swelling or fibrosis may occur. If radiation is to the left chest, the cardiac muscle may be damaged. Radiation may result in damage to the lungs as well. Peripheral lymphedema may occur.
- *Head/Neck:* Hypothyroidism may occur because of damage to the thyroid gland. Some patients may experience long-term or permanent mental changes and emotional problems, especially with radiation to the brain. Xerostomia and increased risk of tooth decay may be a chronic problem. Peripheral neuropathy may occur. Thrombocytopenia may occur, especially if chemotherapy is given concurrently. Damage to the taste buds/salivary glands may affect the ability to taste.
- *Bones:* Osteoporosis may result in fractures.
- *Pelvis:* Infertility may be permanent. Early menopause may occur. Bladder irritation may result in urinary incontinence. Peripheral lymphedema may occur.

Secondary Malignancy and Possible Secondary Malignancies from Chemotherapy Treatment

Secondary (second) cancers are additional cancers that develop years after treatment with chemotherapy and/or radiation for a malignancy. While rare, these cancers may occur, but risk is greatest when chemotherapy is combined with radiotherapy. Chemotherapeutic agents that increase risk include:

- *Alkylating agents* (such as cyclophosphamide, carmustine, and chlorambucil) increases risk of myelodysplastic syndrome (MDS) and acute myelogenous leukemia (AML), usually within 2 to 10 years.
- *Platinum-based agents* (such as cisplatin and carboplatin), increase risk of AML.
- *Topoisomerase II inhibitors* (such as etoposide and mitoxantrone), increase risk of AML, usually within 2 to 3 years. Anthracyclines (such as doxorubicin and daunorubicin) are less likely to cause AML and, if it does occur, it is more easily treated.
- *Targeted therapy* (such as vemurafenib and dabrafenib) increase risk of squamous cell carcinoma.

Secondary Malignancy and Possible Secondary Malignancies Associated with Radiation Therapy

Secondary (second) cancers associated with radiation therapy are varied. Myelodysplastic syndrome (MDS) (a bone marrow cancer that can develop into acute leukemia), acute and chronic myelogenous leukemia (AML, CML), and acute lymphoblastic leukemia (ALL) as well as solid tumors may develop as a result of treatment with radiotherapy, especially if the patient also received chemotherapy. MDS and leukemias tend to develop more quickly than solid tumors, usually peaking between 5 and 9 years. Solid tumors usually don't occur before 10 years but may still occur at 15 to 20 years so the risk persists. Solid tumors are most likely to develop near the area exposed to radiation. Patients treated for Hodgkin's lymphoma may develop a second tumor (especially breast cancer, lung cancer, non-Hodgkin's lymphoma, thyroid cancer, mesothelioma, and soft-tissue sarcoma) up to 40 years after treatment with some patients developing third and fourth cancers. Breast cancer and thyroid cancer are common second cancers associated with radiotherapy in general.

Fever and Chills

Fever is an increase in temperature to at least 100.5°. A temperature below that measurement but above a normal temperature of 98.6° is considered a **low-grade fever**.

When the body's temperature is elevated, the body begins shivering uncontrollably. This causes the production of heat, or energy, and raises the internal temperature. A patient will often complain of feeling cold during this shivering, or chills, period.

The process of fever is brought about by the **immune cells**. Substances are released which cause constriction of the blood vessels. This maintains heat within the body which causes the body's temperature to rise. The **thermoregulatory center** in the hypothalamus, if functioning appropriately, controls the rise and fall of the body's temperature. It will respond by causing dilation of the blood vessels to promote heat loss. Increased energy demands are put on the body during a time of increased temperature with chills. This also results in an increased respiratory rate to supply the tissues with extra oxygen to meet these demands.

Risk Factors of Fever

A disease process, such as a tumor, that impairs the function of the hypothalamus can cause a disruption in the **thermoregulatory process** in the body. If the hypothalamus is not able to control the body's temperature, the modulating response of vasodilation cannot occur to help reduce the body's temperature during fever. This can result in increased chills and increased energy demands by the body's tissues.

Certain types of **cancers** can cause fevers. The tumor cells will secrete substances that stimulate a fever without the immune system's involvement. This is usually seen in cancers involving the lymph system, bone, and the liver.

The most common treatment that can lead to fever is **chemotherapy**. An effect of chemotherapy is suppression of the immune system and the development of an illness similar to the flu. This results in a drug-induced fever.

Surgery and other procedures stress the body and may lead to fever. So can other immune-suppressing drugs and certain antibiotics.

Medical Treatment of Fever

The goal with treatment is to reduce the fever and treat the cause, if known.

- **Acetaminophen** (Tylenol) or **NSAIDs**, such as ibuprofen or naproxen, can be used to reduce the fever. Avoid acetaminophen in patients with liver disease. NSAIDs can cause abdominal distress and GI bleeding when used excessively and should not be used in patients with a tendency for these conditions. NSAIDs can also have blood thinning properties and platelet counts should be assessed before administering.
- **Antibiotics** may be given if an infection is the cause of the fever. Chest x-ray, and sputum and blood cultures can be done to assess for a bacterial cause of infection either in the lungs or systemically.
- If a cancerous tumor is the cause of the fever, assessment and biopsy will need to be done to diagnosis the type of malignancy.

If not treated within a timely manner, or if allowed to become dangerously elevated, fever can lead to extreme weakness and even death if there is damage to the nervous system.

Cardiovascular Toxicity

Cardiovascular toxicity is heart disease caused by therapies used to treat cancer.

Radiation therapy and certain types of chemotherapeutic drugs can cause damage to heart muscle tissue or to the vascular system which can impair cardiac function. Some chemotherapy drugs can even cause spasm of the cardiac vessels which can cause chest pain and cardiac dysrhythmias. This can even lead to an acute MI or cardiac failure.

Patients may be more susceptible to cardiac infections, such as pericarditis or endocarditis, because of a suppressed immune system after receiving chemotherapy treatments. Some medications can be toxic to the cardiac vessels and cause fluid to accumulate around the heart (a cardiac tamponade).

EKG changes can be seen following administration of certain drugs. Atrial dysrhythmias are more common than ventricular, but ventricular fibrillation and death can occur.

Patients who receive certain chemotherapy treatments that are known to potentially cause cardiac toxicity may see affects several years after treatments are completed.

History and Physical Exam Findings

When taking a **history** from a patient with cardiovascular toxicity, ask about any pre-existing conditions that may be present that could potentially exacerbate the situation. Also ask about any current or past treatments they have received for these conditions and for their cancer. Question the patient about any habits they may have, such as smoking or drinking. This includes asking about past history of these habits.

Ask about specific symptoms the patient is experiencing. Question the patient about chest pain, any fluttering feelings in the chest, and any difficulty breathing. Ask about aggravating and relieving factors with these symptoms.

On **physical exam**, assess vital signs for any changes in blood pressure or elevations and irregularities in heart rate. Check all extremities for edema. Listen to heart sounds to assess for any murmurs or a pericardial rub.

Diagnostic tests should include a 12-lead EKG to assess for rhythm irregularities. A chest x-ray should be done to check for cardiomegaly or pleural effusions. Echocardiogram may also be done to check ventricular function.

NCI's Common Terminology Criteria for Adverse Events

The **National Cancer Institute (NCI)** created the **Common Terminology Criteria for Adverse Events (CTCAE v 1.0)** in 1983 to aid in the recognition and grading of adverse effects of chemotherapy. This system has been revised, most recently in 2009 (CTCAE v 4.0) and represents the first comprehensive, multimodal **grading system** for reporting both acute and late effects of cancer treatment. The World Health Organization and Cooperative Oncology Groups also offer criteria for grading toxicities. The purpose of grading toxicities is to provide an objective assessment. The grade of toxicity will determine the reason for **dosage adjustments** or **delays**. The scale ranges from 0-4, with 0 meaning mild toxicity and 4 indicating severe or life-threatening toxicity. Many different types of adverse events are graded on the scale. An example of grading neuropathy would be: Grade 1 peripheral neuropathy is defined as a loss of deep tendon reflexes or paresthesia with the patient being asymptomatic. Grade 2 neuropathy is defined as moderate symptoms with limitations on instrumental ADL's. Grade 3 is defined as severe symptoms that limit self-care activities of daily living. Grade 4 is defined as having life-threatening consequences with urgent intervention needed.

End-of-Life Care

ANA Code for End-of-Life Care

The **ANA code for end-of-life care** states that: "the nurse provides service with respect for human dignity and the uniqueness of the client." It continues by asserting that "nurses individually and collectively have an obligation to provide comprehensive and compassionate end-of-life care which includes the promotion of comfort and the relief of pain, and at times, foregoing life sustaining treatments."

Interdisciplinary Team Support for Cancer Patients and Families Through End-of-Life Care

Members of the interdisciplinary team have vital roles in meeting the needs of the cancer patient during end-of-life care:

- *Pharmacists*: Provide guidance on medications, especially analgesia and antiemetics, including interactions and adverse effects as well as dosage and equianalgesia.
- *Occupational therapists:* Can assist patients to compensate for physical weakness or deficits in order to allow them to remain independent in ADLs as long as possible.
- *Physical therapists:* Can help patients to maintain muscle strength and mobility and can recommend appropriate assistive devices.
- *Nutritionists:* Can provide nutritional guidance and assist patient and family in finding foods that the patient can tolerate and that do not exacerbate symptoms, such as nausea.
- *Spiritual advisor:* Can provide emotional support and help relieve anxiety as well as helping the patient and family members communicate more effectively.
- *Psychologist:* Can provide the patients with tools to help to deal with anxiety, depression, and other responses to disease.

Common Pharmacologic Interventions for End-of-Life Care

Opioid analgesia: Relieves pain and dyspnea

Risks: Excessive sedation, respiratory depression, constipation, confusion, myoclonus, itching.

Antibiotics: Reduce infection

Risks: Prolonged life and suffering, nausea, diarrhea, increased risk of *C. diff* infection.

Oxygen: Reduces dyspnea

Risks: Increases dryness of mucous membranes, interference with ability to communicate, depressed respiratory drive.

Tube feedings/PEG tube: Improve nutrition, hydration

Risks: Infection, local irritation, prolonged suffering, tube leakage, aspiration pneumonia, abdominal discomfort, gastric perforation

Mechanical Ventilation: Relieves dyspnea, prolongs life

Risks: Prolonged suffering, inability to communicate.

Antimuscarinic agents (glycopyrrolate, atropine): Reduces death rattle

Risks: Xerostomia, increased sedation, increased delirium

Glucocorticoids: Reduces intracranial pressure, increases appetite, controls pain, reduces fatigue

Risks: Insomnia, GI upset, delirium, depression, increased risk of infection and hyperglycemia, Cushingoid syndrome, anxiety, increased risk of thromboembolism, myopathy, interference with other medications.

Non-Pharmacologic Comfort Measures for End-of-Life Care

<u>Positioning and Comfort Measures</u>

Non-pharmacological comfort measures include:

- *Self-hypnosis:* Involves invoking an altered state of consciousness in anticipation of nausea and vomiting or pain episodes to decrease frequency, severity, amount, and duration of uncomfortable episodes.
- *Relaxation:* Progressive relaxation of muscle groups often involving imagery, which may be helpful to relieve chemotherapy-induced nausea and vomiting and pain.
- *Imagery:* Mentally removing the focus from unpleasant side effects and refocusing the mind on other images. It increases self-control while decreasing length and perceptions of nausea and vomiting episodes.
- *Distraction:* Diverting attention to other activities such as video games, puzzles, or humor.
- *Desensitization:* Involves relaxation and visualization to decrease perceptions of nausea and vomiting.
- *Acupressure:* A form of massage to increase energy flow and improve emotion.
- *Music therapy:* Often used with other therapies to influence physiological, psychological, and emotional states during and after nausea and vomiting episodes.
- *Positioning:* Allowing the patient to remain in positions of comfort, such as with head elevated, as much as possible. Turning and providing support to prevent skin ulcers.

<u>Environment and Spiritual Support</u>

Non-pharmacological comfort measures for end-of-life care include:

- *Environmental considerations:* The environment should be maintained as quiet and peaceful as possible. Bright lights should be avoided. When possible, alarms on any equipment in the room should be silenced or turned to low volume. If a unit is noisy, closing the door and/or pulling bedside curtains may help to reduce noise and distractions. Chairs should be available at bedside for family members and visitors.
- *Spiritual support*: Kindness and compassion are essential elements of spiritual care. Patients' spiritual needs may vary, but all patients should be provided the opportunity to express their feelings and to have others listen, respond, and bear witness. The oncology certified nurse should help to arrange visits with priests, imams, rabbis, or other ministers according to patient's wishes and should facilitate spiritual procedures, such as healing ceremonies, blessings, and last rites.

Hospice

Hospice helps patients and their loved ones deal with end of life issues while maintaining peace and serenity through the process. They provide medical care, self-care, supportive and emotional care, and bereavement counseling after a cancer patient dies.

Hospice services are available to those cancer patients who have a life expectancy of **6 months or less**. The hospice philosophy looks at death as another phase of life and a passage we all must go through. Their goal is to make this journey as peaceful and comfortable as possible for both the cancer patient and the secondary survivors.

Hospice is comprised of a whole team of healthcare providers from nursing assistants to doctors. Each person has a specific role to provide care for the patient and keep them as comfortable as possible. Many people are under the assumption that cancer treatments are not allowed when a patient is under hospice care. Chemotherapy or radiation may be continued as a form of palliative care to keep the patient more comfortable.

Hospice Care NHO Guidelines

1. The terminal prognosis is determined by the attending physician.
2. The patient and family or significant other are aware of the prognosis.
3. Treatment is toward relief of symptoms not cure.
4. The patient has had a progression of the disease.
5. There have been multiple emergency visits or hospitalizations over the last six months.
6. There has been a decline in the patient's functional status due to terminal illness
7. There are symptoms of impaired nutrition indicated by documented weight loss.
8. The patient refuses further curative medical treatment.

Medicare Coverage of Hospice

Hospice is a healthcare program that provides support and comfort to patients and the families dealing with the final stages of terminal illness. The goal is to provide care at home, although specialized hospice facilities exist in many locations. **Medicare** covers hospice care if:

1. A physician certifies the patient is terminally ill with 6 months or less to live.
2. The patient or family requests hospice assistance.
3. The provider is Medicare-certified.

The physician's hospice referral can be made from either a home or hospital setting. To receive hospice care coverage, a patient must waive standard Medicare benefits for the illness/condition causing the hospice referral; however, care for other conditions unrelated to the hospice referral condition are covered by standard Medicare benefits. Medicare Part A pays for two 90-day and unlimited 60-day benefit periods, with recertification being subject to a doctor's (or nurse practitioner's) re-evaluation of the patient.

Resources for Living Expenses, Lodging, and Travel

There are many agencies that provide **resources** for living expense, travel, and lodging for cancer patients.

- **Agencies** such as the Salvation Army, Catholic Social Services, The United Way, Jewish Social Services, and the National Association of Area Agencies on Aging have programs in place to help financially support cancer patients and their families.
- The **American Cancer Society** offers housing in Hope Lodges for patients undergoing treatment and their families. Hope Lodges are located throughout the United States.
- **Ronald McDonald houses** are also located throughout the United States and provide low cost or free housing to pediatric cancer patients and their families. Often, cancer treatment centers offer short-term housing options or discount programs for local hotels/motels.

- The American Cancer Society has a **road to recovery program** that assists patients with travel to their treatment center. Trained volunteers drive patients and families to and from treatment.

Home Care Benefits

Private insurance plans usually will cover some of the costs of home care on an acute basis; however, **long-term service benefits** may vary among different plans. They usually pay for skilled professional care services with the provision of cost sharing. Few private insurers may pay for personal care services. Most private insurers will pay for comprehensive hospice care. Some people have to buy Medigap coverage or purchase long-term care insurance to meet home care needs. Long-term care insurance originally protected individuals from huge costs that come with a prolonged nursing home stay. Currently, some long-term care insurers have increased coverage to include some in-home services.

Kübler-Ross's Stages of Grief

Grief is a normal response to the death or severe illness/abnormality of a patient. How a person deals with grief is very personal, and each will grieve differently. Elisabeth Kübler-Ross identified **five stages of grief** in *On Death and Dying* (1969), which can apply to both patients and family members. A person may not go through each stage but usually goes through two of the five stages:

- **Denial**: Patients/families may be resistive to information and unable to accept that a person is dying/impaired. They may act stunned, immobile, or detached and may be unable to respond appropriately or remember what's said, often repeatedly asking the same questions.
- **Anger**: As reality becomes clear, patient/families may react with pronounced anger, directed inward or outward. Women, especially, may blame themselves and self-anger may lead to severe depression and guilt, assuming they are to blame because of some personal action. Outward anger, more common in men, may be expressed as overt hostility.
- **Bargaining**: This involves if-then thinking (often directed at a deity): "If I go to church every day, then God will prevent this." Patient/family may change doctors, trying to change the outcome.
- **Depression**: As the patient and family begin to accept the loss, they may become depressed, feeling no one understands and overwhelmed with sadness. They may be tearful or crying and may withdraw or ask to be left alone.
- **Acceptance**: This final stage represents a form of resolution and often occurs outside of the medical environment after months. Patients are able to accept death/dying/incapacity. Families are able to resume their normal activities and lose the constant preoccupation with their loved one. They are able to think of the person without severe pain.

Supporting Families of Dying Patients

Families of dying patients often do not receive adequate support from nursing staff that feel unprepared for dealing with families' grief and unsure of how to provide comfort, but families may be in desperate need of this support:

Before death	Stay with the family and sit quietly, allowing them to talk, cry, or interact if they desire.
	Avoid platitudes, "His suffering will be over soon."
	Avoid judgmental reactions to what family members say or do and realize that anger, fear, guilt, and irrational behavior are normal responses to acute grief and stress.
	Show caring by touching the patient and encouraging family to do the same.
	Note: Touching hands, arms, or shoulders of family members can provide comfort, but follow clues of the family.
	Provide referrals to support groups if available.
Time of death	Reassure family that all measures have been taken to ensure the patient's comfort. Express personal feeling of loss, "She was such a sweet woman, and I'll miss her" and allow family to express feelings and memories. Provide information about what is happening during the dying process, explaining death rales, Cheyne-Stokes respirations, etc.
	Alert family members to imminent death if they are not present. Assist to contact clergy/spiritual advisors.
	Respect feelings and needs of parents, siblings, and other family.
After death	Encourage parents/family members to stay with the patient as long as they wish to say goodbye.
	Use the patient's name when talking to the family.
	Assist family to make arrangements, such as contacting funeral home.
	If an autopsy is required, discuss with the family and explain when it will take place.
	If organ donation is to occur, assist the family to make arrangements. Encourage family members to grieve and express emotions.
	Send card or condolence note.

Oncology Nursing Practice

Scientific Basis

Cancer and Pathophysiology of the Formation of Cancer Cells

Cancer is a potentially life-threatening disease that occurs due to irregular cell growth and reproduction. These cells can develop into a tumor that can occupy an area where normal body cells are usually found. Cancer cells also have the ability to **metastasize**, or extend, into other areas of the body.

Cells within the body are constantly being replaced by normal cells. During this process, an abnormality in a cell's DNA can occur, which causes it to become a **malignant** cancer cell. The body's immune system will usually attack and destroy this cell, but sometimes there can be a failure of the immune system to do this or the immune system is not able to destroy the cell. When this happens, the cancer cell can continue to reproduce itself until a tumor is formed. Some cancers can even attack normal, healthy cells within the body and alter their DNA so they will begin to reproduce as cancer cells.

Categories of Carcinogenesis

Carcinogenesis is defined as the process by which normal genes are damaged so that the cells lose control mechanisms and thereby proliferate out of control. Categories include:

- *Familial carcinogenesis* is based on cancer-suppressor genes that are present normally but when changed cause cancer by their absence. Breast cancer is a common example of this.
- *Viral carcinogenesis* in humans has been identified only in a small number of instances (e.g. hepatitis B virus, human T-cell leukemia-lymphoma virus, human papillomaviruses, and Epstein-Barr virus).
- The *bacterial carcinogenesis* by helicobacter pylori is associated with mucosa-associated lymphoid tissue lymphoma.
- *Chemical carcinogenesis* is induced by chemical/toxin exposure for example, lung cancer from the smoking of tobacco.
- When secondary smoke causes lung cancer this is an example of *environmental carcinogenesis.*
- An example of *physical carcinogenesis* is squamous cell cancer caused by exposure to ultraviolet radiation of the sun.

Main Causes of Cancer

1. **Radiation** can cause cancer by altering a cell's DNA. If the body is not able to repair the damages, the cell can reproduce as a cancer cell. Radiation exposure can be accidental or from diagnostic testing. UV light exposure is a form of radiation, also, and it causes skin cancer. Asbestos is considered a form of radiation, also, and causes mesothelioma tumors within the lungs.
2. **Chemical carcinogens** can alter a cell's DNA to cause cancer. An example of this is cigarette smoke and exposure to tar within cigarettes.
3. **Viruses** can cause cancer. Viruses that alter a cell's genetic material can stimulate the production of cancer cells.

4. The **immune system** may be unsuccessful in repairing or destroying cells with altered DNA, which can lead to cancer. Certain cancer cells have the ability to alter the immune system so that it cannot recognize the formation of malignant cells within normal tissues.
5. Cancer can also occur because of **inherited factors**. A person can inherit oncogenes responsible for causing certain types of cancer.

Steps in Metastatic Sequence

1. Tumor growth and neovascularization.
2. **Tumor cell invasion** of the basement membrane and other extra-cellular matrices.
3. **Detachment** and **embolism** of tumor cell aggregates.
4. **Arrest** in distant organ capillary beds.
5. Extravasation.
6. **Proliferation** within the organ parenchyma.

Invasion, Angiogenesis, Metastasis, and Tumor Heterogeneity

- **Invasion** is the process in which cancer cells continue to reproduce and effectively take over an area of the body's normal, healthy tissue.
- **Angiogenesis** is the process in which a tumor causes the body to produce blood vessels that enable the tumor to survive and grow.
- **Metastasis** is extension of cancer cells to other parts of the body. This occurs when the cancer cells continue to reproduce and spread into other tissues in the area where the original cancer started. It can also occur through the blood or lymph stream by carrying cancer cells to other tissues within the body. Certain cancers have a propensity for metastasizing to specific areas of the body. For example, prostate and breast cancers are more likely to metastasize to the spine.
- **Tumor heterogeneity** is the term used to describe the dissimilarities found between cancer cells within a tumor. The more heterogeneous a tumor is, the more difficult it can be to treat and the more types of treatments may be required to treat it.

Stages of the Development of Cancer

1. **Initiation** is the action of a cancer-causing substance entering the body. Examples include cigarette smoke, radiation exposure, etc. This substance can alter the DNA within the body's cells. The body may respond by fixing the damage and halting the process of cancer cells forming; or the body may not be able to repair the damage that is done, and the DNA can go on with these changes without cancer cells being produced; or the DNA can be changed and go on to replicate cancer cells.
2. **Promotion** is the process in which the body is repeatedly exposed to the cancer-causing substance. This repeats the process mentioned above and increases the likelihood of cancer cells being reproduced.
3. **Progression** occurs when the malignant cancer cells begin to outnumber the normal, healthy cells because of continued replication within the body. At this point, the body is no longer able to attempt to repair the damage done to DNA by the cancer-causing agents and the normal cells continue to replicate as cancer cells.

Characteristics of Cancer Cells Terms

- **Pleomorphism** means that the cells are of different dimensions and forms.
- **Polymorphism** is the ability of the cell's nucleus to expand and change its form.

- **Hyperchromatism** refers to chromatin within the cell's nucleus that is seen clearly when staining is done for studies.
- **Translocations** are changes in the chromosomes in which genetic information is swapped.
- **Deletions** occur when portions of a chromosome's genetic information is obliterated.
- **Amplification** refers to multiple reproductions of a section of DNA.
- **Aneuploidy** refers to an atypical quantity of chromosomes.

Growth Characteristics of Cancer Cells

Just like normal cells, cancer cells are constantly changing, dying, and reproducing. Different types of tumors grow at different rates. This is measured in a percentage of cells that are actively being reproduced at any given time and is called the **growth fraction**. Tumor growth can also be measured in the amount of time it takes for tumor cells to double in quantity. This is called the **tumor volume doubling time**. Tumors require proper nutrition in order to thrive and continue to grow. To receive the necessary nutrients, there must be blood supply to the tumor. This blood supply is produced through angiogenesis. If the blood supply is not available to the tumor, the tumor cells will die. **Gompertzian growth** is a term that refers to a generality that is made regarding tumor growth. It is thought that tumors grow rapidly early on, but then growth slows down as the tumor enlarges. This most likely occurs because of not having the nutrients necessary to thrive.

Hyperplasia, Metaplasia, Dysplasia, and Anaplasia

- **Hyperplasia** is the process in which the quantity of cells within a certain tissue multiplies. This occurs in healthy tissue and in cancerous tissue.
- **Metaplasia** is when one type of cell is interchanged with another within a specific tissue. This occurs in response to chronic damage inflicted on a certain type of cell.
- **Dysplasia** is a change in normal cells. This can involve a change in any of the cell's characteristics.
- **Anaplasia** is used to explain cancer cells. It means that certain cells hold the characteristics that are seen with cancer cells.

Oncogenes

Oncogenes are present within the body's cells and play a role in the development of cancer. They are altered portions of the cells' DNA that function to promote the reproduction of cancer cells. The body does have ways of preventing oncogenes from reproducing cancer cells, though:

- *Proto-oncogenes* make up a portion of the DNA within cells. They are responsible for the replacement of normal cells and also play a role in fixing cells that have been damaged. If proto-oncogenes are altered by cancer cells, they can no longer perform their job of replacing and mending normal cells. These functions will no longer be performed, allowing cancer cells to attack the normal cells in order to produce more cancer cells.
- *Tumor suppression genes* are responsible for halting the replication of cells. They can also function to stop the reproduction of cancer cells. If tumor suppressor genes are altered or damaged, cancer cells will be able to reproduce without any interference.

Immunology

Immunology is the field of medicine that examines the body's ability to fight off infection. The body has a complicated system of cells and certain substances that react when an unknown agent attempts to cause an infectious process within the body.

When a cell is altered to form a cancer cell, the body usually recognizes it as abnormal and attacks it. This prevents its replication and the development of more cancer cells. If **immune cells** are not functioning properly, the cancer cell could go on to reproduce more cells to eventually form a tumor that can potentially invade the surrounding tissues.

Immunology also focuses on treatment research and ways in which the immune system can function more effectively in preventing cancer cell formation.

Two Categories of Immunity

The **two categories of immunology** are nonspecific immunity and specific or acquired immunity.

- Examples of ***nonspecific immunity*** are the skin along with the mucous membranes the skin provides a physical barrier; the epithelial lining of the respiratory tract that traps and sweeps away bacteria, the flushing action of the urine, the large quantity of lysozyme, an enzyme that destroys bacteria.
- ***Specific immunity*** is the immune system's response to an invader or antigen recognized by the body as nonself. Once recognized as nonself the antigen exerts a response in which an army of cells is activated to destroy and dispose of the antigenic material.

Groups of Specific Immunity

Specific immunity may be divided into two groups: **humoral immunity** and **cell-mediated immunity**. This group is made of two serum proteins derived from stem cells in the bone marrow (1) **antibody molecules** (immunoglobulins or Ig) and (2) **complement molecules**. Immunoglobulins are specific in that they bind to one and only one particular antigen. The first exposure to an antigen is followed by a latent phase during which time the detection of antibodies is low. Then there is a rapid response to the antigen then a plateau then a decline is antibody detection. On a second exposure the response time is very rapid, with high concentrations of the antibody detected.

Primary and Secondary Lymph Organs

Primary lymph organs are responsible for the development of lymphocytes. They also form the receptors to which cancer cells will bind. Primary lymph organs include bone marrow, where B-cells are formed, and the thymus within the mediastinum, where T-cells are developed. The thymus is very active in young people, but becomes inactive later on in adulthood.

Secondary lymph organs are the locations at which cancer cells frequently attempt to take over normal tissues. These include the tonsils, the spleen, organs that can develop cancer, lymph nodes, and bone marrow. The tonsils and organs are able to defend themselves against cancer using lymphatics within the mucosal lining of the organ. The spleen acts as a filter of blood and attempts to destroy abnormal cells as they pass through the organ. Bone marrow is the only lymphatic substance that functions as both primary and secondary lymph tissue.

Dendritic Cell Functions

Dendritic cells are formed from lymph tissue but most of them come from mononuclear phagocyte cells. They are responsible for **activating T cells** in fighting foreign cells. It is thought that they are most valuable in immunity against viruses and tumors.

When a foreign cell is present in the body, dendritic cells take the antigen proteins from the cell and travel through the lymph vessels to deliver the information to the T cells. This stimulates the T cells to formulate an immune response against the foreign cell. If dendritic cells are not functioning correctly, the T cells cannot receive the antigen protein information from the foreign cell in a timely manner, which can result in a delay in the immune system triggering a response against them. This can result in the development of an infection or the possibility of cancer cells developing and reproducing to form a tumor.

Lymphocytes, Phagocytes, and Basophils Functions

- **Lymphocytes** are necessary for the body's immune system to function. They are divided into B cells and T cells. B cells are formed in the bone marrow. When a foreign object enters the body, the B cells begin to duplicate and produce immunoglobulins to help function in immunity. T cells mature within the thymus gland and function to produce substances that assist the immune system, help B cells with an immune response, and destroy foreign cells that are present.
- **Phagocytes** are responsible for enclosing foreign substances and destroying them. There are mononuclear phagocytes, polymorphonuclear granulocytes, and eosinophils that aid in this function. Polymorphonuclear granulocytes are the most prevalent type of white blood cells and comprise over 50% of the total number of white blood cells.
- **Basophils** are responsible for traveling to areas where there is tissue injury and causing the release of substances that stimulate an allergic reaction.

Mast Cell Functions

Mast cells are granulocytes. They have many factors that stimulate the immune system to cause an inflammatory reaction with the tissues where foreign cells or damage has occurred. Mast cells usually reside near blood vessels and can also be found throughout the body within tissues. They appear very similar to basophils and are often mistaken for basophils under the microscope. The mast cells located within organs are called **mucosal mast cells** because they are located within the mucosa of the organ. Mast cells that reside near the blood vessels are called connective tissue mast cells.

Types of Null Cells

Null cells are derived from lymph tissue, but they do not function to activate T cells or B cells. Once they are fully formed, null cells possess an affinity for working with macrophages and neutrophils to trigger an immune response. The two types of null cells are natural killer cells and lymphokine-activated cells.

1. *Natural killer cells* hold material that functions as enzymes to destroy foreign cells. When the immune response is triggered, natural killer cells function even more efficiently to kill the cells. They have an affinity for virus cells and some tumor cells.

- 41 -

2. ***Lymphokine-activated cells*** are formed outside of the circulatory system by combining lymphocytes with interleukin-2 and then replacing the cells in the patient's body. This creates cells that are much more affective in destroying foreign cells. They do not trigger activation of other substances within the immune system and must be directly in contact with the foreign cell in order to be affective.

Cytokines

- **Cytokines** refer to a group of cells that function to promote maturity of white blood cells and other substances responsible for immunity. They can also trigger other cells within the immune system to function and work with the immune system when necessary.
- **Interferons** are activated in response to viral invasions within the body. They are released early on after exposure to viral agents.
- **Interleukins** are created by T cells, though they are also found within certain tissues.
- **Hematopoietic growth factors**, or colony-stimulating factors, work in organizing and leading cell reproduction. They also trigger the process that distinguishes stem cells from white blood cells.
- **Tumor necrosis factors** are activated in response to inflammation and actions that lead to cell death.
- **Chemokines** are produced by white blood cells and work to direct white blood cells through the body in response to an antigen's presence.

Complement System

The **complement system** is made up of proteins that function in immunity. When a foreign object enters the body, antibodies will attach to it if it is recognizable to them. This activates the complement proteins to travel through the vascular system to the tissue affected. The foreign object, or antigen, is altered when the antibody attaches to it and undergoes changes that allow the complement protein to attach to it, also. The ***complement protein*** causes several activities to occur once it attaches to the antigen:

- First, neutrophils and macrophages are activated and they begin to travel to the antigen-antibody article.
- Other substances are released to cause damage to the cell membrane of the antigen.
- Enzymes are released to begin breaking down the antigen.
- The complement system also causes activation of basophils and mast cells which will stimulate the inflammatory process to further stimulate the immune system into attacking the antigen.

Characteristics of Families with Familial Cancer Syndromes

- Cancers of the same general type (breast or ovarian) tend to occur in the same lineage (paternal or maternal).
- Cancer is diagnosed at an early age.
- Multiple cancers in the same person (e.g. colon and uterine).
- Rare tumors occur.
- Cancer in organs that occur in heirs.
- Nonmalignant manifestations of familial cancer.

Types of Genetic Mutations

- A **frameshift mutation** is a protein that has been modified because it has at least one base attached or deleted from it.
- A **missense mutation** occurs when an amino acid is replaced by a different amino acid within a protein. This can result in an alteration in performance of the protein or it may not have any effect on performance.
- A **nonsense mutation** is an alteration in the construction of protein because the amino acids are "told" to quit constructing a protein. This results in a protein that is incomplete and cannot function normally.
- **RNA-negative mutations** are proteins that do not have RNA because of an error in duplication.
- **Splicing** results when unnecessary DNA is preserved or when necessary DNA is omitted. This causes a frameshift mutation.
- **Polymorphisms** usually do not result in any visible changes in a person. They are alterations in the DNA sequence.

Research Protocols for Cancer

A **research protocol** is the "blueprint" of a clinical trial or research study for the treatment of cancer. The National Cancer Institute defines a research protocol as "a detailed plan of a scientific or medical experiment, treatment, or procedure." Research protocols include a description of the study, the duration of the study, how the study will be executed, and why it is being done. The protocol will explain how many participants will be in the study, eligibility criteria for the study (including inclusion and exclusion criteria), any medications or other interventions that will be given during the course of the study (including testing), the frequency of the intervention, and how the data gathered throughout the study will be collected. Nursing staff caring for the oncology patient have a critical role in the orchestration of the research protocol. It is vitally important that the protocol be followed thoroughly and accurately to ensure the patient has the greatest chance of the intervention(s) being successful in the cancer treatment.

Clinical Trials Phases

Clinical trials for new drugs must undergo extensive review by the FDA's institutional review board. The job of these review boards is to make sure that the study is ethical, that the patients involved in the trial are being protected from any harm, and that all patients involved in the trial are aware and have consented to all risks. There are 4 phases involved in clinical trials: **Phase 1** has a primary focus on patient safety and is the phase in which the maximum tolerated dose is determined. The most frequent and serious adverse effects are recorded as well as how the drug is metabolized and excreted. Phase 1 clinical trials work to establish an effective drug administration schedule. **Phase 2** is where the preliminary data on the drug's effectiveness is established. Short-term adverse reactions are studied. In **Phase 3** of a clinical trial, the overall benefit versus the risk of the drug is evaluated and more data regarding safety and efficacy is established. **Phase 4** occurs after the drug has been approved by the FDA for marketing purposes. Additional information regarding safety and efficacy are established, with the goal of refining the protocol to determine the optimal treatment use of the new drug.

Clinical Trials for Cancer Drugs

A **clinical trial** is a research-driven study conducted to test the safety and efficacy of new treatments or to discover alternate ways of preventing, screening, or diagnosing a disease.

Treatment trials are utilized for patients who have cancer with the purpose of evaluating the effectiveness of a new treatment or procedure. Clinical trials are designed in a series of phases. The aim of **phase 1** trials is to determine the maximum tolerated dose and strength of the therapy and its safety. The clinical pharmacology is studied as well as the how the tumor responds to the treatment. In **phase 2**, the value of the new treatment is compared with that of standard treatment. Tumor response rates are measured in phase 2. In **phase 3**, a complete experimental test of the treatment is conducted with the goal of establishing whether the new treatment is superior to that of the standard treatment. In phase 3, a large sample of patients is involved and the use of randomization is employed to ensure reliable results. **Phase 4** clinical trials occur once the decision has been made to adopt the new treatment. The focus of phase 4 trials is the long-term effects of the new treatment, including benefits and adverse effects.

Site-Specific Cancer Considerations

Prognosis

Prognosis is defined as the likely course or outcome of a disease process. In cancer, there are many factors that can affect a patient's prognosis. **Type of cancer**, **location**, **stage**, and **grade** are all factors used in determining a patient's prognosis. The stage of cancer is directly related to a patient's prognosis. Often, medical staff use statistical data based on patients with a similar disease presentation to help determine a prognosis. Other factors such as the biological and genetic properties of the cancer cells may be used to determine prognosis. These "biomarkers" can be determined through laboratory and diagnostic testing. In addition, the age and overall general health of the patient are considered in determining prognosis. Patients with other comorbidities have the potential to have a poorer prognosis. How a patient responds to treatment is also a prognostic indicator.

Tumor Classifications

1. **Carcinoma**: Cancer of epithelial tissue cells/
2. **Sarcoma**: A malignant tumor growing from mesodermal tissue.
3. **Lymphoma**: Cancer coming from the nodes or glands of the lymphatic system.
4. **Leukemia**: Cancer of the bone marrow stopping the marrow from producing normal blood cells.
5. **Myeloma**: Cancer in the plasma cells of the bone. In many bones it is called multiple myeloma.

Terms

- **Invasive**: The tumor can invade the tissues surrounding it by sending the cancerous cells of the tumor into the surrounding normal tissue.
- **Metastatic**: Cancer cells from the tumor that have migrated to other tissues near or far from the original tumor.
- **Primary tumor**: The original tumor.
- **Secondary tumor**: New tumors of the same identical tumor cells located in far organs there by cancer cells circulating through the blood circulatory system or through the lymphatic system.

Tumor Grade and Classification

Tumor grade is a description of how the tumor appears under microscopic examination. It is a determining factor in how likely the tumor is to grow and spread. Different grading systems exist for each type of cancer.

- "Well-differentiated" tumor cells appear the most like normal cells. These types of cancer cells tend to grow and spread more slowly. Well-differentiated cancer cells may also be referred to as "**low-grade**."
- "Undifferentiated" cancer cells appear more abnormal and are associated with a poorer prognosis. Undifferentiated cancer cells may also be referred to as "**high-grade**."

Based upon their microscopic appearance, pathologists can assign a numeric grade to the cancer cells. This information is then utilized by physicians to help determine the course of treatment and the patient's prognosis. Tumor grade is not considered the same as the stage of the cancer. Staging refs to the size and extent of the cancer and whether or not the cancer has spread to other areas of the body.

Brain Anatomical Structures

The brain is divided into two halves called **cerebrums**. Each cerebrum is further divided into **lobes**; these are the frontal, temporal, parietal, and occipital lobes. The **hypothalamus** is located at the base of the cerebrum and the cerebellum is located underneath the occipital lobes. The **brain stem** is the most inferior portion of the brain and leads into the spinal cord.

The brain consists of **four ventricles** that act as storage units for cerebrospinal fluid (CSF). Blood is supplied to the brain through the carotid and vertebral arteries. A vascular structure called the **Circle of Willis** functions to connect the blood vessels from the front and back of the brain. Blood flow to the brain is monitored by the blood-brain barrier, which selectively allows certain elements to enter the blood stream around the brain and blocks other items.

The most common brain tumors that affect adults are **astrocytomas,** which occur in connective tissue, **oligodendrocytomas,** which occur in the nerve cells that produce myelin, and **ependymomas,** which occur within the ventricles.

Functions of Brain Areas

- The **frontal lobe** is responsible for appropriate social behavior and intellectual thinking. It also controls our mood and memory. Some speech functions are also located within the frontal lobe.
- The **temporal lobe** is responsible for understanding speech and memory. Hearing sensation is also located in this area of the brain.
- The **parietal lobes** are responsible for sensation. This includes differentiating between sharp and dull objects, experiencing pain, and touch.
- The **occipital lobes** are responsible for vision and understanding an object that is observed.
- Motor function is coordinated by the **motor strip** between the frontal and parietal lobes. The right side of the body is controlled by the left side of the motor strip and vice versa. Maintaining balance and performing coordinated movements is controlled by the **cerebellum**.
- The **hypothalamus** is the location of the satiety center (appetite), the thermoregulatory center (temperature control), and the sleep center.
- The **brain stem** is responsible for the regulation of blood pressure, heart rate, and respirations.

Tests for Diagnosing Brain Tumors

Brain tumors are more likely to occur in men than women and the incidence of brain tumors is slowly increasing. More than one-half of all brain tumors are malignant. There is no routine screening done to check for brain tumors.

When suspected, testing usually begins with a **CT scan**. This should be done with and without contrast to assess for uptake within the tissue of the lesion. If the CT shows a suspicious lesion, an **MRI** with and without contrast is done to better visualize the tumor.

Once a tumor is identified, the patient will be scheduled for a **stereotactic biopsy** or **surgery** to remove the tumor. After the patient has been positioned intraoperatively, a special frame is used to hold the head still and isolate the location where the tumor is located. A more specific MRI using stereotactic protocol may be done beforehand to provide an isolated view of the tumor and its exact location within the brain.

Breast Cancer Pathophysiology

The **breasts** are made up of fatty tissue, blood vessels, lymph vessels, and nerves. Behind the breasts are the ribs and intercostals muscles between the ribs. Each breast is made up of 6-10 ducts that are responsible for lactation. They all come together at the nipple. The lymph vessels run through the breast tissue and drain lymph fluid into the lymph nodes located in the axillae.

Most **breast cancers** occur within the **ductal-lobular units**. These areas of the breasts undergo changes due to the normal hormonal changes a woman experiences each month with the menstrual cycle. They also undergo significant changes with pregnancy and childbirth. Cancer cells can form in the tissues that make up the ducts of the breast. These cells can be carried through the lymphatic system or circulatory system to other areas of the body or the cancer cells can form a tumor that is localized within the ducts.

Diagnosing Breast Cancer

Biopsy of the questionable breast tissue is definitive for a diagnosis of breast cancer. This can be done by inserting a thin needle into the lesion and withdrawing some cells for microscopic study.

If Paget's disease is suspected, a ***punch biopsy*** of the skin can be performed for further evaluation. If it is thought that there is an underlying ductal cancer, biopsy may also be done of the ***ductal tissue***. If a tissue lump is palpable, an ***incisional biopsy*** may be done to remove part of the tumor for further testing. An ***excisional biopsy***, or lumpectomy, is done to remove the entire tumor along with some normal tissue surrounding the tumor. ***Stereotactic biopsy*** is done following an advanced mammogram study that better delineates the region in question. If the tissue is not palpable, thin wires may be inserted directly into the tissue under fluoroscopy so that the correct tissue is removed for study.

History and Physical Exam Findings of Breast Cancer Patients

Most patients with breast cancer do not have any symptoms. When taking a **history** from the patient with breast cancer, ask if they have felt a lump within the breast or axilla. If advanced, the patient may have noticed weight loss. Depending on the extent of involvement, there may be a noticeable change in breast shape. They may have noticed a discharge from the nipple when not lactating. If very advanced with metastasis, the patient may complain of back pain or other bone pain.

On **physical exam**, examine the breasts while the patient is sitting upright. They may appear grossly uneven or there may be dimpling of the skin present over the breast. With Paget's disease, the skin may have an orange peel appearance along with skin changes over the nipple and areola. A lump may or may not be palpable on exam. Clinical breast exam should include the axillae to check for any enlarged lymph nodes. The patient's weight should be assessed and compared with previous recordings, if available.

Types of Invasive Breast Cancer

- **Invasive breast cancer** involves the breast tissue, but also extends into adjacent tissues. This type of cancer has the ability to metastasize to distant parts of the body.
- **Invasive ductal carcinoma** makes up most of the cases of invasive breast cancer. It is located within the ducts, but extends beyond the basement membrane to consume surrounding tissues. It may also travel through the blood or lymphatic systems.
- **Invasive lobular carcinoma** begins in the lobe tissue within the breast and invades surrounding tissue. Up to 10% of all invasive breast cancers arise in the lobe tissue.
- **Paget's disease** begins as a malignant lesion around the nipple and areola. The malignancy usually begins as a ductal carcinoma that spreads to include the external features of the breast. This form of cancer is usually very obvious to the patient because of the physical changes visible in the nipple and areola.

Types of Non-Invasive Breast Cancer

Noninvasive cancers are also called *in-situ cancers*. Within the breast, they are restricted to the ductal-lobular units and do not extend into the lymphatic or circulatory systems.

Ductal carcinoma in situ is a stage 0 type of cancer. It is localized within the ductal-lobular units and does not extend into the bottom portion of the tissue. This type of cancer is considered preinvasive and women who develop this are more likely to develop invasive cancer in the future. This is usually detected through a mammogram and is not usually found on breast self-exam. This is removed surgically.

Lobular carcinoma in situ is usually not identified on mammogram or during breast self-exam. It is usually diagnosed as an accidental finding on biopsy of another lesion. The presence of lobular carcinoma in situ indicates an increased risk for invasive breast cancer in either breast in the future.

Pathophysiology of Types of Prostate Cancer

The **prostate** is located around the urethra in males. It functions to produce the fluid present in semen. The outermost area of the prostate, or peripheral zone, is the primary location for prostate cancer. Because of its close proximity to other structures within the pelvic cavity, **cancer of the prostate** can spread to the bladder and rectum. It also has an affinity for metastasizing to the bones and lungs.

As the prostate gland enlarges because of tumor formation, the urethra can be compressed. This causes difficulty urinating and may even cause some blood in the urine. If a tumor is large enough, pressure can be placed on the colon and rectum and cause constipation or an obstruction.

Most prostate cancers are **adenocarcinomas** in nature. Malignancies can also develop within the ducts that lead from the gland or in the epithelial cells of the gland. Normally, prostate cancer is slow growing with a low risk of metastasis if diagnosed early.

Tests for Diagnosing Prostate Cancer

It is recommended that men over the age of 50 undergo annual **prostate specific antigen (PSA) testing** along with a **digital rectal exam (DRE)**. Men with moderate to high risk of developing prostate cancer are recommended to get screened at ages 45 and 40, respectively. These two tests together can help with early detection of the disease. There is some controversy with this, however, because the entire prostate cannot be palpated through the rectal wall. Also, an elevated PSA does not always indicate the presence of prostate cancer. The test indicates that there is growth of the prostate gland, which can occur with benign prostatic hypertrophy (BPH) in the absence of cancer.

If DRE reveals a mass on the prostate gland, a transrectal ultrasound may be performed to differentiate between solid or cystic. A **biopsy** can be performed in conjunction with ultrasound to evaluate the tissue for the presence of cancer cells.

Once the presence of cancer is confirmed, **CT scans** and **MRI** will be performed to assess for any enlarged lymph nodes or metastatic spread to other organs. A **bone scan** will also be performed to check for bony metastasis.

History and Physical Exam Findings of Prostate Cancer Patients

Patients may not have any complaints when they are diagnosed with **prostate cancer**. More often, they will complain of the same symptoms associated with BPH, or an enlarged prostate. There may be difficulty urinating because of the enlarging prostate applying pressure on the urethra. They may also complain of not being able to fully empty the bladder, frequent urination, or painful urination. If bony metastasis has occurred, the patient may have complaints of back or hip pain. The patient may have suffered a vertebral compression fracture, which is very painful, and the prostate cancer is identified at this point.

On **physical exam**, the patient may appear perfectly normal without any outward signs of the disease. DRE may reveal an enlarged or irregularly shaped prostate gland. If urinary retention has been a problem, the bladder may be palpable on abdominal exam. If advanced, the patient may have obvious weight loss or cachexia.

Breast and Prostate Cancer Grading Systems

The most commonly used grading system in breast cancer is the **Nottingham grading system** (also called the Elston-Ellis modification of the Scarff-Bloom-Richardson grading system for breast cancer). This grading system evaluates the breast cancer cells on tubule formation, an evaluation of the size and shape of the nucleus of the tumor cells and the rate of cell mitosis. Each category gets assigned a score between 1 and 3, with 1 meaning that the cells most resemble that of a normal breast cell and 3 meaning that the cells are most abnormal from that of a normal breast cell.

For prostate cancer, the **Gleason scale** is used for tumor grading. Based on the biopsied specimen from the prostate, both the primary and secondary pattern of tissue organization are identified and graded. Each pattern is given a score of 1-5, with 1 most resembling normal prostate tissue and 5 appearing the most abnormal. The scores are added together and assigned a category.

Lung Cancer Pathophysiology

The **lungs** are responsible for providing the blood with an appropriate amount of oxygen in order to supply the body's tissues with the oxygen necessary to function properly. The absorption of oxygen occurs at the cellular level. The lining of the lungs is composed of columnar epithelial cells which contain cilia that function to filter the oxygen within the lungs. There are also cells within the lung's lining that function to secrete mucus which helps to clear the lungs of foreign particles.

When the lungs are continuously exposed to caustic agents, such as cigarette smoke or asbestos, the **columnar epithelium** is permanently damaged and replaced by **simple squamous cells**. With

- 49 -

cells continuously being damaged and replaced, malignant cells can form and invade the tissue within the lungs. This will decrease the lung's capacity to absorb oxygen and can interfere with normal expansion of the lungs with inspiration.

Diagnosing Lung Cancer

Lung cancer is usually discovered after a patient complains of a respiratory illness that lingers and a tumor is detected on chest x-ray.

- Routine *chest x-ray* may also reveal a malignancy that was previously not detected.
- Once a chest x-ray reveals a suspicious lesion, a *CT scan* is performed to further investigate the lesion and assess for any other lesions not seen on x-ray. Studies will also be performed on other organ systems to assess for metastasis.
- *PET scans* are performed to assist with staging the cancer.
- For definitive diagnosis and histological typing, *tissue sample* and *biopsy* will be performed. This can be accomplished with bronchoscopy, fine-needle aspiration of the lesion, or mediastinoscopy.
- Any lymph nodes that are suspicious will also be *biopsied* for the presence of cancer cells.
- If a pleural effusion is present, a *thoracentesis* will be performed to test for the presence of cancer cells.

History and Physical Exam Findings of Lung Cancer Patients

When taking a **history** from the patient with lung cancer, ask about any smoking habits. This includes current or past tobacco use. Document tobacco use in pack years which is the number of years smoked multiplied by the total packs of cigarettes smoked per day. A patient with at least a 20 pack year history is more likely to suffer complications from smoking. Also question the patient about exposure to any environmental hazards, such as asbestos, fiberglass, or coal. Obtain a thorough history about specific symptoms that are present and how long they have been present. Assess whether the patient has a history of other respiratory comorbidities such as COPD, asthma, or pulmonary fibrosis.

On **physical exam**, assess the patient's respiratory rate and pulse oximetry level. Auscultate the lungs and assess for any adventitious sounds or diminished breath sounds. Evaluate the patient for any sputum production with cough and assess its color and consistency. Examine the patient for any accessory muscle use with breathing and any signs of respiratory distress.

Lung Cancer Types

There are three main types of lung cancer: non-small cell lung cancer, small cell lung cancer, and mesothelioma.

- **Non-small cell lung cancer** is further categorized as squamous carcinoma, adenocarcinoma, large cell, or spindle cell. The most common of these types is adenocarcinoma.
- **Small cell lung cancer** comprises approximately less than 20% of all incidents of lung cancer, but it is a more destructive type of cancer.
- **Mesothelioma** occurs due to asbestos exposure and is almost always fatal.

The presentation of lung cancer will vary depending on its location. A tumor located in the main airway, which is the most common, will cause wheezing and difficulty breathing. A tumor in the upper portions of the lungs can cause referred pain to the shoulder and down the arm. A tumor in the mid-lung may cause diminished breath sounds while a tumor in the lower lobe can cause a pleural effusion along with diminished breath sounds.

TNM Classification for Staging Lung Cancer

The **TNM classification** involves rating the tumor size (T), any **lymph node involvement** (N), and the presence of **metastasis** (M). A number rating is also used with the letter classifications ranging from 0 to 4 depending on severity. An X label is used in place of a number if the tumor, node, or metastasis cannot be definitely determined based on diagnostic testing.

- A numerical ranking of 0 indicates that there is no evidence of tumor, lymph node involvement, or metastasis.
- A numerical ranking of 1 indicates that there is a localized tumor, adjacent lymph node involvement, or distant metastasis.
- A numerical ranking of 2 indicates a tumor that involves lung tissue and the pleura lining, but is not through the entire lung.
- A numerical ranking of 3 involves the whole lung plus the chest wall.
- A numerical ranking of 4 involves the entire lung and adjacent structures such as trachea, esophagus, and pericardium.
- A lymph node ranking of 3 involves adjacent nodes.

Pathophysiology of Colorectal Cancer

The **colon** is responsible for absorbing water and electrolytes from solid waste material. Most of this occurs in the ascending and proximal portion of the transverse colon. Solid waste is then transported through the colon to the rectum and anus to be expelled from the body. Once oxygen and other nutrients are delivered to the colon, blood is drained from the area through the portal vein to the liver. Blood from the rectum and anus is drained to the inferior vena cava.

Cancer affecting the colon, rectum, or anus occurs within the cells lining the organs. A malignancy can develop into a tumor structure or involve a lesion that extends through the layers of the organ. Lymph nodes in the area as well as adjacent organs can be sites of cancer, also, through metastasis from the colon. Cancers that occur in the colon, rectum, or anus can result in bleeding, pain, and obstruction of solid waste leading to constipation or obstruction.

Diagnosing Colorectal Cancer

Regular **screening** should be done to assess for the presence of colon cancer. This is accomplished through *digital rectal exams,* which allow the healthcare provider to assess for any masses within the rectum.

Sigmoidoscopy and *colonoscopy* can be performed regularly to assess for any masses or tissue changes that may be present. These studies are usually performed every 5 years, depending on the patient's history.

Biopsy of any suspicious lesions can be obtained during these studies.

Once a malignant lesion has been identified, the section of colon can be *resected* surgically. The patient may require a *colostomy* following surgery, which may be temporary or permanent depending on the extent of involvement within the colon or rectum. *Radiation therapy* can be done to shrink a tumor before surgical removal or can be done following surgery to ensure destruction of cancer cells. *Chemotherapy* can be given along with radiation treatments and is used when there is lymph node or metastatic involvement.

Colon and Rectum Cancer Symptoms

Adenocarcinoma of the colon is usually slow to develop but can be more invasive than other forms of colorectal cancer. It is common to have metastasis to the lymph system with this type of cancer.

- If located in the *ascending colon*, the patient may experience a decrease in weight along with abdominal pain. When advanced, they may complain of diarrhea or constipation.
- When located in the *transverse or descending portion of the colon*, a bowel obstruction may occur. The patient may also experience a cramping pain.
- Cancers located in the *sigmoid colon* cause a narrowing of the diameter of the stool along with constipation.
- Cancers that form within the *rectum* usually cause bleeding and a feeling like the patient is not able to completely pass stool. They may also complain of rectal pain.
- Cancer in the *anus* can be adenocarcinoma, squamous cell, or basal cell. HIV patients may also develop Kaposi's sarcoma in this area. Anal cancers cause bleeding, pain, and the patient may notice a lump near the anus.

Pathophysiology of Cervical Cancer

The **cervix** is the terminal portion of the uterus that extends into the superior end of the vagina. There are several lymph nodes in the tissue that surrounds the cervix. The cervix contains both squamous and columnar epithelial cells. Most cancers occur at the point where these two cell types meet, the **squamocolumnar junction**.

There are several causes of cervical cancer, but one that has gained more attention recently is the **human papillomavirus (HPV)**. This virus is thought to cause cellular changes in the cervix which can result in cellular mutation and cancer cell formation. A vaccination is now available to help prevent HPV infection, thus reducing the risk of cervical cancer.

Most cervical cancers arise from the **squamous epithelium**. Some are classified as adenocarcinomas and these tend to have a poor prognosis. The patients with adenocarcinoma are generally younger and the cancer tends to be more damaging to other tissues.

Diagnosing Cervical Cancer

- **Pap smears** are recommended for women annually as a screening tool for cervical cancer. This test can also detect pre-cancerous cells so that early diagnosis and treatment can be accomplished.
- If a Pap smear shows abnormal cells, a **colposcopy** is performed. This involves applying acetic acid to the cervix and then performing an exam under magnification.
- If a colposcopy has abnormal results, a **biopsy** of the cervical tissue will be done. A cone biopsy is done if a larger section of tissue is necessary for biopsy.
- **HPV testing** can be done to test for a possible cause of abnormal cells on Pap smear. There is no treatment for HPV once it has been diagnosed; however, a vaccine is now available to reduce the risk of contracting the virus.
- If cervical cancer is diagnosed, a **CT scan** of the pelvis and abdomen will be performed to assess for free fluid in the abdomen as well as the presence of lymph nodes or other lesions.
- Other diagnostics may be performed to assess for metastasis.

History and Physical Exam Findings of Cervical Cancer Patients

When taking a **history** on the patient with **cervical cancer**, assess her family history for any relatives with cancer. Also ask about known infection with HPV or a history of abnormal Pap smears. Assess the patient's sexual history as well because HPV is transmissible from sexual partners. Any other cancer risk factors should be recorded, such as smoking.

On **physical exam**, the patient may not notice any symptoms until the disease has progressed. There may be a thin vaginal discharge present or some spotting after intercourse or between periods. They may also notice a change in their period with having it last longer and possibly have more discharge than normal.

Patients may have **complaints** of difficulty urinating or constipation when cervical cancer is advanced. This is due to the tumor tissue compressing the urethra or bowel. They may also complain of some rectal bleeding or visible blood in the urine.

Diagnosing Ovarian Cancer

Unfortunately, **ovarian cancer** is often not detected until it has metastasized to other areas. In women who are not considered high risk, screening procedures are not performed. In women who are known to be high risk with a positive family history, **CA-125 blood testing** for tumor markers and transvaginal ultrasounds can be performed for screening. Ovarian cancer is usually diagnosed after a patient complains of secondary symptoms such as constipation or abdominal pain.

Laparoscopic surgery is performed to obtain tissue samples from the ovaries for definitive diagnosis. If there is free fluid present in the pelvic cavity, samples of this will be obtained, also, to assess for cancer cells. Once a diagnosis is established, testing is done on other body systems to assess for any metastasis of the disease. This will include **CT scans, chest x-ray, and bone scans.** If lesions are found on other organs, more tissue samples may be obtained to definitively diagnose the presence of metastasis.

History and Physical Exam Findings of Ovarian Cancer Patients

When taking a **history** from the patient with **ovarian cancer**, be sure to ask about any family history of ovarian cancer. There can also be an increased risk of ovarian cancer when a family member has a history of colon cancer because of similar tumor markers with CA-125. Ask about reproductive history including total number of pregnancies or any history of difficulty becoming pregnant. Question the patient about regular health screening habits, such as most recent Pap smear and mammogram and whether the results were normal.

On **physical exam**, the patient may or may not appear sick, depending on how advanced the disease has become. Early on, there may be some abdominal tenderness and vaginal bleeding present. With advanced disease, a tumor may be palpable in the lower abdomen. The patient may have substantial weight loss, and the patient may develop constipation or an intestinal obstruction. Laboratory tests include a CA-125 which is a tumor marker for ovarian cancer.

Testicular Cancer Types

The **testes** are responsible for secreting the hormone testosterone and for producing sperm. Without testosterone, normal male maturation can be delayed or hindered, along with development of secondary sex characteristics.

Testicular cancer is usually not bilateral; it usually only affects one testicle. Male babies who do not have normal descent of the testicles into the scrotum are at risk for developing testicular cancer later in life. Other congenital disorders or physical irregularities can result in testicular cancer.

Seminomas comprise about one-half of all cases of testicular cancer. These are relatively slow-growing and can spread into the lymphatic system. These are usually very treatable with radiation therapy.

Nonseminoma germ cell testicular tumors are more destructive and most have already metastasized to the lymph nodes at the time they are discovered. Most of these develop when the male is an embryo and they are not easy to treat with radiation. These frequently metastasize to other organs.

Diagnosing Testicular Cancer

Men need to be taught to perform **testicular self-exams** monthly to evaluate for any abnormalities in shape of the testes or the presence of any lumps. A clinic exam should be performed on the genitals at least annually.

- When a lump is discovered, an **ultrasound** is done to determine whether the mass is cystic or solid. If solid, a biopsy of the tissue is done for definitive diagnosis.
- If positive for testicular cancer, an **orchiectomy** (removal of the testis) is performed. With the removal of only one testis, most men are able to go on and conceive children without difficulty.
- Studies will also be performed to assess for any metastasis of the disease. This will include **chest x-ray, CT scan of other organ systems, and bone scan.**
- **Renal studies** may also be done to assess for any kidney involvement.
- **Blood tests** to measure certain protein and hormone levels can also be performed. These may show some abnormalities with the presence of a testicular tumor.

History and Physical Exam Findings of Testicular Cancer Patients

Testicular cancer is more common in men younger than 35 years old. During the collection of history, questions should be asked to assess whether they perform regular testicular self-examinations. They need to find out if their testicles were delayed in descending as an infant or if they were present in the scrotum at birth. Another risk factor for the disease is that patients with more than one nipple are at a higher risk for testicular cancer.

On **physical exam**, a thorough genital exam will need to be performed. The size and density of the mass should be documented, as well as its ability to be moved or if it is fixed to the surrounding tissue. Exam should include a rectal exam to assess for any changes in prostate size. Testicular cancer has an affinity for lung metastasis, so a respiratory exam should be performed to assess for any adventitious breath sounds. Chest x-ray should also be done to assess for any masses within the lungs.

Bladder Cancer Types

The function of the **bladder** is to store urine before it passes through the urethra and out of the body. **Cancer tumors** form in the wall of the bladder and can cause bleeding because of cell damage. If large enough, a tumor can also cause a blockage in the urethra, which can affect voiding.

Most bladder cancers are described as **urothelial carcinomas** and usually appear in different locations within the bladder. These affect the epithelial lining of the bladder, and if metastasis is present, can extend into the basement membrane of the bladder wall. Most of the urothelial tumors involve only the lining of the bladder wall and do not extend deeper into the tissue.

Papillary tumors are hereditary and specific chromosomal changes have been seen with this type of tumor. These involve the superficial lining of the bladder and the second layer of the bladder wall tissue.

Diagnosing Bladder Cancer

Routine screening is not currently being performed for early diagnosis of **bladder cancer**. The disease is usually diagnosed after the patient complains of frank blood in the urine. Generally, the patient has no complaints of pain or other noticeable symptoms of malignancy.

- *Urinalysis* can detect the presence of blood. Specific studies can be done on the types of cells obtained through urinalysis.
- *Cystoscopy* can also be performed in which a thin catheter is inserted through the urethra into the bladder and a tiny camera is used to visualize the bladder wall. Tissue samples for biopsy can also be obtained through this test.
- An *IVP* (intravenous pyelogram) is used to assess whether the malignancy is located within the bladder or higher in the urinary system.
- *CT scan and MRI* can also be done to assess for the presence of tumors and to check for metastasis to surrounding organs.
- There is *tumor marker testing* available for patients who have a history of bladder tumors to assess for recurrence.

History and Physical Exam Findings of Bladder Cancer Patients

Question the patient about the presence of any of the common risk factors for cancer. Ask about previous employment and possibility of exposure to hazardous chemicals. Also evaluate the patient for any symptoms of dysuria, difficulty urinating, inability to urinate, or the presence of frank blood in the urine.

On **physical exam**, the patient may not show any outward signs of illness. If difficulty urinating has been a problem, an abdominal exam may reveal a palpable enlarged bladder due to retention. There may also be discomfort when examining the abdomen. The patient may have an increase in rectal pain with firm abdominal palpation, also, if the tumor is compressing the rectum.

If the disease is advanced with metastasis, the patient may have visible weight loss or cachexia. Objective signs of pain may also be present with grimacing or guarding. Lymph nodes through the groin (inguinal) may also be palpable if enlarged.

Development of Leukemia

Blood cells are created in the bone marrow, liver, and spleen. Because of the constant process of blood cell production, a cell can develop that is malignant in nature. If the body's immune system does not destroy this cell, it can go on to replicate and leukemia develops. **Leukemia** causes the sites of blood cell production to begin rapidly producing cells. This results in the production of immature cells and a decreased ability of normal cells to be produced. These **leukemic cells** can travel through the blood stream and cause damage in organs throughout the body, impairing the ability of these organs to function properly.

...mia is labeled based on the type of cells that are impaired and how far along the cell has ...ed. Leukemia is either *myelogenous* or *lymphocytic* in nature and can be *acute* or *chronic*. ...leukemia is more common than chronic and it is also the most common type of leukemia that occurs in children, though leukemia is more common in adults than children.

Symptoms of Leukemia Types

- **Acute myelogenous leukemia (AML)** presents with generalized symptoms similar to the flu. Patients may complain of generalized achiness, fever, or fatigue. Symptoms may be more severe and include shortness of breath, weight loss, decreased appetite, vomiting, changes in visual acuity, and seizures.
- **Acute lymphocytic leukemia (ALL)** has symptoms that are very similar to AML. On exam, enlarged lymph nodes and an enlarged spleen may be palpable.
- **Chronic myelogenous leukemia (CML)** can cause the same generalized symptoms as the acute leukemias, but the patient may also complain of left-sided abdominal pain or a feeling of fullness throughout the abdomen. On exam, the liver and spleen may feel enlarged. The patient may also have symptoms of a bleeding disorder due to decreased production of platelets.
- **Chronic lymphocytic leukemia (CLL)** may present with the same generalized complaints as CML, but symptoms may be slower to appear. Once noticeable, the patient may have an enlarged liver and spleen on exam as well as enlarged lymph nodes. Symptoms of anemia and a bleeding disorder may also be present.

History and Physical Exam Findings of Leukemia Patients

When taking a **history** from the patient with leukemia, it is important to assess any past family history of cancer that may be present. Also question them about the risk of occupational exposure to radiation or chemicals, especially benzene. Patients with a positive history of HIV are at risk for developing lymphocytic leukemia that affects the T-cells. Also, patients with genetic diseases such as Down syndrome, Klinefelter's syndrome, and neurofibromatosis are at risk for developing leukemia.

On **physical exam**, the patient may have palpable or even visibly enlarged lymph nodes. If the platelet count is decreased, bleeding may be present at the mucous membranes or bruising may be evident. The patient may also have frank blood present in the urine or the patient may have dark, tarry stools because of occult blood. The patient may have an enlarged liver or spleen on abdominal exam. If the patient is anemic, they may be obviously pale, fatigued, or have an irregular heart rate.

Lymph System Cells and Tissues

Lymph tissue can be primary or secondary:

- **Primary lymph tissues** include the bone marrow and the thymus gland. Lymph cells are originally produced in the bone marrow. Some of these cells remain in the bone marrow to mature into B cells. The thymus gland receives the remainder of the cells to mature as T cells.
- **Secondary lymph tissues** include the lymph nodes, spleen, specialized tissue within the GI tract, and lymph tissue within the respiratory tract. Lymph tissue is actually located in several areas of the body with the exception of the central nervous system.

Lymph cells include T cells formed in the thymus gland, B cells from the bone marrow, macrophages, and monocytes. Specialized lymph cells are found in the lymph nodes and skin. The specialized cells within the lymph nodes function to form the framework for the lymph node and the cells within the skin are called Langerhans' cells.

Hodgkin's and Non-Hodgkin's Lymphoma

Hodgkin's disease is slightly more common in men than women and seems to occur mostly in patients who are in their 20's or over 50-years-old. The cancerous cells with Hodgkin's disease are called **Reed-Sternberg cells**. They attack the lymph system by working to destroy the B-cells and T-cells. The patient may notice lymph node enlargement, especially through the neck or in the supraclavicular nodes. The patient may have some vague complaints of fever, especially at night, and loss of appetite with weight loss.

Non-Hodgkin's lymphoma may occur due to infection with the Epstein-Barr virus or chemical and pesticide exposure. This form of cancer causes the B cells and T cells to develop into malignant cells. Non-Hodgkin's lymphoma is usually not a localized cancer and patients may not be diagnosed until the disease has spread to other areas. It frequently involves bone marrow and liver malignancies. Other lymph nodes may also be affected which contributes to additional metastasis.

Diagnosing Hodgkin's Disease, Non-Hodgkin's Lymphoma, and Multiple Myeloma

- Hodgkin's disease is definitively diagnosed by performing a **biopsy** on the suspected lymph tissue. Cells are examined under the microscope for Reed-Sternberg cells.
- Non-Hodgkin's lymphoma is also diagnosed through **lymph node biopsy**. Lymph nodes need to be examined microscopically to differentiate between characteristics of Hodgkin's or non-Hodgkin's disease.
- Multiple myeloma is diagnosed through testing that assesses the presence of **elevated levels of specific proteins** present with the disease. Electrophoresis is performed on both the blood and urine. With multiple myeloma, heavy-chain M proteins are elevated in the blood and light-chain M proteins are elevated in the urine. **Bone marrow biopsy** is also performed to assess for increased plasma cells.

With all three diseases, additional testing will be performed on other organ systems once diagnosis of the malignancy is confirmed. This includes **scans** of the abdomen, pelvis, thorax, and brain. **Bone scans** may also be performed, especially with multiple myeloma, to check for bone involvement.

Multiple Myeloma

Multiple myeloma primarily affects older adults and has a poor prognosis with approximately 75% of cases becoming fatal. Risk factors for the disease include genetic predisposition, exposure to radiation, and exposure to heavy metals and certain chemicals.

Multiple myeloma affects a specialized B cell that is responsible for the production of *immunoglobulins*. Multiple myeloma is usually a disseminated disease that affects several body systems. It causes elevated levels of monoclonal immunoglobulins and stimulates the activity of osteoclast cells. This can cause destruction of bone tissue and is evidenced by a "punched out" effect on x-rays. Bone tissue is depleted of calcium which weakens the bones and can lead to fractures. Calcium levels may also be elevated. In its early stages, multiple myeloma may not cause any signs or symptoms. However, as the disease progresses clinical manifestations of multiple myeloma include hypercalcemia, renal insufficiency, anemia and bone lesions-often referred to as the *"CRAB" signs* and symptoms. Patients may have complaints of bone pain, but also may not have any clinical symptoms. Renal damage can occur because of elevated calcium levels. Patients may be anemic and may have increased protein levels on laboratory tests.

Functions of the Head and Neck and Cancer's Effect on Them

1. **Respiration** is aided by the upper airways by warming and moistening the air as it is inspired. The nasal passage also contains hairs that filter the air and prevent some particles from being drawn into the lungs. A tumor in the upper airways can prevent oxygen from being drawn in and this normal function cannot be performed.
2. **Speech** is aided because the nasal cavities function as resonating chambers in producing sound. The vocal cords are located in the larynx and they vibrate to produce sound. Laryngeal cancer can prevent the vocal cords from functioning and make it impossible for the patient to speak.
3. **Swallowing** is accomplished through smooth muscle action of the oropharynx. Food is formed into a small ball, or bolus, by saliva and movements of the tongue. Oral or pharyngeal cancer can make it difficult or impossible for the patient to eat normal foods.
4. **Hormone regulation** of the thyroid gland controls the production of thyroid hormones. Thyroid cancer can cause an over-secretion or under-secretion of these hormones.

Diagnosing Head and Neck Cancers

Though there is no screening testing available, a thorough **oral exam** is recommended in patients who are at increased risk for developing head and neck cancers. This includes palpating the oral mucosa, including the area under the tongue, as well as assessing for any cervical and supraclavicular lymph node enlargement. If cancer is suspected, a mirror can be used to view the pharynx and larynx for the presence of any visible lesions. **Endoscopy** can also be performed to view the pharynx, larynx, and trachea.

CT scans are performed to assess for any tumors in the head or neck. This can also be useful in assessing for any lymph node disease or metastasis to other organ systems. If cancer is located in the nasal cavity or nasopharynx, **MRI studies** are preferred for more specific visualization of lesions.

Definitive diagnosis is accomplished through **biopsy** of the suspect tissue. This can be done by fine needle aspiration of cells or incisional biopsy of a tumor.

Signs and Symptoms of Head and Neck Cancers

Symptoms of head and neck cancer will vary depending on the location of the cancer.

- If originating in the **oral cavity**, the patient may notice redness or white patches along the gums, tongue, or oral mucosa. They may also complain of pain or bleeding in the gums, especially while eating or brushing the teeth.
- Cancers in the **nasal cavity** can result in upper jaw pain and headaches. The patient may also experience recurrent sinus infections or the feeling of always having sinus congestion.
- Cancer affecting the **salivary glands** can cause swelling along the jaw along with pain. The patient may also experience a numb sensation over the face or paralysis of the facial muscles.
- Cancers affecting the **oropharynx, nasopharynx, and larynx** can cause ear pain.
  - **Nasopharyngeal cancers** can also cause difficulty breathing and talking or headaches.

- o **Laryngeal cancers** can make swallowing difficult and painful.
- o **Neck cancer** will usually cause constant throat pain or hoarseness.

Scope, Standards, and Related Issues

Standards of Care for Oncology Nursing

1. **Assessment** is a constant process that is performed by the nurse to evaluate the patient's condition and any changes that may occur in their condition. This includes not only physical signs and symptoms, but psychosocial issues as well.
2. **Diagnosis** is formulated based on the information gathered through continual assessment of the patient. This is a nursing diagnosis based on medical information as well as identification of psychosocial needs.
3. **Outcome identification** is forecasting the optimal outcomes for the patient to resolve issues addressed through diagnosis.
4. **Planning** is organizing treatment in a way that focuses on treating the diagnoses established through thorough assessment.
5. **Implementation** is following through on the plan in order for the identified outcomes to be attained by performing the actions set forth in the plan of care.
6. **Evaluation** is assessing the result of the actions that were implemented to evaluate whether the expected outcomes were achieved. This process will continue with assessing the patient again to identify new problems that may arise or evaluate for recurrence of previous diagnoses.

Maintaining Nurse Accountability

Nursing is a very large profession in which individuals care for the vulnerable members of society. Many actions take place by nurses every day on behalf of their patients, and it is important that those actions are not **harmful**. Nursing as a profession focuses on patient care, but it is important to be able to assess the adequacy of that care. For these reasons, several regulating agencies have developed **nursing practice acts, standards of care, recommended practices, and guidelines**. These provide standards to which a nurse's actions can be measured to make sure they are practicing at an acceptable performance standard. The nurse is responsible to uphold these standards.

Joint Commission Accreditation

The **Joint Commission** is an accrediting organization that health care facilities can utilize to **accredit** their organization. The Joint Commission has been granted "deeming status" by the Centers for Medicare and Medicaid Services. This means that during a Joint Commission survey, the survey team will evaluate the health care institution's **compliance** with the conditions of participation required to be met in order to receive payment from Medicare. In addition, the Joint Commission survey team will evaluate compliance with the Joint Commission standards outlined in their respective accreditation manuals. The mission of the Joint Commission is to "continuously improve health care for the public, in collaboration with other stakeholders, by evaluating health care organizations and inspiring them to excel in providing safe and effective care of the highest quality and value." The public has the ability to search for organizations that are accredited by the Joint Commission on the Joint Commission's website.

National Accreditation Program for Breast Centers (NAPBC)

The **NAPBC** is "a consortium of national, professional organizations focused on breast health and dedicated to the improvement of quality outcomes of patients with diseases of the breast through evidence-based standards and patient and professional education." The NAPBC is administered by

Copyright © Mometrix Media. You have been licensed one copy of this document for personal use only. Any other reproduction or redistribution is strictly prohibited. All rights reserved.

the American College of Surgeons. Institutions that provide excellence in breast care and treatment and are in compliance with established NAPBC standards can choose to apply for NAPBC accreditation.

Accreditation through the NAPBC offers national recognition for its accredited organizations as well as the ability to participate in a National Breast Disease database that is utilized to report patterns of care and the effects of quality improvement initiatives. Accredited organizations undergo an on-site review every 3 years to maintain their accreditation and must show evidence of compliance with all of the standards defined by NAPBC.

Oncology Nursing Society Documentation Standards for Cancer Treatment (2017)

The key elements of the Oncology Nursing Society Documentation Standards for Cancer Treatment (2017) include:

- Administration of chemotherapy and biotherapy, includes documentation standards for workup, post-treatment, and follow-up care.
- Radiation therapy, includes documentation standards for planning, treatment, post-treatment, and follow-up care.
- Bone marrow and stem cell transplant, includes documentation standards for history, pretransplant, product preparation, acute (days 1-100) and chronic transplant phase (days 100+).
- Surgical documentation, includes standards for history, preoperative assessment, post-anesthesia, and postoperative follow-up.
- Venous access device, includes documentation standards for workup, insertion, use, and removal.
- Blood product transfusion, includes documentation standards for pre-transfusion, transfusion, and post-transfusion.
- Management of extravasation, includes documentation standards for extravasation and post-extravasation care.

Documentation standards are based on the American Nurses Association's recommended elements and involve documentation that shows elements of the treatment plan were verified, elements were reviewed by the appropriate nurse or healthcare provider, or elements were properly assessed.

Compassion Fatigue

Characteristics

Compassion fatigue can occur when people overly identify with the pain and suffering of others and begin to exhibit signs of stress as a result. These people are often empathetic, tend to place the needs of others above their own, and are motivated by the need to help others. Indications include:

- Blaming others and complaining excessively.
- Isolating oneself from others and having trouble concentrating.
- Exhibiting compulsive activities (gambling, drinking).
- Having nightmares, sleeping poorly, and exhibiting a change in appetite.
- Exhibiting sadness and/or apathy.
- Denying any problems and having high expectations of self and others.
- Having trouble concentrating.
- Questioning spiritual beliefs, losing faith.
- Exhibiting stress disorders: tachycardia, headaches, insomnia, pain.

- 61 -

Healthcare providers who exhibit compassion fatigue may need to take a break from work in order to recover some sense of self and may benefit from stress management programs, cognitive behavioral therapy, relaxation and visualization exercises, and physical exercise.

Stress Management Strategies

While it's not possible to eliminate all stress, oncology certified nurses can learn to manage stress so it has less emotional and physical impact on their lives. **Stress management** strategies include:

- Relaxation exercises:
  - Meditation/Breathing exercises: Slow in and out while repeating a word or phrase.
  - Massage: Self massage or by others.
  - Progressive relaxation techniques.
- *Visualization exercises/Positive thinking*: Use the power of the mind to imagine a more positive outcome.
- *Time management:* Establish priorities, make schedule, and delegate.
- *Exercise:* Increase activity and exercise 20-30 minutes daily.
- *Breaks:* Plan regular breaks from work or other activities, 5-15 minutes.
- *Snacks:* Prepare healthy snacks and avoid high sugar/high fat snack foods.
- *Hobbies or interests*: Find an outlet, such as reading, music, painting, or crafts.

Standards of Professional Performance

Standards of Professional Performance for Oncology Nursing

1. **Quality of care** is continuously evaluated in order for all of the patient's needs to be met.
2. **Practice evaluation** is performed to assess that one is compliant with standards of care as well as legal requirements for nursing practice.
3. **Education** should be ongoing in order to be knowledgeable on current aspects of cancer disease and treatment.
4. **Collegiality** encourages the nurse to work as a member of the medical team to provide effective care for the patient.
5. **Ethics** refers to the fundamental beliefs that are used when serving as an advocate for the patient.
6. **Collaboration** is the function of the nurse to incorporate input from all of the people involved in the patient's care.
7. **Research** is performed based on the oncology nurse's input regarding areas that may require further investigation and data collected by the oncology nurse is vital in performing research.
8. **Resource utilization** is utilizing all means necessary to provide the resources necessary to help the patient.
9. **Leadership** is serving as a role model for other colleagues while providing guidance.

Standards of Oncology Certified Nurse Education

The beginning level **oncology certified nurse (OCN)** must have:

- A current registered nurse license.
- 1000 hours of adult oncology nursing experience within the preceding 30 months.
- 12 months or more experience working as a registered nurse in the preceding 3 years.
- Oncology education equal to at least 10 contact hours of continuing education or academic elective within the preceding 36 months.

Oncology certified nurses may take further certification to specialize in specific areas, such as bone and marrow transplant. Master's degrees are available in oncology nursing as well as post-degree certification programs. Regardless of the level of oncology nursing, the oncology certified nurse's education must include knowledge of health promotion and screening, pathophysiology, different treatment modalities, chemotherapy administration, management of symptoms and oncologic emergencies, survivorship, palliative care, and end-of-life care. The oncology certified nurse should be prepared to provide treatment and support to patients and professional guidance to other nurses.

Providing Sensitive Information Techniques

The **SPIKES strategy** (Beale et al) can be used as a guide to providing sensitive information (bad news):

Set up interview	Make plan for delivering news and arrange for a private space and presence of significant others (such as spouses or children).
Assess patient **p**erception	Question patient/family about what they know about the disease and discover any misperceptions.
Obtain **i**nvitation	Ask patient/family directly if they want information and how much and respect decisions, remaining available for questions.
Provide **k**nowledge	Provide sensitive information or bad news slowly rather than quickly so the patient and family have time to digest the information. Ask if they have questions and avoid technical jargon. Consider psychosocial implications and well as cultural differences.
Address **e**motions	Respond to patient's/family's feelings and emotional response. Attempt to identify emotional response (sad, depressed, angry, confused) and acknowledge (move closer, touch patient, express regret, verbally respond).
Strategy/ **S**ummary	Ask if patient/family ready to discuss treatment plan and present treatment options if "yes" and set up a later time to discuss if "no."

Confidentiality

Confidentiality is the obligation that is present in a professional-patient relationship. Nurses are under an obligation to **protect** the information they possess concerning the patient and family. Care should be taken to safeguard that information and provide the **privacy** that the family deserves. This is accomplished through the use of required passwords when family call for information about the patient and through the limitation of who is allowed to visit. There may be times when confidentiality must be broken to save the life of a patient, but those circumstances are rare. The nurse practitioner must make all efforts to safeguard patient records and identification. Computerized record keeping should be done in such a way that the screen is not visible to others, and paper records must be secured.

Informed Consent

Patients or guardians must provide **informed consent** for all treatment the patient receives. This includes a thorough explanation of all procedures and treatment and associated risks. Patients/guardians should be apprised of all options and allowed input on the type of treatments. Patients/guardians should be apprised of all reasonable risks and any complications that might be life threatening or increase morbidity. The American Medical Association has established **guidelines for informed consent**:

- Explanation of diagnosis.
- Nature and reason for treatment or procedure.
- Risks and benefits.
- Alternative options (regardless of cost or insurance coverage).
- Risks and benefits of alternative options.
- Risks and benefits of not having a treatment or procedure.
- Providing informed consent is a requirement of all states.

Utilitarianism and Deontological Ethical Theories

The **utilitarianism theory** states that activities that bring joy are acceptable, while those that bring sadness are unacceptable. It is based on a cause and effect model that an action will result in a response. The action is considered appropriate or inappropriate based on the result of a good or bad response. This theory promotes the belief that a situation can result in a good or bad outcome with the action used to reach this outcome being the focus of the theory.

The **deontological theory** is based on the belief that not everyone will react the same way in the same situation. Its aim is to individualize each situation to each person rather than try to fit each person into a mold. This helps to bend the "rules" that may be in place to solve a certain dilemma. Use of this theory relies heavily on basic morals and values that are called upon to resolve conflicts.

End-of-Life Care Ethical Challenges

One of the pressing **ethical challenges in end-of-life care** is the access to **hospice care**. Unfortunately, studies regarding access of care show that many patients in the United States are not able to receive hospice care at the end of life. This lack of access may be due to where a patient lives or to lack of awareness of available resources. End-of-life care often involves the use of drugs to alleviate pain and suffering in the terminally ill patient. Physicians are sometimes hesitant to prescribe narcotics to the terminally ill for fear of legal repercussions.

Ethical Issues to Treatment of Terminally Ill Patients

There are a number of **ethical concerns** that healthcare providers and families must face when determining the treatments that are necessary and appropriate for a terminally-ill patient. It is the nurse's responsibility to provide support and information to help parents/families make informed decisions. Common treatments with their advantages and disadvantages:

- **Analgesia** - Provide comfort. Ease the dying process. Increase sedation and decrease cognition and interaction with family. May hasten death.
- **Active treatments** (such as antibiotics, chemotherapy) - Prolong life. Relieve symptoms. Reassure family. Prolong the dying process. Side effects may be severe (as with chemotherapy).
- **Supplemental nutrition** - Relieve family's anxiety that patient is hungry. Prolong life. May cause nausea, vomiting. May increase tumor growth with cancer. May increase discomfort.
- **IV fluids for hydration** - Relieve family's anxiety that patient is thirsty. Keep mouth moist. May result in congestive heart failure and pulmonary edema with increased dyspnea. Increased urinary output and incontinence may cause skin breakdown. Prolong dying process.
- **Resuscitation efforts** - Allow family to deny death is imminent. Cause unnecessary suffering and prolong dying process.

Ethical Assessment

While the terms *ethics* and *morals* are sometimes used interchangeably, ethics is a study of morals and encompasses concepts of right and wrong. When making **ethical assessments,** one must consider not only what people should do but also what they actually do, as these two things are sometimes at odds. Ethical issues can be difficult to assess because of personal bias, and that is one of the reasons that sharing concerns with other internal sources and reaching consensus is so valuable. Issues of concern might include options for care, refusal of care, rights to privacy, adequate relief of suffering, and the right to self-determination. Internal sources might include the

- 65 -

ethics committee, whose charge is to make decisions regarding ethical issues. Risk management can provide guidance related to personal and institutional liability. External agencies might include government agencies, such as the public health department.

Bioethics

Bioethics is a branch of ethics that involves making sure that the medical treatment given is the most **morally correct choice** given the different options that might be available and the differences inherent in the varied levels of treatment. In the acute/critical care unit, if the patients, parents, and the staff are in agreement when it comes to values and decision-making, then no ethical dilemma exists; however, when there is a difference in value beliefs between the patients/parents and the staff, there is a **bioethical dilemma** that must be resolved. Sometimes, discussion and explanation can resolve differences, but at times the institution's ethics committee must be brought in to resolve the conflict. The primary goal of bioethics is to determine the most morally correct action using the set of circumstances given.

Beneficence and Nonmaleficence

Beneficence is an ethical principle that involves performing actions that are for the purpose of benefitting another person. In the care of a patient, any procedure or treatment should be done with the ultimate goal of benefitting the patient, and any actions that are not beneficial should be reconsidered. As conditions change, procedures need to be continually reevaluated to determine if they are still of benefit.

Nonmaleficence is an ethical principle that means healthcare workers should provide care in a manner that does not cause direct intentional harm to the patient:

- The actual act must be good or morally neutral.
- The intent must be only for a good effect.
- A bad effect cannot serve as the means to get to a good effect.
- A good effect must have more benefit than a bad effect has harm.

Autonomy and Justice

Autonomy is the ethical principle that the individual has the right to make decisions about his/her own care. In the case of children or patients with dementia who cannot make autonomous decisions, parents or family members may serve as the legal decision maker. The nurse must keep the patient and/or family fully informed so that they can exercise their autonomy in informed decision-making.

Justice is the ethical principle that relates to the distribution of the limited resources of healthcare benefits to the members of society. These resources must be distributed fairly. This issue may arise if there is only one bed left and two sick patients. Justice comes into play in deciding which patient should stay and which should be transported or otherwise cared for. The decision should be made according to what is best or most just for the patients and not colored by personal bias.

Ethical Decision-Making Environment

An environment for **ethical decision-making** and **patient advocacy** does not appear when it is needed; it requires planning and preparation. The expectation for the institution should clearly communicate that nurses are legally and morally responsible for ensuring competent care and respecting the rights of patients, including allowing informed consent and protecting confidentiality. Decisions regarding ethical issues often must be made quickly with little time for contemplation; therefore, ethical issues that may arise should be identified and discussed. Clearly defined procedures and policies for dealing with conflicts, including an active ethics committee, inservice training, and staff meetings, must be established. Patients and families need to be part of the ethical environment, and that means empowering them by providing patient/family information (print form, video, audio) that outlines patient's rights and procedures for expressing their wishes and dealing with ethical conflicts. Respect for privacy and confidentiality and a nonpunitive atmosphere are essential.

Evidence-Based Guidelines Steps

Steps to **evidence-based practice guidelines** include:

- **Focus on the topic/methodology:** This includes outlining possible interventions/treatments for review, choosing patient populations and settings and determining significant outcomes. Search boundaries (such as types of journals, types of studies, dates of studies) should be determined.
- **Evidence review:** This includes review of literature, critical analysis of studies, and summarizing of results, including pooled meta-analysis.
- **Expert judgment:** Recommendations based on personal experience from a number of experts may be utilized, especially if there is inadequate evidence based on review, but this subjective evidence should be explicated acknowledged.
- **Policy considerations:** This includes cost-effectiveness, access to care, insurance coverage, availability of qualified staff, and legal implications.
- **Policy:** A written policy must be completed with recommendations. Common practice is to utilize letter guidelines, with "A" the most highly recommended, usually based the quality of supporting evidence.
- **Review:** The completed policy should be submitted to peers for review and comments before instituting the policy.

Outcomes Evaluation and Evidence-Based Practice

Outcomes evaluation is an important component of evidence-based practice, which involves both internal and external research. All treatments are subjected to review to determine if they produce positive outcomes, and policies and protocols for outcomes evaluation should be in place. Outcomes evaluation includes the following:

- **Monitoring** over the course of treatment involves careful observation and record keeping that notes progress, with supporting laboratory and radiographic evidence as indicated by condition and treatment.
- **Evaluating** results includes reviewing records as well as current research to determine if outcomes are within acceptable parameters.
- **Sustaining** involves continuing treatment, but continuing to monitor and evaluate.
- **Improving** means to continue the treatment but with additions or modifications in order to improve outcomes.
- **Replacing** the treatment with a different treatment must be done if outcomes evaluation indicates that current treatment is ineffective.

Key Quality Concepts

There are a number of **key concepts** related to quality that must be communicated to all members of an organization through inservice, workshops, newsletters, fact sheets, and team meetings. Quality care/performance should be:

- **Appropriate** to needs and in keeping with best practices.
- **Accessible** to the individual despite financial, cultural, or other barriers.
- **Competent**, with practitioners well-trained and adhering to standards.
- **Coordinated** among all healthcare providers.
- **Effective** in achieving outcomes based on the current state of knowledge.
- **Efficient** in methods of achieving the desired outcomes.
- **Preventive**, allowing for early detection and prevention of problems.
- **Respectful** and caring with consideration of the individual needs given primary importance.
- **Safe** so that the organization is free of hazards or dangers that may put patients or others at risk.

Continuous Quality Improvement (CQI)

CQI emphasizes the organization and systems and processes within that organization rather than individuals. It recognizes internal customers (staff) and external customers (patients) and utilizes data to improve processes. CQI represents the concept that most processes can be improved. CQI uses the scientific method of experimentation to meet needs and improve services, and various tools, such as brainstorming, multi-voting, various charts and diagrams, story boarding, and meetings. **Core concepts** include:

- Quality and success is meeting or exceeding internal and external customer's needs and expectations.
- Problems relate to processes, and variations in process lead to variations in results.
- Change can be in small steps.

Steps to CQI include:

1. Forming a knowledgeable team.
2. Identifying and defining measures used to determine success.
3. Brainstorming strategies for change.
4. Plan, collect, and utilize data as part of making decisions.
5. Test changes and revise or refine as needed.

Maintaining Competency

- Identify **strengths/weaknesses** and knowledge deficits in any area pertinent to patient care including physiological and psychological aspects of care.
- Practice **competencies** necessary for the unit/profession. If new competencies emerge, the nurse can become familiar with them and practice their skills until competency is achieved.
- Make **goals**. The nurse can make goals to develop professionalism on a regular basis, which will help them to have a plan to follow.

- The nurse can reach **professional learning goals** by obtaining certifications, taking classes on pertinent subjects, attending conferences on subjects related to the field, taking a college course to learn the newest information, becoming involved in research projects dealing with aspects of the perioperative setting, etc.

Leadership Styles

Leadership styles include:

- *Democratic:* Presents a problem and asks staff or teams to arrive at a solution although the leader usually makes the final decision. This type of leadership may delay decision-making, but staff and teams are often more committed to the solutions because of their input.
- *Autocratic/Authoritarian:* Makes decisions independently, and strictly enforces rules, but team members often feel left out of process and may not be supportive. This type of leadership is most effective in crisis situations, but may have difficulty gaining commitment of staff.
- *Laissez-faire* (free rein): Exerts little direct control but allows employees/ teams to make decisions with little interference. This may be effective leadership if teams are highly skilled and motivated; but, in many cases, this type of leadership is the product of poor management skills and little is accomplished because of this lack of leadership.
- *Transactional:* Manages by exception and is often punitive, with rewards/punishment based on performance. Tends to take action after problems occur and only intervenes then. This style of leader is very rule-oriented and expects deadlines to be met and tasks to be completed, but morale may be low and staff members may have little motivation to improve nursing practice. Because of this approach, the organization may stagnate and quality improvement measures may suffer.
- *Transformational:* Manages through inspiring and motivating others and is able to communicate vision so that staff members often have the same goals. The transformational leader considers the individuals and their needs as well as the organizational needs and is able to think critically, solve problems, and encourage the exchange of information. This type of leader provides feedback to staff members and shows respect for their opinions and their skills. Because staff members feel valued, they may take active roles in helping to solve problems and improve the quality of care.

Professional Performance Evaluation

Oncology certified nurses are evaluated on their **professional performance** based on:

- *Clinical expertise* and the ability to carry out all steps in the nursing process efficiently and effectively, assessed through observation, supervision, and feedback from patients, team members, and other staff members.
- *Initiative* in carrying out research, sharing research findings, promoting quality improvement, and implementing best practices.
- *Educational preparation and advancement*, including continuing education, required training, and academic classes as well as further certification or degrees.
- *Professional standards,* exemplified by modeling honesty and integrity and advocating for the profession.

- **Self-assessment**, carried out by the individual nurse to help to identify areas of strength and weakness. Self-assessment may be carried out before or after training and as part of routine evaluations. Self-assessments often involve identifying a situation that reflects the nurse's clinical practice and reflecting on how the nurse dealt with the situation.
- **Responsibility**, exemplified by coming to work on time and carrying out expected duties.

Proper Personal Protective Equipment Protocol

Personal protective equipment used during administration of chemotherapy may vary depending on the patient's condition, type of chemotherapy, and route of administration. Typical PPE needs include:

- **Gown:** Must be worn when handling or administering cytotoxic drugs or cytotoxic wastes. The gown should be long-sleeved, disposable, water-repellent, and have tight cuffs. If caring for a number of patients in the same area, the same gown can be worn throughout the shift unless it is soiled or torn, but the gown should not be worn outside of the chemotherapy administration area.
- **Gloves**: Non-latex gloves that are certified as acceptable for cytotoxic drugs should be used in order to minimize patient/staff exposure to latex. Hands should be washed before applying and after removing gloves. Gloves must be changed between patients and when torn or contaminated. Double gloves are usually used for handling and administration.
- **Mask**: Facemask must be worn if patients are immunocompromised or if the nurse may be exposed to aerosolized cytotoxic agents.
- **Goggles/Face guard**: Protective eye/face guards must be used if there is risk for aerosolization of cytotoxic agents or risk of splashing, or when cleaning spills.

Personal Protective Equipment Necessary for Types of Chemotherapeutic Agents

NIOSH classifies chemotherapeutic agents as hazardous drugs because of their carcinogenicity, teratogenicity, reproductive toxicity, organ toxicity and genotoxicity. Safety measures include: using enteric-coated oral medications when possible and avoiding crushing or cutting them, labeling chemotherapeutic agents as hazardous, storing them separately from other drugs in secure storage unit, and following safe-handling guidance provided by manufacturers. Note that eye protection and respiratory protection may not be necessary if a control device is used when preparing the agents.

Required Personal Protective Equipment

Tablets/capsules, cutting or crushing	Double gloves and gown, respiratory protection
Oral liquid administration	Double gloves and gown
Topical drug administration	Double gloves, gown, eye protection, respiratory protection
Ampule, opening	Double gloves, gown, eye and respiratory protection
SQ, IM injection, preparation and administration	Double gloves, gown, eye protection, respiratory protection
IV infusion, Administration	Double glove, gown, eye protection (if splash potential), respiratory protection (if inhalation potential)
Irrigant, administration	Double gloves, gown, eye protection, respiratory protection
Inhalants	Double gloves, gown, eye protection, respiratory protection

Chemotherapeutic Agents

Storage and Disposal

Storage of chemotherapeutic agents classified as hazardous drugs must be in separate closed containers or rooms from other drugs. Negative pressure rooms are recommended but not required for bulk storage. The containers and the drugs must be labeled to identify the agents as hazardous. Chemotherapeutic agents should be stored at the temperature recommended for each drug with most oral preparations stored at room temperature in a cool, dark place. Some parenteral agents must be stored in refrigeration.

Disposal of chemotherapeutic agents classified as hazardous waste pharmaceuticals (HWP) by the Federal Resource Conservation and Recovery Act (RCRA) requires special handling, but state regulations may vary with some states categorizing all chemotherapeutic agents as HWP. Agents that are HWP cannot be disposed of as standard medical waste. Some states allow empty containers with trace amounts of chemotherapeutic agents remaining to be disposed of as medical waste, but others allow no trace amounts at all. Special black rigid containers or secure bag are generally used to dispose of chemotherapeutic waste and are labeled for waste incineration only.

Spills and Contamination/Exposure

Improper contact with **chemotherapeutic agents** may include:

- **Spills:** A spill kit should be readily available near the area where chemotherapeutic agents are prepared and administered. If a spill is greater than 5 mL, an accident report must be filed and the organization's safety director notified of the accident. If the spill occurs outside of the safety cabinet, then people should be cleared from the area and absorbent pads placed on the spill while the nurse is wearing full PPE. Once absorbed, the soiled pads must be place in a hazardous waste disposal bag. The area contaminated by the spill must be scrubbed with water and detergent (not disinfectant).
- **Contamination/Exposure:** Immediately remove any contaminated clothing or PPE and wash the exposed area with detergent, soap, and water. If the eyes are splashed or affected, they must be flushed for at least 15 minutes at an eye-wash station. The organization's safety director must be notified. Medical attention may be necessary in some cases.

Treatment Modalities

Surgery

Surgeries Used for Various Purposes

- **Prophylactic purposes**: the excision of premalignant lesions.
- **Diagnostic purposes**: biopsies for definitive histological diagnosis.
- **Staging purposes**: the extent of the carcinoma must actually be observed inside the patient.
- **Treatment purposes**: the simple removal of the entire carcinomatous tumor for curative reasons.
- **Palliation purposes**: where any therapy given is not going to alter the outcome of the disease, but maintenance of the best quality of life is desired for the patient and to allow death with dignity and maximum comfort.

Surgery Used for Cancer Treatment

When cancer is first suspected, **surgery** is used to establish a diagnosis. This is accomplished through many types of biopsies. **Incisional biopsy** can be performed where a small sample of suspected tissue is removed for testing, or **excisional biopsy** can be performed in which the entire suspected tissue is removed. Biopsy can also be accomplished using a needle with a fine point or larger size to perform a core biopsy. Lymph nodes can also be biopsied using a needle technique. Surgery is used to determine how advanced the disease has become and to stage the disease. This involves removing the malignant tissue and obtaining tissue samples from multiple areas to assess for the presence of disease. Surgery can also be used as a primary **treatment** of the disease with removal of the affected organs. This is accomplished by removing the malignant tumor. Surgery can also help to debulk a tumor and reduce symptoms, though this does not cure the disease and is performed as a palliative treatment.

Types of Cancer Surgery

- **Surgical excision** is done to remove the malignant tissue. This is done with removal of just the involved tissue with a margin of healthy tissue, or may be more extensive with removal of the affected tissue and surrounding lymph nodes and other tissues.
- **Electrosurgery** involves applying an electric stimulus to the area affected by the malignancy and destroying the cancer cells.
- **Cryosurgery** can be performed which involves applying liquid nitrogen to the cancer tissues. This causes destruction of the malignant cells through a freezing process.
- **Laser treatments** can be applied directly to the malignant tissue to cause destruction of the malignant cells. This is performed using a specialized scalpel that emits laser stimulus.
- **Stereotactic surgery** is used with brain tumors to provide an exact location of the tumor in a three-dimensional appearance. Special equipment is used for positioning the patient to utilize this type of surgery.

Surgery can be performed through a scope approach with laparoscopy and endoscopy. Both biopsy and removal of tumors can be performed utilizing this approach.

> **Review Video: L.A.S.E.R.**
> Visit mometrix.com/academy and enter code: 703707

- 72 -

Bone Marrow/Stem Cell Transplants

Bone Marrow Transplant: Infusion of bone marrow into a patient who has been treated previously with high dose chemotherapy or radiation to halt rejection of the transplanted material.

Types of Bone Marrow Transplants:

- **Allogenic** - infusion of bone marrow from one individual to another.
- **Autologous** - infusion of a patient's own bone marrow previously removed and stored
- **Syngeneic** - infusion from one identical twin to another.

Potential Complications from Bone Marrow Transplantations

Graft-versus-host disease occurs when the patient develops a rejection reaction to bone marrow received from a donor that may not be a perfect genetic match. This occurs in as many as one-half of bone marrow recipients. High doses of steroids as well as other medications that decrease immune reactions can be used to try and prevent this from happening.

Interstitial pneumonitis is an inflammation in lung tissue. It is more common in those patients who received radiation treatments to the chest, treatment with bleomycin, or are carriers of the cytomegalovirus. These infections can be caused by viruses, bacteria, or fungi. Antimicrobial medications are used to treat this infection.

Veno-occlusive disease occurs when small veins in the liver are damaged and occurs more often in patients with known liver disease. Anticoagulant therapy with heparin can help to prevent this condition. Patients are on strict fluid restrictions with this condition and are monitored closely for fluid overload.

Allografting Versus Autografting for Bone Marrow Transplants

Allografting is the process by which bone marrow is obtained from a donor and transplanted into the cancer patient. This can also be done with blood stem cells or umbilical cord blood that has been stored. Specialized tests need to be completed to confirm that the donor and patient will be a match to prevent a rejection reaction by the recipient. Identical twins are ideal donors for each other, but other family members or donor bone marrow may be used if the match is close enough.

Autografting of bone marrow involves removing bone marrow cells from the patient and returning the cells to them. This can be performed if a matched donor cannot be found. It is also used in patients who are at increased risk for developing a rejection reaction to donor bone marrow. There is a risk of the bone marrow cells containing cancer cells, so this needs to be ruled out before this procedure could be performed.

Hepatic Sinusoidal Obstruction Syndrome

Hepatic sinusoidal obstruction syndrome (SOS), previously known as **veno-occlusive disease**, is a life-threatening complication that occurs in 15-20% of hematopoietic stem cell transplant patients. It occurs when fibrous material accumulates, resulting in obstruction of venules in the liver, which in turn causes portal hypertension and destruction of the liver cells. Clinical manifestations include hyperbilirubinemia, weight gain, ascites, right upper quadrant pain, hepatomegaly, splenomegaly, and jaundice. SOS should be considered in any patient that has these symptoms after stem cell transplant, especially in the first three weeks. Veno-occlusive disease is treated by maintaining intravascular volume and renal perfusion and minimizing fluid accumulation. Prevention includes minimizing risk factors, such as decreasing exposure to hepatotoxic medications, and iron chelation for those patients who already have liver disease related to increased iron levels. Prevention also includes prophylaxis, usually with ursodeoxycholic acid for allogenic transplants, beginning the day before stem cell transplant, and continuing three months after the procedure.

Radiation Therapy

Target Theory

Target theory states that radiation damage results from direct and indirect hits on the DNA chain. Ionization affects either the molecules of the cell or the cell environment. As a result of direct hits:

1. There is a change or loss of a **base** (thymine, adenine, guanine, or cytosine).
2. The breakdown of the **hydrogen bond** between the two chains of the DNA molecule.
3. Breaks in one or both chains of the **DNA molecule.**
4. **Cross-linking** of the chains after breakage.

These four events lead to mutations that lead to impaired cellular function or cell death of the cancer cells. An indirect hit refers to the ionization of water, the medium surrounding the molecular structures within the cell, which causes a change in the cellular environment.

Radiation Physics and Radiobiology

Radiation physics is the study of the effects of radiation exposure on cells. Radiation treatment for cancer involves treating malignancies with a focused beam of ionizing radiation. This causes changes within the cancer cells that result in their destruction. Ionizing radiation can be electromagnetic or particulate. ***Electromagnetic radiation*** is effective using energy waves. An example of this is a regular x-ray. ***Particulate radiation*** involves the smallest elements of cells, such as electrons, protons, and neutrons.

Radiobiology is the study of the living cell after radiation treatment has been applied to the cell. It examines the specific actions that occur to promote cell destruction, as well as the length of time necessary for this to occur. It also examines the various doses necessary to destroy cells, with the minimum dosage required to destroy a cell effectively being the most desirable. It also examines the effects that radiation treatment has on normal tissues.

Radiation Potential Side Effects

- The **skin** can be burned by radiation and exhibit redness, other changes in color, death of normal cells, or loss of hair. There can also be visible changes to the vascular supply to the skin.
- Radiation treatments can damage the mucous membranes of the **mouth, nasal cavity, and pharynx or larynx**. This can result in dryness, inflammation, irritation, and even bleeding. The salivary glands can also be affected which may increase the dryness.
- The skin over the **chest wall** can be affected by radiation, but internal structures may also be damaged.
- Radiation therapy can cause inflammation and tissue damage within the airways, esophagus, and in the sac that surrounds the **heart**. Scarring can also occur in these areas.
- Radiation to the abdomen can result in skin damage over the **abdominal wall**.
- The **organs** may also suffer damage due to radiation.
- Tissue damage in the stomach and intestines can lead to problems with absorption of nutrients and inflammation. Scarring can cause stenosis of the intestinal lumen and lead to obstructions.

Relation of Cure, Control, Adjuvant, and Palliation to Radiation Treatment

- **Cure** – Radiation treatment for a cure has a primary goal of eliminating all cancer cells so that growth of the cancer cannot occur. It is also hoped that normal, non-cancerous cells will not be damaged from radiation exposure.
- **Control** – While a cure is not the expected outcome, the radiation treatment should control further development of cancer cells. This allows the patient to be without symptoms of the cancer.
- **Adjuvant** – This type of radiation treatment is performed before surgery to decrease the size of a tumor and make it more easily resected, or it is performed after surgery to destroy any existing cancer cells that may be present.
- **Palliation** – This type of radiation treatment is aimed at helping to control the symptoms from cancer. This is done when there is no hope for a cure, but the patient is experiencing unpleasant symptoms from the disease, such as pain. The goal is to make the patient more comfortable.

> **Review Video: Adjuvants**
> Visit mometrix.com/academy and enter code: 178200

Chemotherapy

Relation of Cell Cycle, Cell-Cycle Time, Growth Fraction of Tumor, and Tumor Burden to Chemotherapy Treatment

- **Cell cycle** is the action of cell reproduction. This occurs in all cells, including cancer cells. Certain cancer treatments can be targeted to affect cancer cells at specific points within the reproductive cycle.
- **Cell-cycle time** is the length of time required for a cell to complete an entire reproductive cycle. This is important in formulating cancer treatments because some cancer cells will have a longer cell-cycle time than others. This can affect the length of time the cell spends in each phase of the reproductive cycle.
- **Growth fraction of tumor** is the number of cancer cells that are going through the reproductive cycle. This is measured in a percent. The percentage of dividing cells at any time is important for treatments that target specific phases of the reproductive cycle.
- **Tumor burden** is the size of a tumor measured in the number of cells that comprise it. This helps to determine the difficulty in treating a cancer because the smaller the tumor, the more responsive it will be to treatment.

Major Classifications of Chemotherapy Drugs

Chemotherapeutic agents are **classified** as to how they work in conjunction with the various phases of the cell cycle. They are known as either **cell cycle specific**, meaning they work at a particular phase of the cell cycle or as **cell cycle nonspecific**, meaning they are active throughout all phases of the cell cycle. Chemotherapeutic agents can be further classified into the following major categories: alkylating agents, anti-metabolites, anthracyclines, anti-tumor antibiotics, camptothecins, epothilones, vinca alkaloids, taxanes, and platinums. Anti-metabolites are active in the "S" phase of the cell cycle and are considered cell cycle specific. Epothilones, taxanes, and vinca alkaloids are specific to the "M" phase of the cell cycle. These agents are also known as mitotic inhibitors. Alkylating agents, anthracyclines, and platinums are all considered cell cycle nonspecific agents. In addition to these classes, additional cancer therapies include hormone therapy, monoclonal antibodies, immunotherapy, and targeted therapies.

Cell Cycle Phase Specific Drugs

Certain chemotherapeutic agents are designed to work at a particular phase of the cell cycle. These agents are known as **cell cycle phase specific**. The **anti-metabolite** class of chemotherapeutic agents interferes with DNA and RNA growth by substituting for the normal building blocks of RNA and DNA. Damage to cancer cells occurs during the "S" phase of the cell cycle. Examples of anti-metabolites include 5-FU, 6-MP, fludarabine, methotrexate, hydroxyurea, and pemetrexed. **Mitotic inhibitors** are another class of chemotherapeutic agents that are considered cell cycle specific. This class includes the taxanes, epothilones, and vinca alkaloids. Mitotic inhibitors arrest mitosis or inhibit the enzymes needed for cell reproduction from making proteins. They work during the "M" phase of the cell cycle; however, they can damage cells in all phases of the cell cycle. Examples of mitotic inhibitors include vincristine, vinblastine, paclitaxel, and ixabepilone.

Anti-Metabolites

Anti-metabolites were among the first chemotherapeutic agents noted to be effective in treating cancer. They are **cell cycle specific**, attacking at specific phases of the cell cycle. Anti-metabolites work by interfering with specific substances within the cell, thereby impairing their ability to divide. The anti-metabolites are further classified by the substances in which they interfere. Anti-metabolites are used in the treatment of leukemia, breast, ovarian, and GI cancers. Examples of anti-metabolites include methotrexate (a folic acid antagonist), 5-FU, cytarabine, capecitabine, gemcitabine (pyrimidine antagonists), 6-mercaptopurine (a purine antagonist), and cladribine and fludarabine (adenosine deaminase inhibitors). Cytarabine is an anti-metabolite used in the treatment of leukemia and lymphoma. 5-FU is an anti-metabolite used in the treatment of colon, rectal, breast, GI, head and neck, and ovarian cancers. Capecitabine is an anti-metabolite used in the treatment of breast and colorectal cancers. Fludarabine is used to treat chronic leukemia and non-Hodgkin lymphoma.

Mitotic Inhibitors

Mitotic inhibitors include the plant alkaloids and taxanes as well as the epothilones. They work by stopping **mitosis** and are **cell cycle specific**, working in the "M" phase of the cell cycle. With the arrest of mitosis and inhibition of necessary enzymes, the proteins needed for cellular reproduction are not made. Mitotic inhibitors are used in the treatment of breast and lung cancers, as well as in the treatment of myeloma, lymphoma, and leukemia. Paclitaxel is a plant alkaloid and taxane that is used in the treatment of breast, ovarian, lung, bladder, prostate, melanoma, and esophageal cancer. Ixabepilone is used in the treatment of metastatic or locally advanced breast cancer. Vinblastine is a plant alkaloid used in the treatment of testicular, breast, lung, head and neck, and bladder cancer. It is also used in the treatment of sarcoma, lymphoma, and choriocarcinoma.

Cell Cycle Phase Nonspecific Classes of Drugs

The cell cycle is composed of **four phases**: G1, S1, G2, and M. Many chemotherapeutic agents are active in the "S" phase of the cell cycle in which DNA replication is most active. Chemotherapeutic agents that work in all phases of the cell cycle and are not specific to one particular phase are known as **cell cycle phase nonspecific agents**. The **alkylating agents** work by directly damaging cell DNA to prevent the cancer cell from reproducing. Alkylating agents work in all phases of the cell cycle and are most active in the resting phase of the cell cycle. Examples of alkylating agents include nitrogen mustard, carmustine, lomustine, busulfan, thiotepa, and cyclophosphamide. The **platinum class** of chemotherapeutic agents are also cell cycle phase nonspecific. These agents work by inhibiting DNA synthesis, transcription, and function by cross-linking DNA subunits. Agents in the platinum class include cisplatin, carboplatin, and oxaliplatin.

Anti-Tumor Antibiotics

Anti-tumor antibiotics are **cell cycle nonspecific agents** that act during multiple phases of the cell cycle. Anti-tumor antibiotics are derived from byproducts of the species of soil fungus *Streptomyces*. They work by binding with DNA to prevent the synthesis of RNA. They also prohibit cell growth by preventing DNA replication. Anthracyclines, chromomycins, and a few miscellaneous chemotherapeutic agents make up the anti-tumor antibiotic class. Doxorubicin, daunorubicin, epirubicin, mitoxantrone, idarubicin, dactinomycin, plicamycin, mitomycin, and bleomycin are examples of anti-tumor antibiotics. Common side effects with anti-tumor antibiotics include neutropenia, thrombocytopenia, alopecia, fever, headache, nausea and vomiting, anorexia, peripheral neuropathy, cardiac toxicity (with anthracyclines), pulmonary toxicity (with bleomycin), skin rash, photosensitivity, and changes in urine color (with mitomycin). Lifetime dose limitations of the anthracyclines are recommended due to the risk of permanent cardiac damage. Anti-tumor antibiotics are used in the treatment of leukemias, lymphomas, and solid tumor cancers.

Common Anti-Tumor Antibiotics Medications

Anti-tumor antibiotics are used in the treatment of leukemias, lymphomas, and solid tumor cancers. Anti-tumor antibiotics are **cell cycle nonspecific agents** that act during multiple phases of the cell cycle. Anti-tumor antibiotics are derived from byproducts of the species of soil fungus *Streptomyces*. They work by binding with DNA to prevent the synthesis of RNA. They also prohibit cell growth by preventing DNA replication. Anthracyclines, chromomycins, and a few miscellaneous chemotherapeutic agents make up the anti-tumor antibiotic class. Doxorubin, daunorubicin, epirubicin, mitoxantrone, idarubicin, dactinomycin, plicamycin, mitomycin, and bleomycin are examples of anti-tumor antibiotics. Doxorubicin is an anthracycline anti-tumor antibiotic used in the treatment of stomach, testicular, prostate, uterine, bladder, breast, head and neck, liver, ovarian, pancreatic, and lung cancers. It is also indicated for the treatment of some lymphomas, multiple myeloma, and sarcoma. Epirubicin is an anthracycline anti-tumor antibiotic used in the treatment of breast cancer. Mitomycin is an anti-tumor antibiotic used to treatment adenocarcinoma of the stomach or pancreas. It is also indicated in the treatment of anal, bladder, breast, cervical, colorectal, head and neck, and non–small cell lung cancer.

Alkylating Agents

The **alkylating agents** are the oldest class of chemotherapy drugs. They work by interfering with the cell's DNA and inhibiting cell growth. Because of the way these agents interfere with a cell's DNA, there is a risk of long-term damage to the **bone marrow** and subsequently the development of **leukemia**. The risk of leukemia development is at its highest 5-10 years post treatment and is also increased with higher doses administered. Alkylating agents include the nitrogen mustards, nitrosoureas (including carmustine and streptozocin), alkyl sulfonates (including busulfan), triazines (including dacarbazine), and the ethyleneamines. The alkylating agents are used in the treatment of leukemia, lymphoma (including Hodgkin lymphoma), multiple myeloma, sarcoma, lung, breast, brain, and ovarian cancers. Dacarbazine (DTIC) is an alkylating agent used in the treatment of melanoma, Hodgkin lymphoma, sarcoma, and neuroblastoma. Carmustine (BCNU) is an alkylating agent used to treat primary brain tumors, Hodgkin lymphoma, melanoma, and lung and colon cancer.

Chemotherapy Medications

Chemotherapy medications can target cancer cells during their reproductive cycle or can interfere with the way the cells function. Those that act upon the cell during the **cell cycle** can be very specific and target cells only during certain phases of reproduction or during any phase of the cycle. Those that target cells at specific points in the cycle are either given in small doses or on a constant basis. Those that are **non-specific** are usually given in large boluses.

There are several different types of chemotherapy medications that attack cells at any given phase of the reproductive cycle. They can interrupt the duplication of DNA within the cancer cell causing a breakdown in cell reproduction. Some medications can interfere with the proteins that form the building blocks of cell DNA. Different phases of the DNA replication cycle can be interrupted resulting in formation of irregular DNA and, ultimately, cell destruction.

Oral Leukemia Chemotherapeutic Agents

1. Busulfan
2. Chlorambucil
3. Hydrea

4. 6-Mercaptopurine
5. 6-Thioguanine

Chemotherapy Agents

Paclitaxel: Paclitaxel is classified both as a plant alkaloid and taxane chemotherapeutic agent. It is administered intravenously and is classified as an irritant agent. It is used in the treatment of breast, ovarian, lung, prostate, and esophageal cancers, as well as melanoma.

Carboplatin: Carboplatin is an alkylating agent used in the treatment of ovarian, lung, head and neck, endometrial, bladder, breast, and cervical cancers. It is also used in the treatment of central nervous system tumors and sarcomas. It can be administered intravenously and also given as an intraperitoneal infusion for the treatment of ovarian cancer.

Cisplatin: Cisplatin is the sister agent of Carboplatin. It is an alkylating agent used in the treatment of testicular, ovarian, bladder, head and neck, esophageal, lung, breast, cervical, stomach, and prostate cancers. It is also used in the treatment of lymphomas, multiple myeloma, neuroblastomas, melanoma, and mesothelioma. Cisplatin is considered an irritant agent. It can be administered intravenously or as an intraperitoneal infusion.

Cytarabine: Cytarabine is an anti-metabolite chemotherapeutic agent used in the treatment of leukemias (including AML, CML, and CLL) and lymphomas. It can be administered intravenously, intramuscularly, or subcutaneously. Cytarabine is one of only a few chemotherapeutic agents that can be administered intrathecally, for direct administration into the cerebral spinal fluid.

Topoisomerase Inhibitors

Topoisomerase inhibitors are substances that block the action of the topoisomerase enzymes. **Topoisomerase enzymes** are substances that break and rejoin DNA strands that are needed for cells to divide and grow. Blocking of these enzymes then leads to cellular death of the cancer cells. Topoisomerase inhibitors are divided into topoisomerase I and topoisomerase II. Camptothecin and its derivatives (including irinotecan) are examples of **topoisomerase I inhibitors**. Doxorubicin, etoposide, and mitoxantrone are examples of **topoisomerase II inhibitors**. Irinotecan is a plant alkaloid and topoisomerase I inhibitor used in the treatment of metastatic colon or rectal cancer. Etoposide is a plant alkaloid and topoisomerase II inhibitor used in the treatment of testicular, bladder, prostate, lung, stomach, uterine, and brain cancers. It is also indicated for the treatment of some lymphomas, sarcomas, and neuroblastoma. Mitoxantrone is an anti-tumor antibiotic and topoisomerase II inhibitor used in the treatment of prostate and breast cancer, as well as leukemia and lymphoma.

Vein Selection for the Administration of Chemotherapeutic Agents

1. The selection should begin with a critical assessment of all available veins of the patient.
2. All equipment for venipuncture should be assembled before any attempt is made.
3. During vein selection, avoid any arm with known or proven compromised circulation.
4. To preserve venous integrity over time the nurse should begin distally and alternate venipuncture sites.
5. If there is no site available by observation, use of a tourniquet is permissible.
6. A cannula should be selected that is appropriate for both the length of the therapy and the patient's available veins.
7. If the drug is to be given via a freely-running side arm the dressing should not hinder visualization.

8. When injecting a vesicant do not use an infusion pump.
9. If a drug in combination is known to be associated with rapid onset of nausea and vomiting, it is given <u>last</u>.
10. The entire course of the vein should be visible during the injection or infusion.
11. A vesicant should not be injected distal to a previous site.
12. Vesicant agents should not be infused as a mini-infusion or continuous infusion into a peripheral vein

Biotherapy

Biotherapy is a form of treatment that is created from natural components. Biotherapy treatments may be capable of changing the way the human body reacts to cancer cells. Most biotherapy agents are formed from **cytokines** which trigger the immune system to attack malignant cells. These agents are used to interrupt normal cell functions that occur within malignant cells. They can interfere with cell growth, production of necessary proteins by the cancer cells, and can interrupt the production of enzymes by cancer cells.

Examples of biotherapy include specialized **antibodies and vaccines**. These antibodies are not only used to treat cancer, though. Because they target cancer cells, they may also be used for diagnosing and staging cancer. Radioactive material can be attached to the antibodies and scans can be performed to detect the areas of antibody distribution. This can identify specific areas of the body that are affected by cancer and how advanced the disease may have become.

Types of Biological and Molecular Treatments

1. **Cytokines** make up the largest group of biotherapy agents. They are proteins that are produced by immune cells that interfere with normal actions of a cell. Examples include interferon, interleukins, tumor necrosis factor, and blood growth factors.
2. **Monoclonal antibodies** recognize specific antigens on the outside of cancer cells and trigger an immune response targeted at these cells.
3. **Fusion proteins** function to cause destruction of cancer cells.
4. **Effector cells** are specialized immune cells that are taken from the patient and then given by IV infusion.
5. **Immunomodulators** are less specific than some other biotherapy agents, but function to trigger an immune response.
6. **Retinoids** are produced by vitamin A and function in cell growth and function.
7. **Vaccines** introduce the body's immune system to a specific antigen in order to form antibodies against the foreign agent.
8. **Molecular targeted therapies** are comprised of various agents that interfere with normal function of cancer cells.
9. **Gene therapy** is still considered an experimental treatment. Its goal is to directly interfere with a cancer cell in order to destroy it.

Immunotherapy, Hormonal Therapy, and Targeted Therapy

Classifications, Purpose, and Risk Factors of Interferon

Interferons are a naturally occurring protein found in the body. When used in medicine, interferon belongs to the classification cytokines, and their function is to change the **response** of the cells of the immune system, thereby slowing the growth of cancer cells. There are three classifications of interferons, alpha, beta, and gamma. Interferons can increase the effectiveness of the medication zidovudine, which increases risk of toxicity. Interferon can interfere with excretion of theophylline, so levels should be closely monitored. Commonly used in cancer treatment, interferon alpha-2 B can cause hepatotoxicity as well as hypertriglyceridemia. A normal triglyceride level is less than 150 mg/dl with levels of 500 mg/dl or higher considered in the very high range. If hypertriglyceridemia remains persistent and severe, treatment with interferon should be discontinued. Other side effects of interferon alpha-2 B include flu-like symptoms such as fever, myalgia and fatigue. Interferon can also cause neutropenia, anemia, and thrombocytopenia. Hematologic effects should be monitored and dosages adjusted or held according to severity.

Monoclonal Antibodies

Monoclonal antibodies can be divided into two types: unconjugated and conjugated.

Unconjugated monoclonal antibodies are those not bound to a drug, toxin, or radioactive substance. Unconjugated MAbs may also be referred to as naked MAbs and are the most commonly used monoclonal antibodies. Trastuzumab is an example of an unconjugated MAb. Gemtuzumab, ibritumomab, and iodine-131 tositumomab are all examples of conjugated MAbs.

Conjugated MAbs are joined to radioactive isotopes, chemotherapeutic agents, or toxins to poison the cancer cells they are targeting. Conjugated MAbs work by transporting the associated anticancer agents directly to the cancer cells. Conjugated MAbs do not attach to hormones. Ibritumomab is indicated in combination with rituximab in the treatment of relapsed or refractory low-grade, follicular or transformed B-cell NHL. Gemtuzumab is indicated for the treatment of CD33 positive acute myeloid leukemia. Iodine-131 tositumomab is indicated for the treatment of CD20 positive, follicular NHL (not used in combination with rituximab). Alemtuzumab is indicated for the treatment of B-cell chronic lymphocytic leukemia. Ipilimumab is for the treatment of unresectable or metastatic melanoma. Treatment with ipilimumab can result in severe and fatal immune-mediated adverse reactions as a result of T-cell activation and proliferation. The most common manifestations of these reactions include enterocolitis, hepatitis, dermatitis, neuropathy, and endocrinopathy.

Epidermal Growth Factor Receptor Inhibitors

Epidermal growth factor receptor is a protein that influences cancer growth in different types of cancers. It is found in abnormally high levels on the surface of many types of cancer cells, causing them to excessively divide in its presence. Increased EGFR is associated with more aggressive tumors, recurrence, poorer prognosis, and resistance to endocrine therapy.

EGFR inhibitors are classified as either tyrosine kinase inhibitors or monoclonal antibodies, depending on the way they are used to treat the cancer. Epidermal growth factor receptor inhibitors that are classified as monoclonal antibodies work by blocking the epidermal growth factor receptor protein present on the surface of the cancer cell that causes excessive cell division and subsequent tumor growth. EGFR inhibitors are used to treat breast, colon, pancreatic and non-small-cell cancers. Lapatinib is an epidermal growth factor receptor inhibitor used in the treatment of metastatic breast cancer. Gefitinib is an EGFR inhibitor commonly used in non-small-cell lung cancer. Because EGFR inhibitors are targeted agents, they can have less side effects than traditional chemotherapy, but cutaneous side effects are seen frequently. These include acneiform eruptions, xerosis, paronychia, and eczema.

Cancer Treatment Hormones

Hormone therapy in cancer treatment works by slowing or stopping the growth of hormone-sensitive tumors. This is accomplished either by **interference** with the action of the hormone or by **blocking** of the body's ability to produce hormones. Tumors that are not hormone sensitive will not be affected by hormone therapy. In the treatment of hormone-sensitive breast cancer, ovarian suppression agents such as goserelin acetate or leuprorelin may be utilized. Ovarian suppression agents work by interfering with the signals the pituitary gland sends to the ovaries to produce estrogen. In the treatment of prostate cancer, antiandrogens may be used in combination with an orchiectomy or in combination with a luteinizing hormone–releasing hormone agonist. Antiandrogens work by competing with androgens for binding to the androgen receptor, thereby decreasing the ability of the androgens to promote or accelerate prostate cancer growth. Examples of antiandrogen agents include flutamide, enzalutamide, bicalutamide, and nilutamide.

Targeted Therapies

Targeted therapies are a type of cancer treatment that "targets" specific molecules involved in cancer cell growth and survival. Targeted therapies differ from traditional chemotherapy in that traditional chemotherapy acts on all rapidly dividing cells, including both normal and cancerous cells. Targeted therapies only interfere with specific molecules, thereby lessening some of the side effects commonly associated with traditional chemotherapy. They are considered "**cytostatic**," meaning they focus on blocking tumor cell proliferation, as opposed to cytotoxic. Targeted therapies may be a small molecule drug or a synthetic antibody designed to attack certain targets on cancer cells. Targeted therapies act in a variety of different ways. Some prevent growth signaling in the tumor cell, some interfere with the development of tumor blood vessels, some promote cell death, others stimulate the immune system to destroy cancer cells, and others deliver toxic drugs to the cancer cells themselves. Much focus and attention have been aimed at the further advancement and development of targeted therapies for many diseases, including cancer.

Targeted Therapies Types

Targeted therapies in cancer treatment are continuing to emerge as researchers continue to narrow in on and better define the genetic changes in cancer cells. Targeted therapies work differently than traditional chemotherapy. They are more specific in their mechanism of "targeting" cancer cells and therefore tend to cause less damage to normal cells. New targeted therapies are being researched and discovered every day in the treatment of diseases, including cancer.

Imatinib mesylate is a type of targeted therapy used to treat gastrointestinal stromal tumors and chronic leukemia. Imatinib works by inhibiting the cellular enzyme tyrosine kinase, thereby inhibiting cell growth. **Gefitinib** is another example of a targeted therapy used in cancer treatment. Gefitinib works by blocking epidermal growth factor receptor, which is often found in higher quantities on a cancer cell. Epidermal growth factor receptors signal cells to grow and divide. When this signal is blocked, the cancer cell will cease to grow and divide. Gefitinib is used in the treatment of advanced non–small cell lung cancer.

Targeted Therapies Limitations and Side Effects

One of the limitations of **targeted therapy** is that, over time, cancer cells can become **resistant**, rendering the targeted therapy less effective or ineffective. Resistance can occur in one of two ways:

1. The target can change through mutation so that the targeted therapy no longer interacts well with it.
2. The tumor itself can find a new pathway for it to grow that does not depend on the target.

To combat the issue of resistance, combination therapies may be used.

Another limitation of targeted therapy is that it may be difficult to **identify** particular targets for drug development due to the target's structure or its function within the cancer cell.

Although some of the side effects associated with traditional chemotherapy may be less with the use of targeted therapies, there are still significant and substantial **side effects** associated with targeted therapies. Diarrhea, liver problems, skin problems (including acneiform rash, dry skin, nail changes, and hair depigmentation), problems with blood clotting and wound healing, hypertension, and in rare instances gastrointestinal perforation have been reported with the use of targeted therapies.

Treatment Administration

Professional Qualifications Needed for Administration of Chemotherapy Agents

1. Current license as a registered nurse.
2. Certification in CPR.
3. Skill in intravenous therapy.
4. Educational preparation and demonstrated knowledge in all areas related to neoplastic drugs, including preparation, disposition, elimination and interactions.
5. Demonstrated knowledge of preparation of medication errors and skill of drug administration.
6. Ongoing acquisition of updated information and verification of continuing knowledge and skills.
7. Policies and procedures that govern specific actions for chemotherapy administration.

Pretreatment Considerations

1. Make sure the patient is completely informed about the treatment plan.
2. Make sure there is a **signed** informed consent form.
3. Check the drug dosage against the physician's order.
4. Check the patient's last laboratory results.
5. If the WBC is low, calculate the AGC (absolute granulocyte count) [(% of neutrophils) + bands X total WBC = AGC].
6. Consider the way each drug is metabolized and eliminated. If an impaired organ is involved, toxicity may result.
7. Consider any pretreatment antiemetics, hydration, or measures to eliminate resulting alopecia.
8. Make sure that emergency equipment is near at hand to counter any allergic reaction or extravasation of drug or vesicant.
9. Ensure adequate lighting and patient comfort.
10. Review the patient's entire medication history (for incompatibilities, interactions, and toxicities).

Types of Venous Catheters

- **Short-term venous catheters** can be inserted into peripheral or central veins and are generally utilized for less than 2 weeks. These can be used for multiple medications, including chemotherapy or total parenteral nutrition (TPN). Because they are more often used in smaller peripheral veins, damage to these vessels can occur with infusion of more caustic agents.
- **Long-term venous catheters** are inserted when infusion is necessary for longer than 2 weeks. These are generally inserted into larger veins, such as the jugular or superior/inferior vena cava, and are used for infusion of medications and TPN. A sterile dressing is required and the patient can frequently go home with these lines to administer medications on their own.
- **Medication ports** can be implanted under the skin when regular infusion of chemotherapy is desired. These can also be used to obtain blood samples. These are frequently used to prevent frequent venipuncture.
- **Arterial catheters** are also used when arterial access is necessary. These are frequently used when high doses of chemotherapeutic medications must be given.

Venous Catheters Common Complications

Blockage of the catheter can occur without regular flushing of the line. Regularly flush the line with normal saline. Flushes should also be performed before and after all medication administrations to prevent accumulation of the medication in the line. If a clot is the cause of the blockage, a clot-busting medication, such as urokinase, should be given to dissolve the clot. Certain medications can build up within the catheter and cause a blockage of the system. Follow instructions from the physician or pharmacist to breakdown the buildup of medication using another medication that causes it to dissolve.

Infection is always a risk with a venous catheter and sterile technique needs to be followed to avoid this serious complication. If an infection does occur, antibiotics will be ordered to prevent sepsis.

Venous catheters can **pull out or move** from their ideal location. This will need to be readjusted by the physician and the line re-secured in the correct location.

Infusion Systems

Large volume infusion systems are used for infusions that will take longer to administer. They can be electric IV pumps or pumps that control multiple infusions at once. These are used primarily when infusing blood or various medications, including antibiotics and chemotherapy.

Small volume infusion devices are used for medications that will be infused quickly. These are frequently used for antibiotics and may be electronically controlled or pressure released.

Patient-controlled infusions allow the patient the ability to administer their own medication. These are frequently used for IV analgesics through patient-controlled analgesic pumps (PCA pumps). The IV pump is programmed to allow only a certain amount of medication to be delivered with each dose with a total amount to be given within a certain time period. This prevents any problems with overdosing. The pump can also be set with a basal rate which automatically provides a specific amount of medication to be delivered.

Guidelines for Administering Antineoplastic Agents

- **Oral** - Emphasize the importance of complying with the prescribed schedule. Plan for drugs with emetic potential to be taken with meals; drugs that require hydration to be taken early in the day.
- **Subcutaneous or intramuscular** - Demonstrate and require the patient to perform a return demonstration to ensure the patient understands if doing self-injections. Encourage rotation of injection sites.
- **Topical** - Cover surface with a thin film of the medication. Instruct the patient to wear loose-fitting cotton clothing. Wear gloves and wash hands thoroughly.
- **Intra-arterial** - This method requires catheter placement in an artery near the tumor; administer in a heparinized solution through an infusion pump. Monitor the patient throughout treatment. Instruct patient and/or significant other on the use of the pump if medication is to be given at home. **Intracavitary** - Instill the drug into the bladder through a catheter or chest tube into the pleural cavity. Follow instructions carefully.
- **Intraperitoneal** - Place the drug into the abdominal cavity through an implantable port or external suprapubic catheter. Warm the solution to body temperature before giving.

- **Intrathecal** - Reconstitute all medications with preservative free sterile normal saline or sterile water. (Usually a physician administers intrathecal drugs.)
- **Intravenous** - Drugs may be given through intravenous catheters or peripheral vein access. Follow the institution guidelines for administration of drugs.

Disease Specific Treatment Modalities

Localized Treatments Available for Breast Cancer

Localized treatments involve surgery or radiation treatments.

- **Surgical procedures** performed for breast cancer include lumpectomies, segmental resection, or mastectomies. Mastectomies can remove just the breast tissue (subcutaneous mastectomy), breast tissue plus some of the skin over the lesion (skin-sparing mastectomy), breast tissue plus skin and glands (total mastectomy), breast tissue and skin plus axillary lymph nodes (modified radical mastectomy), or breast tissue and skin along with lymph nodes and pectoral muscle (radical mastectomy). Sometimes just the first lymph node to be affected by the cancer (the sentinel node) is removed. This is still investigative, though.
- **Radiation treatments** may be done to ensure destruction of all cancer cells. It can be done along with chemotherapy or on its own. Radiation usually begins 2-4 weeks following surgery and may be done for palliative treatment of bony lesions. Side effects include irritation of the overlying skin, tissue and nerve damage, and fatigue.

Systemic Treatments Available for Breast Cancer

The goal with **systemic treatment** is to treat the whole body in an attempt to destroy any cancer cells that may have migrated from the primary cancer site. **Chemotherapy** is the main type of systemic treatment that is used. Some of the more common chemotherapy drugs used to treat breast cancer include Cytoxan, Adriamycin, Taxol, and Mexate. Very often, multiple chemotherapy drugs will be given for more effective treatment. Most patients will receive 4-6 treatments with chemotherapy, if side effects are tolerable enough to continue treatment. Increasing the length or dose of treatment has not been found to be more effective in treating breast cancer. Many people will try homeopathic treatments, such as herbal treatments or treatment with vitamins and minerals. These have not been medically-approved. Other treatments that patients use to help with treating the effects of cancer include hypnosis, massage therapy, reflexology, and biofeedback.

Mastectomy Postoperative Care

Postoperative nursing care for a patient who has undergone a mastectomy for the treatment of breast cancer includes a combination of high priority interventions that focus on assessment, support, and patient education. Wound care and remobilization of the affected side are a focus of physical recovery. In the **immediate postoperative period**, the arm should be positioned so that it is slightly elevated. Exercises to regain full range of motion can begin within 3-5days after surgery and should be gradually increased. The patient should be educated on the positioning and care of the arm on the affected side, drains, pain management, IV lines and tubing, and ambulation. Early ambulation and the importance of coughing and deep breathing should be emphasized. The incision should be assessed for inflammation, tenderness, swelling, and drainage. If the patient has a drain in place, the fluid should be assessed and measured and the drain secured to the skin or clothing. Patients may struggle with feelings of sadness at the loss of their breast. Additionally, the patient may feel anxious while awaiting the final pathology of the breast tissue and learning about the possible involvement of more lymph nodes.

Brain Tumors Treatments

- **Surgical resection** is done to remove the tumor if possible. This is done through a procedure called a **craniotomy**. The same positioning techniques are used as with a biopsy and all or as much of the tumor as possible is removed. Along with the malignant tumor, some healthy tissue may also be removed. The patient may suffer alterations in function in relation to the area of the brain in which the tumor is located and surgery is performed.
- **Radiation therapy** may be performed after surgery or may be used if surgery is not possible. Many brain tumors have microscopic strings of cancer cells that spread throughout the brain tissue but are not visible on MRI. Radiation is aimed at destroying any of these remaining cancer cells. This can cause edema of the surrounding brain tumor and destruction of some of the healthy brain tissue that remains.
- **Chemotherapy** can also be given, but it is not considered a primary therapy for malignant brain tumors.

Postoperative Nursing Care for a Craniotomy

Postoperative care of the **craniotomy** patient is complex because the patient is at risk for a multitude of postoperative complications. A thorough and accurate **neurological assessment** is paramount. **Hemodynamic stability** is critical and should be regularly assessed. Hypertension in the postoperative craniotomy patient increases the risk of hemorrhage. Hypotension may cause hypoperfusion and brain ischemia. Postoperative interventions include DVT prophylaxis, incision and drain care, early ambulation, and prevention of atelectasis through incentive spirometry. Physical and occupational therapy should be involved in the evaluation and treatment of the patient postoperatively. Nursing staff should be aware of the risk of postoperative complications and assess the patient for early signs of these complications. Meningitis, brain abscess, and wound infection may manifest with signs and symptoms including fever, headache, malaise, redness, warmth or purulent drainage from the incision site, nausea and vomiting, and altered level of consciousness. Additional complications may include endocrine complications such as diabetes insipidus or syndrome of inappropriate antidiuretic hormone secretion, postoperative hemorrhage, seizures, or a leak in cerebral spinal fluid.

Prostate Cancer Treatments

If the cancer is detected early, the patient may have some options with treatment:

- **Surgery** can be performed for removal of the prostate and surrounding lymph nodes. In certain instances, the testicles can also be removed which stops the production of testosterone and can help to decrease the progression of the disease. There are risks with surgery and the patient can develop incontinence or impotence following surgery.
- **Radiation** can be performed to destroy the cancer cells within the prostate gland. There is the risk of damage to surrounding healthy tissues, though. Radiation can also be delivered through brachytherapy in which radiation seeds are implanted within the prostate.
- **Cryosurgery** can be performed in which extreme cold is applied to the lesions on the prostate to destroy them.
- With advanced prostate cancer, **hormonal treatments** may be given to reduce the amount of testosterone produced. The patient can develop feminizing side effects, though, such as enlargement of the breasts and hot flashes.

Postoperative Nursing Care for a Transurethral Resection (TUR)

Postoperative nursing care for a patient who has undergone a **transurethral resection of the prostate** (TURP) includes a through and accurate assessment of the patient. Patients who have had a TURP are at risk for hemorrhage. Vital signs should be monitored closely and an accurate intake and output record maintained. The patient's **urinary catheter** should be assessed for patency regularly. Urinary catheters can become occluded with clots, which can increase the risk of hemorrhage. **Urine** should be assessed for color and character and recorded. Increasing fluids helps to decrease the burning sensation patients may feel with the urinary catheter and also lessens the chance for the development of a urinary tract infection. Patients may experience incisional pain, pain caused by bladders spasms, or abdominal cramping postoperatively. **Analgesics** and **nonsteroidal anti-inflammatory agents** are used to manage incisional pain. **Belladonna** and **opium suppositories** may be used for the management of bladder spasms.

Lung Cancer Treatments

- **Surgery** is the most common treatment for **lung cancer**. Given the poor prognosis with the disease, most patients are enrolled in an experimental study to try all treatments available. Removal of the lobe of the lung that is affected by the cancer is the most conservative surgical treatment available. Removal of the entire lung can be done, though there are several complications that can occur. Out of the patients that are able to survive surgery, only about 50% of them have the complete surgery performed because metastasis is often detected after surgery is started.
- **Radiation therapy** can be performed to treat a tumor. This is usually performed as a palliative measure or to reduce the size of a tumor before surgical resection.
- **Chemotherapy** can be performed along with radiation and is usually done to help with symptom control.

Symptom control includes medications to control pain, nebulizer treatments to attempt to open the airways and assist with breathing, and steroids to control inflammation.

Postoperative Nursing Care for a Thoracotomy

A traditional **thoracotomy** for the treatment of lung cancer involves an open incision with skin closure via subcutaneous sutures of staples. A chest tube is inserted to facilitate fluid drainage and lung expansion. A minimally invasive procedure known as video-assisted thoracoscopy surgery (VATS) may also be an option for patients. Two to three smaller incisions are made into the chest wall and a videoscope and other small surgical tools are utilized. Patients undergoing traditional thoracotomy have a longer hospitalization, longer recovery time, and higher morbidity, and they experience more pain than those undergoing a VATS.

Postoperative care includes incisional care, pain management, and a bowel regimen to combat the constipation that goes along with opioid use, ambulation, and care of the chest tube. In addition, pulmonary hygiene should be performed aggressively to decrease the likelihood of pneumonia, atelectasis, and respiratory failure. Deep breathing in the postoperative period decreases the likelihood of pulmonary complications.

Colorectal Cancer Treatments

Most patients undergo **surgical treatment** for **colorectal cancer**. The extent of the surgery depends on how much of the colon is affected by the malignancy.

A **colostomy** may be required following surgery and this may be permanent or temporary.

Radiation therapy can also be used to treat colorectal cancer. This can be done before surgery to help shrink a tumor so that it can be surgically removed or it may be done following surgery to destroy any cancer cells that may remain. Permanent tissue damage can result from radiation therapy and this will be dependent upon the dose and number of treatments.

Chemotherapy is usually done along with radiation treatments. This is usually done if there is some extension of a malignancy beyond a localized tumor.

Other medications are being studied to target growth factors and help the body develop antibodies against cancer-causing cells. These are still in the clinic phase.

Postoperative Nursing Care for a Colostomy

Postoperative assessment of the cancer patient who has undergone a **colostomy** includes assessment of vital signs and lung and bowel sounds. The stoma site should be assessed for color and size. The stoma should appear pink and moist. Intake and output should be accurately recorded including drainage from a nasogastric tube, urinary catheter, and stoma. Coughing and deep breathing exercises should be encouraged as well as early ambulation. Pain should be proactively managed. A thorough skin assessment should be performed to ensure adequate wound healing. Body image and sexuality concerns are likely and should be discussed with the patient postoperatively. Sexual counseling should begin while the patient is in the hospital. Patients often struggle with viewing the stoma and learning to care for it. The nurse will need to provide the patient with education on ostomy care and supplies as well as dietary needs.

Cervical Cancer Treatments

There are a couple of factors to consider when deciding which treatment to pursue for **cervical cancer**. The patient may still be interested in having children, so treatments that will preserve the function of the uterus and cervix would be desired. The extent of the cancer will also be considered when deciding on a treatment plan.

- If childbearing is not a factor, a total **hysterectomy** along with removal of lymph nodes will be performed. Some surgeons can perform a procedure that only removes the cervix in patients who still wish to have children.
- **Radiation therapy** is usually performed to ensure destruction of cancer cells. When lymph nodes are involved, chemotherapy will also be performed.
- **Chemotherapy** can be done palliatively or when distant metastasis is involved.
- The best treatment is **screening** with regular Pap smears. The incidence of cervical cancer has decreased because of the increased awareness of the importance of early detection.

Ovarian Cancer Treatments

- Surgical removal of the ovaries, an **oophorectomy**, is necessary. In some cases, just the malignant tissue is removed from the ovary, but only if it is very localized and isolated. Surgery can also be helpful in determining the extent of metastatic lesions present in the pelvic and abdominal cavities.
- **Radiation therapy** can be done to treat metastatic lesions. This can cause permanent tissue damage with multiple side effects, though. It is possible for radioactive treatments to be inserted in the abdomen to deliver a steady dose of radiation therapy to metastatic lesions.

- **Chemotherapy** can also be given, but is usually used with an early diagnosis or palliatively in end-stage disease. Like the radioactive treatments, chemotherapy can also be given directly into the abdomen to provide more direct treatment to tumors. This also decreases the risk of side effects that are normally seen when chemotherapy medications are given orally or via IV.

Postoperative Nursing Care for a Hysterectomy

Postoperative assessment of the cancer patient who has undergone a **hysterectomy** includes assessment of vital signs and lung and bowel sounds. **Hemorrhage** is a postoperative risk factor and women who have undergone a vaginal hysterectomy are at a higher risk. Nursing staff should assess the incisional site for redness, warmth, edema, or drainage, and report any signs or symptoms of infection. Patients should be encouraged to cough and breathe deeply by splinting the abdomen with a pillow. Pain should be proactively managed. Intake and output should be accurately recorded. Fluid intake should be encouraged. **Deep vein thrombosis (DVT) prophylaxis** is critically important in patients who have undergone abdominal surgery. Patients are at a higher risk of developing a pulmonary embolus. The patient should be educated on perineal care. Patients who have undergone a hysterectomy may experience a negative self-concept and have misconceptions after their surgery. Nursing staff can help to clarify any misconceptions patients may have postoperatively through education and support.

Testicular Cancer Treatments

A cure is usually possible with **testicular cancer**. Awareness of the disease has increased over the past several years, which has promoted self-examination and earlier treatment.

- Usually the treatment of choice is an **orchiectomy** to remove the affected testicle. Depending on the severity of disease, lymph nodes from the pelvic cavity may also be removed for testing. If a single testicle is removed and the other is left and there is no presence of disease, the patient should not have any problems with normal sperm production in the future.
- **Radiation therapy** can be used to treat metastasis to the lungs. Permanent tissue damage can result from radiation treatments so the risks are weighed against the benefits.
- **Chemotherapy** may also be used with end-stage disease or a recurrent episode of testicular cancer. This is usually accomplished by using multiple drugs versus a single drug for treatment.

Postoperative Nursing Care for an Orchiectomy

Postoperative assessment of the cancer patient who has undergone an **orchiectomy** includes assessment of vital signs and lung and bowel sounds. Hemorrhage is a postoperative risk factor. **DVT prophylaxis** should be initiated. The patient should be encouraged to cough and breathe deeply. The patient should be educated to avoid lifting and straining. **Hemodynamic status** should be carefully assessed postoperatively. The incision should be assessed for redness, warmth, edema, or drainage, and any signs or symptoms of infection reported. Pain should be proactively managed. Patients who have undergone an orchiectomy may experience a negative self-image. Discussions regarding body image concerns and sexuality should be encouraged. Patients who undergo more extensive surgery including bilateral orchiectomy with lymph node dissection are at a greater risk for sexual dysfunction. Patients may also have concerns regarding fertility. Patients should be educated on fertility-sparing measures prior to surgery as cryopreservation of sperm preoperatively is the most effective means of fertility preservation.

Bladder Cancer Treatments

The goals of treatment are to remove the cancer and prevent metastasis, as well as maintain appropriate bladder function.

- Resection is frequently accomplished through a procedure called a **transurethral resection** (TUR). The tumor is usually burned electrically or with lasers in this procedure, but bleeding and healthy tissue damage can also occur.
- **Chemotherapy** is used by implanting the medications within the bladder to treat the tumor. Some of the common chemotherapy drugs used can cause a severe depression of the immune system.
- **Surgery** can be performed to remove the bladder and prostate and create a urinary diversion to be used for voiding. A *hysterectomy* is also performed in female patients. This surgery commonly causes sexual dysfunction.
- **Radiation** can also be performed to attempt destruction of the tumor cells. Damage can occur to healthy tissues as well, though. Radiation therapy is usually used when the bladder cancer is advanced.

Postoperative Nursing Care for a Cystectomy

The standard treatment for bladder tumors that invade the muscle is surgical removal of the bladder by **radical cystectomy**. Postoperative nursing care includes assessment of vital signs and lung and bowel sounds. Urinary output should be closely monitored and maintained at a minimum of 30 mL/hour. The surgical site should be assessed for redness, warmth, edema, or drainage, and any signs or symptoms of infection reported. Signs of peritonitis related to an anastomotic leak include fever, leukocytosis, abdominal distension, and tenderness. The stoma should be assessed as well as the surrounding skin. Pain should be proactively managed. Patients who have undergone a cystectomy may experience a negative self-image. Patients should be encouraged to discuss their feelings regarding body image and sexuality. Patient education on cleansing and care of the stoma should be performed. Patients with a continent reservoir who will perform self-catheterization will need education on how to complete the catheterization.

Head and Neck Cancer Treatments

For newly diagnosed head or neck cancer, **surgery and radiation** are used for treatment.

- *Chemotherapy* is usually used to treat cancer that is recurrent or due to metastasis from a different primary site.
- *Surgery* can involve removal of the tumor or can be more extensive with removal of surrounding lymph nodes and muscle tissue. Major vascular and nervous system structures may be located in the area where the cancer is located. Careful dissection may be performed or some structures may need to be removed. Extensive neck surgery may result in anatomic deformities from muscle removal. Major oropharyngeal surgery could result in removal of a portion of the mandible which can lead to anatomic defects in the facial structure.
- *Radiation* destroys the malignant cells in the area of the tumor. Damage can occur to healthy tissue as well, though. This can result in permanent alterations in taste or speech. Damage can also occur to the salivary glands or facial nerves.

Postoperative Nursing Care for an Oropharyngeal Surgery

For patients with advanced laryngeal cancer, extensive glottic carcinomas, subglottic tumors, and advanced tumors of the base of the tongue that involve the larynx, a total **laryngectomy** may be indicated in conjunction with radiation therapy. Postoperatively, careful assessment of the patient's **airway** is critical. The patient should be closely observed for signs of respiratory distress. Suctioning may be necessary to help the patient clear secretions. The head of the bed should remain elevated to promote ventilation and decrease swelling. Tracheostomy care should be provided as needed to maintain patency of the stoma. Pain should be managed proactively and the patient should be placed on a bowel regimen to prevent constipation. The surgical site should be assessed for redness, warmth, or edema. Patient education regarding care of the tracheostomy should be completed early in the postoperative period to allow time for the patient to learn how to complete it independently. A dietitian should be involved with patients to ensure they are receiving the nutritional formula and number of calories that meet their needs.

Acute Myelogenous Leukemia (AML) Treatments

The primary treatment for **AML** is high dose **chemotherapy**. Survival rates are improving for patients with AML because of advances made in drug treatment of the disease. Some agents that are now produced not only work to destroy the leukemic cells, but also help to promote the growth and maturity of normal blood cells. If there is metastatic spread of the disease into the brain, radiation is often used to treat the cranial lesions.

Once remission is achieved, the chemotherapy agents that were originally used may be given once a month to provide maintenance therapy. This is to help prevent return of the disease and prolong the remission state.

Bone marrow transplant can be used if chemotherapy treatment does not prevent recurrence of the disease. About one-half of patients have a successful result from bone marrow transplant. A match must be found to be a donor of bone marrow and there is a risk of rejection by the patient.

Chronic Myelogenous Leukemia (CML) Treatments

Chemotherapy is the primary treatment used to treat **CML**. The most common drugs used are given orally and help to cure the disease by decreasing the production of white blood cells. If the disease worsens, chemotherapy doses are usually increased, but this does not usually result in better results.

CML can cause a condition called a **blastic crisis**. Repeat doses of chemotherapy may be used to treat this condition and radiation may also be used to help slow down the progression of any lesions forming within the bones. Chemotherapeutic medications may be given intrathecally to treat the development of disease within the central nervous system.

Bone marrow transplant can be used with approximately one-half of patients having successful long-term results. Autologous bone marrow transplant has varying results. Bone marrow transplant can be used to treat a blastic crisis, but this has not had extremely successful results.

Acute Lymphocytic Leukemia (ALL) Treatments

Chemotherapy is also used to treat **ALL**. Cranial radiation is performed if spread of the disease includes the central nervous system. Chemotherapy may be continued after remission is achieved and medications that were not used before may be used for this maintenance therapy.

Bone marrow transplant from a matched donor can also be performed to treat ALL. There is the risk of rejection of the donor marrow by the patient. Bone marrow transplants have been attempted in which the marrow is removed from the patient and the leukemic cells are removed before the marrow is replaced in the patient.

In children, the **maintenance therapy** of chemotherapeutic medications may continue for 2 to 3 years following remission. Bone marrow transplant can also be attempted in children. Using autologous bone marrow may not be an option, though, for those patients with advanced disease.

Each of the chemotherapeutic agents has its own side effects and the patient should be educated on these potential effects.

Chronic Lymphocytic Leukemia (CLL) Treatments

With **CLL**, the patient is not usually treated until they begin to exhibit symptoms from the disease. Some of the symptoms that warrant treatment included enlarged lymph nodes that are painful, anemia, decreased blood counts, or enlarged liver or spleen.

- **Chemotherapy drugs** can be used to slow down the production of immature lymph cells and to decrease the production of leukemic lymph cells.
- **Steroids** may be helpful if the white blood cell count is elevated or if all cell types are decreased.
- In severe cases, the **spleen** may be removed if medications are not helpful in controlling symptoms.
- **Radiation** can be helpful when the spleen or lymph nodes are enlarged and causing pain. The aim of this treatment would be to decrease production of immature lymph cells.
- Right now, bone marrow transplant is not generally used to treat CLL but studies are being conducted to assess the effectiveness of this treatment.

Non-Hodgkin's Lymphoma Treatments

- Treatment is often delayed until the patient develops symptoms. In early stages of non-Hodgkin's lymphoma, **radiation treatments** are used in localized areas where the affected lymph nodes are present.
- **Chemotherapy** may also be used as a treatment. A medication that supplies antibodies against the disease may also be used to treat the disease.
- With advanced disease, multiple **chemotherapeutic medications** are used and **radiation** may be given at the same time. **Antibody medication** may also be given to try and induce a state of remission.
- In the patient who has a relapse of the disease after a state of remission, **chemotherapy** is frequently given using medications that have not been given in the past. **Stem cell treatments** are also effective at treating recurrent non-Hodgkin's lymphoma.
- Treatment is usually quite aggressive with non-Hodgkin's lymphoma and patients should be closely monitored for side effects from the multiple medications used to treat the disease.

Hodgkin's Disease Treatments

- In early stages of the disease, **radiation** alone can be tried to control the disease in localized areas. **Chemotherapy** may also be given in the early stages of disease followed by radiation treatment. Multiple chemotherapeutic agents may be given for the most effective treatment coverage.

- With more advanced disease, **chemotherapy** is the mainstay of treatment. This may be done alone or may be followed up with **radiation therapy**. Multiple chemotherapeutic medications may be given, especially with end-stage disease.
- For patients who have a relapse of multiple myeloma after a period of remission, different **chemotherapy** drugs from those used previously may be given. If the patient has been in remission for at least one year, the same medications that were used before may be given again. **Autologous bone marrow transplant** has proved effective in treating disease at this stage, also. Though controversial, **blood stem cell treatments** are also very effective at inducing a remission state.

Multiple Myeloma Treatments

- **Multiple myeloma** is treated with **chemotherapy**. **Steroids** are often frequently given with the chemotherapy medications. **Interferon** can also be used to decrease the production of plasma cells when bone marrow biopsy reveals elevated levels of plasma cells.
- If there is bony involvement with lesions present, **radiation treatment** may be performed and directed at the specific sites involved.
- **Stem cell treatment** has had excellent results with almost one-half of patients entering remission following treatments. This is most effective in patients under 70-years-old.
- **Bisphosphonates** such as Fosamax have shown some effectiveness at treating multiple myeloma when used in conjunction with standard treatments. This helps to promote calcium deposition in the bones to improve bone strength and decrease the risk of pathologic fractures.
- Thalidomide has been given to some patients who have not responded to other treatments of multiple myeloma. It works by decreasing the levels of certain proteins that are elevated with the disease.

Symptom Management and Palliative Care

Anatomical and Surgical Alterations

Surgical Anatomic Changes Resulting in Impairments in Ventilation

Surgery may be done to remove a section of a lung, or the entire lung, which is invaded by cancer. This decreases the amount of **oxygen** that can be inspired with each breath. During the post-op period the patient may have a chest tube present, which will also affect **lung expansion** during breathing. Cancer involving the chest wall may require removal of ribs and muscle tissue, which will impair a patient's ability to take deep breaths.

Patients who have cancer of the trachea may require surgical excision of the tumor. This may result in a permanent **tracheostomy site** which requires special care and serves as another path through which air can escape before reaching the lungs.

Frequent surgeries that are performed on patients with lung cancer include a **pneumonectomy** to completely remove a lung, a **lobectomy** to remove one lobe of a lung, or various-sized **resections** to take just a small portion of the lung.

Anatomic Changes Resulting in Impairments in Ventilation

Cancer tumors located within the pleural cavity can invade the space usually occupied by lung tissue. This may compromise lung expansion during breathing. Tumors within the lung tissue can destroy normally healthy tissue and decrease the lung capacity for oxygen as well as decrease the surface area necessary for air exchange if the alveoli are involved. Any tumors within the airways can cause compression and decreased flow of oxygen into the lungs.

Allergic reactions to **medications** given to treat cancer can cause swelling of the smooth muscle lining the airway and lead to blockage of the airway.

Radiation treatments can cause permanent damage to lung and airway tissues, which can decrease expansion, decrease elasticity, and prevent proper functioning for oxygen to be absorbed into the blood stream.

Damage to the lungs can result in air, blood, or infected fluid accumulating within the pleural space. Air within the space is called a pneumothorax, the presence of blood is a hemothorax, and the presence of infected fluid is an empyema.

Types of Stomas

- **End stomas** are created by cutting the bowel and then diverting it through the abdominal wall. The rest of the bowel that is left distally may be removed from the body or sewn off.
- **Loop stomas** involve bringing a section of the colon out onto the abdomen. This is usually a temporary situation when a bowel obstruction is present or to help with symptom treatment at the end of a patient's battle with cancer. Another surgical procedure can be performed in the future to correct the colostomy so that the bowel will function normally.

- **Double-barrel stomas** are two stomas present in the abdominal wall. The stoma that is formed from the proximal portion of bowel will excrete stool while the distal portion only secretes mucus. The consistency of the stool from the proximal end will vary depending on its location. If more distal in the bowel, the proximal stoma will secrete stool that is more formed, but if more proximal in the bowel, the stool will be more watery.

Types of Colostomy

A **colostomy** is a hole that is created through the abdomen to connect with a portion of the colon. This is usually created after a portion of the colon is removed because of invasive cancer. A colostomy can be temporary or permanent.

- *Temporary colostomies* are created when it is believed that the colon will be able to function normally in the future and the patient will once again be able to have regular bowel movements. This is used after a tumor is removed that is causing obstruction of the colon or to allow a temporary diversion for stool while the bowel mends after surgery is performed.
- A *permanent colostomy* is created when a large enough portion of the bowel is removed that it is believed the patient will no longer be able to have regular bowel movements on their own. This usually occurs when a tumor invades the area from the colon and distally.

Urinary Diversion

A **urinary diversion** is a surgical re-routing of the flow of urine so that urine is usually no longer excreted through the urethra, but rather through another opening or through the abdominal wall, and usually into a collecting device.

Urinary diversions are needed with urine flow is **blocked**. Common reasons for blockage include: birth defects to the urinary system, kidney or bladder stones, trauma to the urethra, an enlarged prostate, or tumors in the pelvic cavity. A diversion may be needed when cancer invades the bladder and a cystectomy, or bladder removal, is necessary.

When a patient has a urinary diversion, they should be assessed for any changes in skin integrity because of the potential for skin breakdown when urine is in contact with it.

Urinary Diversion Types

There are **two major types of diversions**: continent and noncontinent.

- *Noncontinent diversions* are diversions that do not allow the patient to have control over the times at which they void. They are connected to a drainage bag and urine generally drains into the bag as it is made. Noncontinent diversions are created from a portion of the small intestine. A stoma is created with the small intestine and the ureters are attached to the section of intestine to drain urine from the body. Urinary reflux can occur and the patient is at a high risk for developing infections in the urinary tract. This also places the patient at an increased risk of developing kidney infections.
- *Continent diversions* are diversions which allow the patient to have control of when they will void. One way to create this type of diversion involves connecting the ureters from the kidneys to a section of the large intestine. This allows urine to flow through the intestine and colon to be exited through the anus. A valve is created which allows the patient to maintain continence.

- *Orthoptic neobladders* are a type of continent diversion. These involve making a bladder from a portion of the stomach or intestine and connecting the ureters to it to collect urine. The urethra is also attached to enable urine to flow normally out of the body. This procedure is usually performed when there is bowel disease or damage from disease.

Lymphedema

Lymphedema is an accumulation of lymph fluid that causes edema. This is due to a blockage within the lymph system preventing lymph fluid from flowing as it normally would.

Lymphedema can be primary or secondary. **Primary lymphedema** may occur without reason. This can frequently be a congenital problem due to impairment in the vascular system that either prevents lymph fluid from draining properly or a problem with the venous system in reabsorbing lymph fluid.

Secondary lymphedema is caused by a primary disease or treatment:

- **Cancer surgery** that requires removal of lymph nodes or obliteration of some of the lymph vessels can disrupt the normal flow of lymph fluid and cause edema.
- **Radiation treatments** can cause damage or destruction to lymph structures which impair the flow of fluid. Cancers that invade the lymph nodes can also impair the normal function of the lymph system.
- Lymphedema of the lower extremities is very common following **removal of lymph nodes** in the lower abdomen or groin.
- Lymphedema can be common in the upper extremities following **mastectomy** surgery when the lymph nodes are removed.

Physical Exam Findings for Lymphedema Patients

During **physical exam** on patients with lymphedema, observe how their clothes are fitting and if waist bands and seams of clothing leave indented marks on their body. Examine all of the extremities for edema and document whether it is pitting or nonpitting. Also look for changes in the texture of the skin, such as a thickened or dimpled appearance. Assess the color of the patient's skin for any duskiness or darkening. Also assess all extremities for motor or sensory deficits. Measure all four extremities to check for any discrepancies between limbs. Record this and re-measure regularly to assess for any increases or decreases in circumference. Daily weight checks should be done to assess for any increase due to fluid accumulations.

Diagnostic tests should include a CT scan to assess for fluid accumulations and any pathology that may be causing the lymphedema. Vascular studies should be performed to assess for venous stasis disease.

Pharmacologic Interventions

Penicillin Group of Antibiotics

Penicillin-type antibiotics are used to fight more common types of bacteria. These include *Staphylococcus, Streptococcus, E. coli, Salmonella, Klebsiella, Enterobacter,* and *H. influenzae.*

More **common side** effects include nausea, vomiting, and diarrhea. Many patients are ***allergic*** to penicillin antibiotics and this reaction can range from itching and a rash to anaphylactic shock. An overall decrease in the blood count can occur as well as hypokalemia. Some penicillins can also cause an increase in bleeding time.

Nursing interventions include monitoring for an allergic reaction by assessing respiratory function and performing regular skin checks. Regular monitoring of lab tests should be done to assess for changes in blood count, electrolyte levels, and coagulation or bleeding studies. Also monitor lab tests for any affects the antibiotics may have on liver or renal function. Evaluate for any GI symptoms of nausea, vomiting, or diarrhea and affects these can have on the patient's nutritional status.

1st Generation Cephalosporin Antibiotics

First generation cephalosporins are used to treat infections caused by common organisms such as *Streptococcus, Staphylococcus, Klebsiella,* and *E. coli.* These treat many of the same organisms that the penicillins are affective against.

Patients who are allergic to penicillins can have an **allergy** to this class of antibiotics, also. These should be avoided in these patients, especially if they have had a previous anaphylactic reaction to penicillins. Patients can have an allergic reaction to cephalosporins ranging from rash to anaphylactic shock.

Other **side effects** are similar to those of the penicillins including GI symptoms of nausea, vomiting, and diarrhea; a decrease in blood count; and changes in liver or renal function.

Nursing interventions include monitoring for any allergic reactions and checking for previous penicillin allergy in the patient. CBC should be monitored for a decrease in blood cell counts, liver function tests monitored for change in liver function, and BUN and creatinine monitored for a change in renal function.

2nd Generation Cephalosporin Antibiotics

Second generation cephalosporins are effective in treating infections caused by *E. coli, Klebsiella, Proteus, Enterobacter,* and *Haemophilus influenzae.*

Potential **side effects** from this class of drugs include allergic reactions ranging from itching and a rash to anaphylactic reaction. GI side effects of nausea, vomiting, and diarrhea can occur. The second generation cephalosporins can also cause elevations in BUN and creatinine with impairments in renal function. Though rare, a reaction similar to that of Antabuse that occurs in those who drink alcohol can occur. This causes malignant hypertension, flushing, and nausea and vomiting. Patients need to be advised to avoid alcohol when taking second generation cephalosporins for an infection.

Nursing interventions include monitoring for any allergic reactions by doing respiratory and skin checks. Also assess for any impairment in nutritional status due to continued nausea, vomiting, or diarrhea. Lab results should be monitored for any change in renal function.

3rd Generation Cephalosporin Antibiotics

Third generation cephalosporins are used to fight infections caused by *Enterobacter, Proteus, Strep. pneumo, E. Coli, Klebsiella*, and *Proteus*.

Potential **side effects** include allergic reactions, which can range from itching and hives to anaphylactic shock. Nausea, vomiting, and diarrhea are also potential effects. A temporary decrease in WBCs and platelets can occur. These antibiotics can be caustic when given IV and can cause a localized irritation at the infusion site. This is evidenced by edema, erythema, and tenderness at the IV site.

Nursing interventions include assessing for any allergic reaction to the medication and assessing for any changes in nutritional status due to nausea, vomiting, or diarrhea. A CBC should be assessed for any decrease in WBCs or platelets. Also monitor the IV site when giving third generation cephalosporins by this route. Stop the medication if irritation should occur and apply a warm compress to help relieve the pain and swelling

β-Lactam Antibiotics

Beta-lactam antibiotics are used to treat many of the infections that are also treated by third-generation cephalosporins. In addition, they are effective against *Pseudomonas, Staph.*, and *Enterococcus*.

Potential **side effects** include allergic reactions, but these do not have the same cross-reactivity with the penicillin antibiotics that can be seen with the cephalosporins. An increase in WBCs can occur along with some changes in coagulation studies. Temporary elevations in the liver enzymes can also occur. As with other antibiotics, GI symptoms of nausea, vomiting, and diarrhea can occur. Very rarely, seizures can occur in the patient taking these antibiotics.

Nursing interventions include assessing for allergic reactions and monitoring for any GI side effects. A CBC should be assessed for any changes in the WBC. PT/PTT should be monitored for any changes in coagulability. Liver enzymes should also be assessed for any elevations, though this is usually temporary. Also assess the patient for any seizure activity.

Fluoroquinolone Antibiotics

Fluoroquinolone antibiotics are used to treat infections caused by *Chlamydia, Mycoplasma*, and *Klebsiella*. Some are effective against *Strep* and *Staph*, while others are not.

Potential **side effects** of the fluoroquinolones include allergic reactions and GI symptoms similar to other antibiotics. They can also cause a decreased effectiveness of antacids that are not in the H$_2$-blocker family. These antibiotics can affect the nervous system by causing headaches or dizziness when mild or can have serious nervous system affects with seizures. Patients may complain of hypersensitivity to light while taking fluoroquinolones and may show signs of increased or decreased blood sugar. Very rarely, serious kidney damage can occur.

Nursing interventions include monitoring for side effects and GI effects. Patients who take oral antacids may want to switch to an H$_2$-blocker while taking these antibiotics. Monitoring should be

- 102 -

done for any seizure activity. Labs should be assessed for any changes in glucose levels or kidney function.

Aminoglycoside Antibiotics

Aminoglycoside antibiotics are used to treat infections caused by *Enterococcus*, *Proteus*, and *Pseudomonas*.

The **side effect profile** of these antibiotics can be quite severe. The usual allergic reaction or GI symptoms can occur, as with other antibiotics. Aminoglycosides can also have effects on the auditory system which can lead to deafness or chronic vertigo. Blood dyscrasias can occur that affect WBCs, RBCs, and platelets. Kidney damage can also occur when taken in high doses. Liver function can also be impaired while taking aminoglycosides. Cardiovascular effects include a drop in blood pressure and an increase in heart rate.

Nursing interventions are focused on assessing for any of these potential side effects. Labs will need to be monitored for changes in blood counts, BUN and creatinine to assess renal function, and liver function tests to monitor hepatic function. Be cognizant of any symptoms of hearing loss the patient may experience. Monitor vital signs regularly to assess for a drop in blood pressure or an increase in pulse.

Antifungal Medications

Antifungals are used to treat infections caused by *Candida*, *Aspergillus*, *Cryptococcus*, and *Histoplasmosis*.

Potential **side effects** are broad and depend upon the type of antifungal used. Allergic reactions and GI symptoms can occur. Antifungals can affect renal and liver function. Blood dyscrasias can occur affecting all blood cells. Electrolyte imbalances and changes in the blood's ability to clot can be affected. Cardiovascular affects include arrhythmias, an increase or decrease in blood pressure, or EKG changes with a prolonged QT interval. There are also multiple drug interactions that can occur with antifungals and the patient's medications will need to be reviewed before beginning these drugs.

Nursing interventions are going to focus on assessing the patient for any potential side effects. Laboratory tests should be assessed for a drop in blood counts, renal studies and LFTs should be assessed for impairment in function, and coagulation studies should be assessed for changes. Electrolytes should be assessed for any changes and an EKG should be performed to assess for QT changes.

Antiviral Medications

Antivirals are used to treat herpes simplex virus, varicella zoster virus, and cytomegalovirus. There is viral resistance with some of the drugs in this class and others are used to provide cross coverage.

Potential **side effects** include allergic reactions and GI symptoms. Effects can also be seen in liver and renal function. Change in electrolyte levels and a decrease in WBCs can occur. Anemia may also be present with a decrease in RBCs. Nervous system effects include peripheral neuropathy and pain or even seizures. Patients may experience joint pain while taking antivirals.

Nursing interventions will focus on assessing for any of these side effects. Labs should be monitored with a CBC for change in blood counts, and renal and liver studies should be done to assess for a change in function. Monitor the patient for complaints of pain, either neuropathic or joint pain. As always, assess for any change in nutritional status due to possible GI symptoms or nausea, vomiting, and diarrhea.

Anti-Inflammatory Medication

Anti-inflammatory medications are used to treat fever and pain, usually due to an inflammatory process somewhere in the body. **Inflammation** occurs as a result of a series of events. Some type of external or internal stimulus affects the body's tissues and causes damage. This causes activation of the COX (cyclo-oxygenase) pathway. As a result of this inflammatory process, prostaglandins are released, which are responsible for contributing to the perceived sensation of pain. Anti-inflammatories function by disrupting the COX pathway, which avoids the production of prostaglandins and prevents the pain that accompanies inflammation. This allows the tissue to heal and prevents activation of the immune system. If anti-inflammatories are not given, or are not effective, inflammation will continue to be present in the affected area of the body.

If the production of prostaglandins is not blocked, the body will eventually respond by producing opioid-like substances to help block the sensation of pain.

Anti-Inflammatory Medications

Anti-inflammatory medications frequently used in cancer patients are classified as NSAIDs (non-steroidal anti-inflammatory drugs), COX-2 inhibitors, and corticosteroids. The COX-2 medications are metabolized following the cyclooxygenase-2 pathway which results in fewer side effects.

- The most common **NSAIDs** used include ibuprofen, naproxen, etodolac, and indomethacin. All of these can cause GI side effects from nausea to GI bleeding. They are also renal metabolized so care should be given to a patient with compromised kidney function.
- The only **COX-2 medication** currently on the market is Celebrex. It does have potential to cause GI side effects, but not as frequently as the NSAIDs. The risk of GI side effects is reduced by 50% when compared with NSAIDs. It is also metabolized by the kidneys.
- Some common **corticosteroids** include cortisone, prednisone, and dexamethasone. These are all renal metabolized. Cortisone and prednisone can cause sodium and water retention, while dexamethasone is less likely to cause this side effect in low doses.

Anti-Inflammatories Side Effects

Cardiovascular effects of anti-inflammatory medications include water and sodium retention which can lead to congestive heart failure. Peripheral edema and hypertension can also occur. Fluid retention can also lead to lung congestion with dyspnea and shortness of breath. If edema becomes severe enough and lasts for an extended period of time, stasis changes can become evident in the lower extremities with development of stasis ulcers.

Nursing interventions include monitoring the patient for any changes in cardiovascular status. Regularly monitor vital signs including blood pressure and report any increase in pressure. Educate the patient on the importance of restricting sodium in the diet to prevent additional fluid retention. Extremities should be assessed for any developing edema, including stasis changes. Skin integrity should also be examined. Regularly assess lung sounds for any signs of fluid accumulation. Listen to the patient speak to see if they are having any difficulty completing sentences without having to stop and take a breath.

Potential Digestive System Side Effects

Most commonly, **GI upset** with nausea, vomiting, GERD symptoms, and gastric ulcer formation can occur with anti-inflammatories. These symptoms are more likely in patients who use these medications on a regular basis. Pancreatitis can occur with certain NSAIDs and patients with a history of liver disease can develop hepatotoxicity with regular anti-inflammatory use.

Nursing interventions with patients who take anti-inflammatories on a regular basis include monitoring labs to assess for any changes in amylase or lipase levels which could indicate pancreatic effects. Also assess for signs or symptoms of pancreatitis such as severe abdominal pain with intractable vomiting. Liver function tests should also be regularly assessed for any changes in liver function. Be especially cautious in patients with a history of liver disease. Monitor for GI side effects such as dark, tarry stools, hematemesis, nausea, and vomiting. If GERD-type symptoms develop, the patient may be at risk for developing an alteration in nutritional status.

Potential Renal and Electrolyte Side Effects

Anti-inflammatories are metabolized by the renal system and can be toxic to the kidneys. **Acute renal failure** can occur, especially in those patients who already have altered renal function. Malfunction of the kidneys can cause **electrolyte imbalances** because of an alteration in metabolism. Certain electrolyte imbalances can cause mental status changes and cardiac effects.

Nursing interventions include closely monitoring the patient's intake and output. Assess for any signs of edema. Patients with renal impairment will not complain of pain. Laboratory tests should be closely monitored for any changes in electrolyte levels. This includes mainly changes in sodium and potassium levels. Hypo- or hypernatremia can cause mental status changes. An increase or decrease in potassium can cause EKG changes and may lead to cardiac dysrhythmias. Elevations of glucose levels can occur and this can be especially dangerous in diabetic patients. Closely monitor blood glucose levels and report any increases to the physician.

Potential Side Effects and Nursing Interventions

Phenothiazine Anti-Emetics

The most common **phenothiazine anti-emetics** are prochlorperazine (Compazine) and chlorpromazine (Thorazine).

Common **side effects** include sedation and a decrease in blood pressure. Dizziness and changes in vision can also occur. Anticholinergic effects, such as hypotension, dry mouth, and constipation can be significant with chronic use.

Nursing **interventions** include closely monitoring the patient for orthostatic hypotension. Educate the patient to rise slowly from sitting or laying positions. Anticholinergic effects can be potentiated if the patient is also taking other medications with these side effects. Advise the patient to not get out of bed without assistance because of the risk of falls with dizziness and changes in vision. Closely assess for any changes in mental status with increased anticholinergic effects. Dry mouth can cause alterations in nutritional status. Encourage frequent sips of water, if not contraindicated, and offer hard candy to decrease dryness. If anticholinergic side effects become severe, Benadryl can be given to counteract the effects of phenothiazine medications.

Promethazine (Phenergan)

Phenergan is a very common anti-emetic medication given to patients undergoing cancer treatment. Its most common **side effect** is sedation. The patient may also experience decreases in blood pressure. Anticholinergic effects of dry mouth and urinary retention can occur along with

- 105 -

orthostatic hypotension. Very rarely, a patient may experience seizures. Other potential side effects include a sensitivity to light and possible allergic reaction with a rash. Patients may complain of increased anxiety or restlessness with Phenergan. This can be decreased with Benadryl.

Nursing interventions include closely monitoring the patient for anticholinergic side effects. Educate the patient to rise slowly from a sitting or lying position. Offer frequent sips of water and hard candy, if allowed, to counter sensations of dry mouth. Assess intake and urinary output. Keep the room dim if the patient complains of light sensitivity. Assess for seizure activity and report this to the physician immediately if it should occur. Deep I.M. is the preferred route, but at times IV is needed. Phenergan is a vesicant. Ensure proper IV placement before and during infusion. When giving IV, make sure to dilute the solution to at least 25 mg/mL and give over 10-15 minutes.

Narcotic Analgesics

Cardiovascular and Respiratory Side Effects

Cardiovascular side effects with **narcotics** include hypotension due to dilation of peripheral blood vessels. There may also be an increase or decrease in heart rate. This can be exacerbated by dehydration in the patient who is not taking in many fluids because of nausea and vomiting. Respiratory depression can also occur with narcotic analgesics and may result in respiratory failure or even death if the medications are given in doses that are too high. Along with this comes an accumulation of pulmonary secretions because of a decrease in the cough reflex.

Nursing interventions include closely monitoring blood pressure and respiratory rate. Increasing IV fluids can help to raise the blood pressure by increasing fluid volume. Helping the patient with deep breathing and coughing exercises can help to clear pulmonary secretions. Caution should be used for choking hazards with a patient, especially if they already have some dysphagia because of the loss of the cough reflex and decreased gag response.

GI and GU Side Effects

Nausea, vomiting, and constipation are the most common **gastrointestinal side effects** of **narcotic analgesics**. If nausea and vomiting should develop, anti-emetics can be given if the patient is not too sedated from the narcotics. Constipation can be quite severe with narcotics and may even lead to a bowel obstruction. A **genitourinary side effect** includes decreased urinary output due to retention. This can also be quite uncomfortable for the patient and may require catheterization.

Nursing interventions include monitoring the patient for common GI and GU side effects. If the patient is very nauseous to the point of vomiting, nutritional status should be assessed and the patient should be monitored for signs of dehydration. Anti-emetics can be given, but these can have an additive sedating effect with the narcotics. Constipation can be relieved with regular stool softeners and occasional laxative use. The patient should also drink more fluids and have more bulk in their diet, if tolerated. Urinary retention may be severe enough to warrant catheterizing the patient.

CNS Side Effects

Narcotic analgesics depress the central nervous system and can cause effects such as sedation, mental status changes, confusion, decreased concentration, and hallucinations. Narcotics cloud a patient's sensorium and can even affect their mood causing mood swings from extreme happiness, almost mania, to depression or anger. Though rare, seizures can even occur.

Nursing interventions include monitoring for any sedation or lethargy in patients taking narcotics. If a patient is confused, try to orient them to their surroundings to decrease anxiety. Try to calm them if mood swings are exhibited and explain the cause of mood swings to family members to decrease any anxiety they may have. Do not allow patients to get out of bed without assistance if hallucinations are occurring or if they are very sedated or lethargic as a result of the narcotics. Monitor the patient for any type of seizure activity and alert the physician if this should occur.

Barbiturates

The most common **side effect** with **barbiturates** is sedation and lethargy. Allergic reactions can also occur with a mild rash to a severe rash condition called Stevens-Johnson syndrome. Barbiturates are metabolized by the liver and can cause hepatotoxicity, especially in those who already have liver disease. Rare effects include anemia due to a decrease in blood cell production and a decrease in folate levels. Patients can build a drug tolerance to barbiturates, which leads to needing an increase in drug dosage in order to achieve the same effects.

Nursing interventions are aimed at monitoring the patient for excessive sedation and lethargy. Frequently orient the patient to their surroundings and do not allow them to get out of bed without assistance to prevent falls. Do regular skin assessments to check for any rash reactions or Stevens-Johnson syndrome. Monitor liver function tests and CBC for any changes. Also assess the patient for any decrease in effectiveness of the medication at current dosages.

Tricyclic Antidepressants

Anticholinergic effects can occur with **tricyclic antidepressants**. These include a decrease in blood pressure, especially orthostatic hypotension, dry mouth, urinary retention, and constipation. The patient can also have extrapyramidal side effects. Rarely, cardiac dysrhythmias and anemia can occur. Because they are metabolized by the liver, hepatotoxicity can occur. Patients may complain of drowsiness and sedation.

Nursing interventions include monitoring for any anticholinergic effects and treating these symptomatically. Have the patient increase their fluid intake if dry mouth and constipation are problems. Educate the patient in rising slowly from a sitting or lying position. Assess vital signs and heart sounds for any decreases in blood pressure or the presence of an irregular heart rate. Monitor CBC and liver function tests for any changes. Assess the patient for sedation or any changes in mental status. Assist the patient when rising to prevent falls if they are sedated or if they are suffering from orthostatic hypotension.

Benzodiazepines

Sedation, confusion, and lethargy are the most common **side effects** with **benzodiazepines**. These can be severe enough to cause a patient to become disoriented or have difficulty concentrating. These effects are more common in very young patients and in elderly patients. Benzodiazepines can also have severe withdrawal symptoms if they are stopped suddenly after extended use. The patient can experience a decrease in blood pressure and an irregular heart rate. Rarely, anemia can result due to a decrease in blood cell production and liver enzymes can be elevated.

Nursing interventions include closely monitoring the patient for any mental status changes and lethargy. Continue to orient the patient to their surroundings and implement fall precautions. Regularly assess vital signs to check for hypotension. Assess CBC and liver function tests to monitor for any changes. Educate patients on tapering their benzodiazepine usage and how to wean off the medication without stopping abruptly to avoid withdrawal symptoms.

<u>SSRI Antidepressants</u>

Generally, the **SSRI antidepressants** are safer and have a lower **side effect** profile than the tricyclic antidepressants. Constipation can occur with SSRIs along with a decrease in urinary output due to retention. A decrease in blood pressure can occur, especially orthostatic hypotension when the patient rises from a sitting or laying position. Sedation may also occur. Rarely, cardiac dysrhythmias can occur. The patient may also rarely develop anemia or hepatotoxicity.

Nursing interventions include assessing the patient for constipation and having them increase their fluid intake or increase fiber in the diet to prevent this. Stool softeners can also help. Monitor vital signs and heart sounds to assess for any decrease in blood pressure or irregularities in the heart sounds. Educate the patient to rise slowly from a sitting or laying position to prevent orthostatic hypotension. Assess for any sedation or mental status changes. Monitor the CBC for anemia and liver function tests for elevations.

Single Lineage vs. Multilineage Factors Growth Factors

Growth factor medications can be classified as single lineage or multilineage:

- **Single lineage factors** include those affecting granulocyte production, erythropoietin, those that increase platelet production, and stem cell factor. The granulocyte factors cause an increase in neutrophils, which help with immune function and help to prevent infection. Erythropoietin is naturally produced by the kidneys and stimulates production of red blood cells. This usually occurs in response to a decrease in blood cells due to anemia. The platelet growth factors function in the same way, but to increase the production of platelets to help with blood clotting. Stem cell factor helps to increase the production of all blood cells by stimulating primitive cells.
- **Multilineage growth factors** work on increasing the granulocyte cells to help boost the immune system and resist infection. This includes stimulating production of certain other cells, such as tumor necrosis factor (TNF), which helps to fight cancer cells.

Nursing Interventions with Blood Growth Factors

The **CBC** should be regularly **assessed** to evaluate the effectiveness of treatment with the growth factors. These medications can cause bone pain due to activity of the bone marrow to increase blood cell production. Assess the patient for pain and record pain levels. Administer analgesics as ordered. Also assess the patient for any signs of fluid overload, such as peripheral edema and adventitious breath sounds. Monitor electrolyte levels for any changes. Rarely, blood clots can develop in the legs or an embolus may travel to the lungs. ***Closely monitor the patient for these possibly fatal side effects.***

There may be pain at the injection site. Monitor the IV site for redness, warmth, induration, or swelling. Apply warm compresses to the site if irritation should develop.

Rarely, a patient who has had a past allergic reaction to medications derived from *E. coli* bacteria may have cross-reactivity to certain growth factors. Obtain an accurate history of any past drug reactions the patient may have had.

Complimentary and Integrative Modalities

Complimentary or Alternative Medicine

Complimentary or alternative medicines (CAMs) are "Interventions not taught in medical schools or not available in US hospitals." It is not relevant that the nurse be a practitioner or believer of these methods of cancer therapy, but remembers that the patient does. This is the reason that these methods need to be known by the nurse and medical practitioner and more importantly accepted and respected. If the patient believes this will aid in recovery, they may affect the outcome if they are accepted by faith

Alternative Therapies, Complementary Therapies, and Integrative Therapies

Complementary and alternative medicine refers to the whole field of treatments that are available outside of the entire realm of traditional medical treatments. It is thought that over one-half of all cancer patients utilize some form of complementary or alternative medicine. Unfortunately, there is minimal scientific data to support the safety and true benefit of these treatments.

- **Alternative therapies** are those treatments that are used instead of traditional medical treatments. People who use these believe they work better and are safer than traditional treatments. These may include herbal treatments or medical rituals.
- **Complementary therapies** are treatments that are used along with traditional medical treatments. These include herbal supplements and other treatments that may help with side effects from traditional treatments.
- **Integrative therapies** are used along with traditional medical treatments and are supported by the medical team in providing some benefit to the patient. These can include acupuncture, massage therapy, or some vitamin supplementation.

Types of Cancer Alternative Treatments Cancer

- **Dietary treatments** involve supplementing the regular diet with items that are thought to be richer in certain nutrients, such as anti-oxidants, with the belief that these items can interfere with cancer cell reproduction. Anti-oxidants and some vitamins can interfere with certain cancer treatments and cause them to be less effective.
- **Folk medicines** include special teas and potions, topical ointments, and rituals that are believed to help cure or prevent cancer. Many of these are deeply rooted in cultural beliefs.
- **Pharmacologic and biologic treatments** include toxin eliminators, immune "boosters," or hyperbaric oxygen treatments. These have not been proven to be effective in treating cancer.
- **Herbal remedies** are widely used with the belief they can cure cancer or to help treat the side effects of conventional treatments.
- **Mind and body techniques** utilize meditation and other forms of relaxation to help with decreasing stress and providing pain relief.
- **Manual healing** is the belief that touch can help to treat the disease. This includes massage therapy and acupuncture.

Acupuncture, Massage, and Reflexology

- **Acupuncture** is based on an ancient Asian technique of disrupting an energy flow in the body. The belief is that there are certain pathways, or meridians, in the body through which energy travels. Acupuncture creates a blockage in this energy flow to help reduce certain symptoms, such as pain, and promote relaxation.
- **Massage** is used to reduce pain and promote relaxation. This can promote increased blood flow to a certain area of the body, help to decrease blood pressure, and even stimulate the release of endorphins, which can decrease pain. Massage therapy can be individualized depending on the patient's needs and disease process.
- **Reflexology** is a specialized type of massage therapy that focuses on the feet. It is based on a belief that there are certain portions of the feet that can be massaged to treat symptoms elsewhere in the body. The foundation of reflexology is that each area of the body affects other areas.

Imagery, Meditation, and Biofeedback

- **Imagery** is a technique in which the patient is instructed to imagine a pleasant experience and use this concentration to dissociate themselves from unpleasant sensations they may be experiencing. This involves imagining sensations as they affect the whole body from "seeing" a different place to "tasting" or "smelling" a pleasant experience.
- **Meditation** involves clearing the mind and focusing on the present situation in a calm fashion. This relies on focusing on current symptoms, even if unpleasant, but altering perception of these symptoms so they are not interpreted as being unpleasant. Meditation may draw upon spiritual beliefs.
- **Biofeedback** is the process of being fully aware of subtle physiologic changes in the body in order to respond to them in a positive way. This can be subtle changes in body temperature or muscle tightness with pain and a conscious act of relaxation to help dispel these symptoms and prevent the unpleasant sensation.

Communication with the Patient

Alternative medicine includes mind-body techniques, herbal remedies, and alternative medical systems like Chinese medicine and India's Ayurvedic medicine. The oncology nurse is required to deal realistically with subtle and enticing aspects of **alternative medicine** while continuing to involve the patient in his own care and therapy. The nurse must keep open every channel of communication with the patient, motivate the patient, and keep open the idea that the patient is in charge of their own health care. The nurse must be nonbiased, nonjudgmental and respectful of the patient's own ideas of his/her care.

Pain and Palliative Care

Pain

Pain is the uncomfortable physical and emotional sensation associated with an actual or perceived unpleasant stimulus that affects the body.

Pain can be acute, chronic nonmalignant, or cancer (malignant) in nature.

- *Acute pain* lasts less than 6 months. It often has a known cause and individuals who suffer from acute pain frequently show outward signs of being in pain such as grimacing, increased respirations, sweating, or crying.
- *Chronic nonmalignant pain* lasts longer than 3 months. It often has no known cause and can have a profound effect on a person's life. Individuals who suffer from chronic nonmalignant pain frequently exhibit signs of fatigue, depression, and hopelessness.
- *Cancer pain* can be further subdivided into two types: acute cancer pain due to the cancer itself or from treatments for the cancer and chronic cancer pain due to progression of the disease or ongoing treatments. It is important to remember that cancer patients can also suffer from psychological pain.

Risk Factors for Pain

Risk factors for pain are related to the disease process, the treatment the patient is undergoing, or to psychosocial factors:

- When related to the *disease*, pain is localized to the site of the cancer. For example, bone pain when bony metastasis is involved, visceral pain when an organ is involved, or neuropathic pain when a tumor causes nerve compression.
- *Treatment-related pain* occurs with chemotherapy, radiation, or cancer surgery. Several chemotherapeutic medications can cause neuropathic pain. Chemotherapy also causes immunosuppression, which can lead to other illnesses, such as herpes zoster (shingles). Radiation can cause pain at the site radiated or neuropathic pain at the site. Chronic pain related to surgery can be caused by a mastectomy for breast surgery, a thoracotomy, or with a radical neck dissection.
- *Personal and psychosocial factors* that cause pain include resistance to taking narcotics for fear of becoming "addicted," or unwillingness of the healthcare provider to administer narcotics for fear of overmedicating or promoting addiction. Elderly patients are more susceptible to chronic pain and are frequently under-medicated.

Major Body Systems Changes Caused by Pain

- **Respiratory** – There can be a decrease in respiratory rate if taking a deep breath is painful. But the patient may also have an increase in respiratory rate if he or she is starting to hyperventilate with anxiety.
- **CNS** – Pain may cause the patient to have a change in mental status ranging from unconsciousness to confusion. Coordination and mood may also be affected by pain.
- **Cardiovascular** – An increase in heart rate may be present. The patient may be hyper- or hypotensive, depending on the cause of the pain.
- **GI** – Nausea is a common symptom experienced by a person in pain. Constipation may also be present.

- **GU** – Decreased urinary output may be present, due to urinary retention.
- **Dermatologic** – Sweating, flushing, and itching may all be present with pain. A patient may also experience skin reactions similar to hives.

Physiologic Process of the Perception of Pain

There are four main stages in the physiologic process that results in the perception of pain. These are **transduction**, **transmission**, the **perception of pain**, and **modulation**:

1. First, some type of stimulus occurs that causes damage to cells and stimulates the body's pain receptors to react *(transduction)*. Inflammatory substances, such as prostaglandins and substance P, are released at the time this damage occurs.
2. During *transmission*, these substances travel to the dorsal horn of the spinal cord and attach to receptors that are located there. At the same time, opioid receptors within the spinal cord are stimulated.
3. This signal is then sent to the brain where it is interpreted. This causes a person to *perceive the discomfort of pain*.
4. In *modulation*, nerve cells in the brainstem release opioid-like substances which travel to the spinal cord and attach to the opioid receptors there. This is part of the body's defense mechanism and a way to naturally decrease pain.

> **Review Video: Pain Perception and Influences**
> Visit mometrix.com/academy and enter code: 297039

Nociceptive Pain

- **Nociceptive pain** occurs as a result of stimulation to pain fibers within body tissues. This can be further subdivided into somatic pain and visceral pain:
- *Somatic pain* is derived from bones, joints, or connective tissues and an individual can usually pinpoint the location of the pain. The point of most severe pain is at the location where the injury is present, but it may radiate away from that site, also. It is usually described as a nagging, aching sensation. Examples of somatic pain would be the pain that occurs due to a fractured arm or a torn ligament in the knee.
- *Visceral pain* is organ pain. It is due to damage to the tissue that makes up the body's organs. It is usually vague in location and is described as an aching or cramping pain. Examples of visceral pain would be the pain that is present with pancreatitis or a bowel obstruction.

> **Review Video: Visceral Pain**
> Visit mometrix.com/academy and enter code: 430402

Neuropathic Pain

Neuropathic pain occurs as a result of compression/entrapment or injury to nervous tissue. This includes the peripheral nerves, sympathetic nerves, or the central nervous system. It can further be described as peripheral neuropathic pain, centrally mediated pain, or sympathetically maintained pain:

- **_Peripheral neuropathic pain_** is caused by damage to the peripheral nerves. It is usually described as a numb or tingling sensation. Examples of peripheral neuropathic pain include the sensation a person feels with carpal tunnel syndrome or diabetic peripheral neuropathy.
- **_Centrally mediated pain_** causes a burning or aching sensation with the sensation of a sharp pain that radiates away from the site of aching pain. An example of centrally mediated pain is the sciatic nerve pain a person can feel with lumbar degenerative disk disease.
- **_Sympathetically maintained pain_** is due to an injury that causes a disruption in the mechanism responsible for controlling the nerve. An example of this would be complex regional pain syndrome, formerly known as reflex sympathetic dystrophy (RSD).

> **Review Video: Neuropathic Pain**
> Visit mometrix.com/academy and enter code: 780523

Major Characteristics of Pain

- **Location** – The patient points to the area where the pain is felt. He or she may be able to pinpoint the exact location or the location may be vague and cover a broad area. This is useful in assessing if the patient has bone pain, visceral pain, or neuropathic pain.
- **Intensity** – Have the patient rate his or her pain on a scale of 0-10 with 0 being no pain and 10 being the worst pain ever experienced. This allows healthcare providers to objectively assess a patient's pain.
- **Quality** – The pain is described in terms of sharp, dull, aching, shooting, radiating, etc. This can help with diagnosing the problem.
- **Temporality** – This describes if the pain is constant, intermittent, or brought on by certain activities. Again, this can be helpful in diagnosing the problem. Temporality is also helpful in determining what type of analgesic may be helpful in relieving the pain (long-acting or short-acting).

Assessing Pain in the Young and Elderly

Assessing pain can be difficult in very **young patients** because of possible barriers to communication if a child is not able to describe the location, intensity, or quality of their pain. A *Faces pain scale* may need to be used to help a child answer questions regarding his or her pain. This allows them to select a picture of how they feel, from a smiling face for no pain to a crying face for the worst pain. Nonverbal communication can also be helpful when assessing a child in pain. Are they crying, consolable, withdrawn, moving spontaneously?

When assessing pain in **elderly patients**, consideration needs to be given to co-morbidities that may be present. Many elderly patients take multiple medications, so a detailed history needs to be obtained to avoid any drug-drug interactions. Also make note of the patient's mental status and if there is any confusion or dementia present. *The Faces scale* may be helpful in elderly patients, also, if there is difficulty with communication.

McGill Pain Questionnaire

The McGill Pain Questionnaire: A multidimensional clinical tool based on 20 sets of words for patients to describe their pain based on a chart-sized diagram for insertion into the patient's record. (This takes about 5-15 minutes to complete)

There has been recognition of sociocultural variables in patient's response to pain descriptions. Females and non-Caucasians have significantly lower scores on the McGill Questionnaire than males or Caucasians. African Americans and older patients had less pain and depression. Also, specific ethnic identities conditioned the individual expression of pain, even though assimilation into the American population had occurred.

Oncology Nurse's Role in the Assessment of Pain

The nurse has responsibility for **identifying** the cause of pain; **eliminating**, as much as possible, pain due to nursing care; **treating** pain symptomology; **relieving** any environmental factors that exacerbate pain; and **recommending** the type, route, and schedule of pain alleviating agent; also **monitoring** the patient's relief of, or continued presence of, pain symptomology. Plus evaluate the appearance of any and all side effects and any family concerns.

Cancer pain has been long recognized as an enormous problem. The Oncology Nursing Society's position on pain management emphasized the pain is often managed inadequately. An understanding of this requires **knowledge** of its prevalence, its significance, and the professional issues involved in its management. The nurses' role is one of a part of a team effort. The nurse has the task of **identifying** the type of pain by their professional assessment skills; identify nurse care related pain, recognizing psychosocial causes, identifying conditions in the physical environment that leads to patient pain. Also, recommending the correct analgesics or other appropriate pain medications for correct pain management. In the **assessment** of pain keep in mind that pain is a symptom, not a diagnosis. If you get the assessment wrong, the treatment you formulate will be wrong. Anything that the patient notices that increases or relieves pain adds to the information the nurse has and can add to effective pain therapy.

Nonopioid vs. Opioid Analgesics

Because **non-opioid analgesics** are usually better tolerated with fewer potential side effects than opioid analgesics, it is better to use them whenever possible. However, a patient's pain should not be undermedicated. Non-opioid analgesics are typically used for mild pain, as an additional medication with opioids, or together with some narcotics as a combination drug. Examples of these include acetaminophen (Tylenol) and non-steroidal anti-inflammatories drugs, or NSAIDs (ibuprofen, naproxen, or aspirin).

Opioid analgesics should be used for moderate to severe pain and when pain is not responding to non-opioid medications. These should also be used when pain is increasing in severity. Examples of opioid analgesics include hydrocodone/acetaminophen (Lortab), oxycodone/acetaminophen (Percocet), meperidine (Demerol), or morphine. Propoxyphene (Darvocet) should not be used to treat cancer pain because it may accumulate in the patient's system and cause toxicity. The patient should be assessed for his or her reaction to various pain medications to avoid over medication and potential unwanted side effects.

Other Classes of Drugs to Treat Pain

- **Stimulants**, such as methylphenidate (Ritalin), may be given to treat sedation and lethargy. Side effects include nervousness, restlessness, increased heart rate, hypertension, insomnia, and anxiety.
- **Anticonvulsants**, such as phenytoin (Dilantin) and gabapentin (Neurontin), may be used to treat neuropathic pain. They can also be helpful in treating postherpetic neuralgia that may occur following shingles. Side effects include sedation, bone marrow depression, and nausea.
- **Antidepressants**, such as amitriptyline (Elavil) and venlafaxine (Effexor), may be used to treat neuropathic pain and postherpetic neuralgia. Side effects include sedation, dry mouth, sexual side effects, and orthostatic hypotension.
- **Antihistamines**, such as hydroxyzine (Vistaril) and diphenhydramine (Benadryl), may be used for pruritus, anxiety, or nausea. Side effects include sedation, dizziness, tachycardia, and blurred vision.
- **Benzodiazepines**, such as alprazolam (Xanax) and lorazepam (Ativan), may be used for anxiety and severe muscle spasms. Side effects include sedation, hypotension, respiratory depression, and dizziness.
- **Corticosteroids**, such as dexamethasone (Decadron) and methylprednisolone (Solu-Medrol), may be used to help with nerve compression, severe inflammation, and increased intracranial pressure.

Breakthrough Pain, Incident Pain, and End-of-Dose Pain

- **Breakthrough pain** – A period of intense pain that occurs in addition to chronic pain. Short-acting analgesics are helpful in treating this kind of pain. If not already taking, a patient needs to be started on a long-acting analgesic to keep the pain level more tolerable before breakthrough pain occurs.
- **Incident pain** – Occurs during a specific movement or activity, for example, deep breathing and coughing after abdominal surgery. Short-acting analgesics are helpful in treating this type of pain. It is important to anticipate activities that cause pain and medicate the patient before he or she will be performing these activities. For example, give an analgesic before the patient participates in physical therapy.
- **End-of-dose pain** – Pain that occurs before the next dose of medicine is due to be given. A long-acting analgesic may be helpful in providing a steadier state of pain relief. Short-acting analgesics can also be used to relieve this pain.

Analgesic Tolerance, Physical Dependence, and Addiction

- **Analgesic tolerance** develops after a patient has been on narcotic analgesics for an extended period of time and the dose of medication is no longer effective in reducing his or her pain. An increased dose of medication is necessary to achieve the same pain relief previously obtained from a lower dose. This can occur over and over again while the patient is on narcotics.
- **Physical dependence** occurs when the medication is necessary for a patient to avoid withdrawal symptoms. These withdrawal symptoms will occur if the medication is abruptly stopped or if an antagonist agent, such as Narcan, is administered. Physical dependence commonly occurs after extended use of narcotic analgesics and benzodiazepines.

- **Addiction** is psychological dependence to a drug. There are both genetic and environmental influences that cause some people to be predisposed to addiction. Addiction is characterized by the behavior of continuing to take a drug despite the fact that it is causing harm to one's self.

Goal of Palliation

The term "terminal" used to be synonymous with cancer and was the major focus of therapy. In the last 20 or so years, with increasing 5-year survival rates, improved early diagnosis, and better surgical and drug treatments, terminality has been relegated to the status of a phase of cancer treatment. This is the **palliative phase**. The object of palliation is to relieve pain and suffering. In the palliative phase of cancer treatment (which is different than the general concept of *palliative care*), the most powerful pain medication is used in this phase. The patient is dying, so only comfort and pain relief is the goal. The overall goal of palliation is to manage primarily pain and to maximize the quality of life conditions in the patient's terms.

Principals of Palliative Care

- Death is regarded as a natural process, to be neither hastened nor prolonged.
- The patient and family are the unit of care.
- Invasive medical procedures and diagnostic tests are minimized, unless they are likely to result in the alleviation of symptoms.
- Use of "heroic" life-prolonging treatment measures are not recommended, unless to improve or maintain quality of life.
- When managing pain with opioid analgesics, the correct dose is the dose that provides pain relief without unacceptable side effects.
- The patient is the "expert" on whether pain and symptoms have been adequately relieved.
- Fluids and feeding are not forced or artificially induced. Patients eat if they are hungry or for the social benefit of sharing food.

Alterations in Functioning

Neutropenia

Neutropenia is defined as a neutrophil count less than 1,000 cells/mm³; a normal neutrophil level is 2,500 to 6,000 cells/mm³. **Neutrophils** are a form of granulocyte that functions with the other components of the immune system to fight infection. They are the most common type of white blood cell and are necessary to fight infection. Neutrophils are formed by stem cells within the bone marrow.

The other types of white blood cells are **eosinophils and basophils**, which are also formed by stem cells within the bone marrow.

Malfunction of the bone marrow can cause a decreased production of neutrophils by the stem cells and can result in an infection in the patient because of a decreased ability to fight organisms. If the number of neutrophils within a person's blood stream is reduced, bacteria cells are more apt to cause an infection, either localized or systemic. Neutrophils serve as the primary source of defense for the immune system.

Risk factors for neutropenia:

- A patient's **age** and overall **health** can cause them to be more susceptible to developing neutropenia. Elderly patients are more likely to have impairments in blood cell production than younger patients.
- **Poor nutritional status** can affect the body's ability to produce blood cells because the nutrients that are necessary for overall health are not present.
- The **presence of other diseases**, such as diabetes, can also impair function of the immune system.
- Cancer affecting **bone marrow function** can impair the production of neutrophils. Examples include leukemia and multiple myeloma. Bone cancers can also affect the function of bone marrow.
- **Chemotherapy** suppresses bone marrow function and decreases neutrophil production.
- High doses of **radiation** to the bones can also affect the function of bone marrow and decrease neutrophil production.
- **Steroids** used for cancer treatment affect the function of neutrophils by preventing them from detecting bacterial cells and fighting infection. This impairs the immune system by allowing bacteria to reproduce without neutrophils present to destroy them.

History and Physical Exam Findings in Neutropenia Patients

When taking a **history** on a patient with neutropenia, find out which treatments the patient has undergone up to this point. This not only includes chemotherapy and radiation, but also any medications they may be taking. Be sure to ask what treatments for neutropenia, if any, have been used in the past. Also find out if there were any complications or side effects from taking these medications.

On **physical exam**, assess vital signs to check for an elevated temperature, which could indicate an infection. Also evaluate for an elevated heart rate or decreased blood pressure which can indicate an infection. Assess the patient for muscle wasting or excessive weight loss. Be sure to do a thorough skin exam to assess for any localized infections. Breath sounds should be evaluated for any signs of fluid accumulation in the lungs or any adventitious breath sounds. Overall, look for a sign that may point to a cause of the neutropenia if there is not an easy explanation for this.

Neutropenia Treatment

If an infection has occurred, **antibiotics** are given. Blood cultures or localized cultures can be done to identify the causative bacteria and sensitivity testing is done to determine which antibiotic is most effective for treatment. If the infection is not bacterial in nature, **antivirals** or **antifungals** may be given.

Growth factors can also be given to stimulate increased production of neutrophils for the stem cells within the bone marrow. These will increase production of all of the granulocytes and help to return the immune system to a normal functioning status. This can help to decrease the chance of developing an infection. Neutrophil counts need to be monitored regularly while receiving this treatment until a desired level is attained.

A patient's **nutritional status** should be considered and a dietary consultation may be necessary to ensure the patient's diet is adequate to meet the demands of the body. Dietary changes may need to be made for the body's tissues to receive the necessary nutrients to produce blood cells normally.

Myelosuppression

Myelosuppression is impaired blood cell production because of dysfunctional bone marrow. This results in *pancytopenia*, or a decrease in all blood cells. This can occur because of a primary blood dyscrasia that causes the bone marrow to not function the way it should. It can also occur as a result of cancer treatment, such as chemotherapy, which suppresses blood cell production in an effort to cure cancer.

- When the *red blood cell count* is less than normal, anemia and decreased energy occurs. This can also cause the other effects of anemia, such as increased heart rate, palpitations, and a decrease in the amount of oxygen and nutrients delivered to the body's tissues.
- A low *white blood cell count* causes the immune system to not function correctly. This causes the patient to be more susceptible to infections and illness.
- When the *platelet count* is reduced the capability of the blood to clot is affected. This puts the patient at risk for bleeding, possibly even severe hemorrhage and hypovolemic shock.

Thrombocytopenia

Thrombocytopenia is the condition in which the **platelet level** drops below a normal level, generally *less than 100,000* platelets per microliter. A normal platelet count is 150,000 to 350,000 platelets per microliter. Platelets usually regenerate every 7 to 10 days so they are constantly changing and being produced.

Platelets are produced in the bone marrow and travel through the circulating bloodstream. Any impairments of the bone marrow can affect the production of platelets. This can occur with bone cancer, chemotherapy, or radiation to the bones.

The main *function of platelets* is to join with other platelets to cause blood clots and prevent hemorrhage. They can also accumulate within blood vessels to cause a thrombus. When this blood clot breaks free and travels through the blood stream, it is called an embolism. This can go on to block blood vessels in the lungs, heart, and brain which can lead to a pulmonary embolism, a myocardial infarction, or a cerebrovascular accident.

- 118 -

Thrombocytopenia Risk Factors

Thrombocytopenia can result from diseases or treatments that result in an increased destruction, decreased production, or increased usage of platelets. Diseases that cause the development of purpura, or bruising, are due to an increase in destruction of platelets.

- **Cancers that affect the bone marrow** can cause a decrease in the production of platelets, leading to a decreased platelet count.
- Diseases that cause **increased blood clotting** can use the platelets faster than they are produced, which will result in a decreased platelet count.
- **Chemotherapy** and **radiation** can both cause destruction of the cells from which platelets are derived. This will cause a decrease in the number of platelets that are produced in the bone marrow.
- Certain **medications**, especially blood thinners, can lead to a decrease in the function of platelets, which causes the blood to be less likely to clot. Some infections can also lead to an increase in platelet destruction and alter the function of platelets.

History and Physical Exam Findings in Thrombocytopenia Patients

When taking a **history** on a patient with thrombocytopenia, find out which treatments the patient has undergone up to this point. This not only includes chemotherapy and radiation, but also any medications they may be taking. Be sure to ask what treatments for thrombocytopenia, if any, have been used in the past. Also find out if there were any complications or side effects from taking these medications.

On **exam**, examine the patient for any bleeding. The gums and the nose should be checked for bleeding, and stool should be assessed for occult bleeding. Do a thorough skin exam to assess for any bruising or petechiae which are small pinpoint hemorrhages. If severe, a patient can develop bleeding within the brain, such as a subdural hemorrhage. Assess for any mental status changes, changes in gait, or slurred speech. Assess laboratory tests to evaluate for changes in the platelet level. Continue to monitor this after treatment is started to assess for improvement.

Thrombocytopenia Treatment

If the platelet count drops to a level that is extremely low, a **platelet transfusion** can be done to raise the level back to normal. This involves using platelets from a blood bank and infusing them into a patient. There are risks with this similar to the risks present with a blood transfusion. At times, patients may develop a resistance to platelet transfusions and they may need to receive plasma transfusions to replace lost platelets.

There are **medications** available which can be given to stimulate the production of platelets. Similar to erythropoietin, thrombopoietin is used to stimulate production and maturation of platelets.

Treatments can also be aimed at treating the **cause of thrombocytopenia**. If a patient has a congenital clotting disorder due to decreased platelet production, regular injections of medication to stimulate platelet production can be given. If there is a problem with destruction of platelets, steroids can be used to treat thrombocytopenia.

Thrombotic Events

Thrombotic events can include blood clots that occur in the venous or arterial systems that cause a blockage of blood flow. Some type of tissue injury occurs. This can be related to treatment with medications that are caustic to the vessels or tissues, radiation treatment that causes damage to vessels or tissues, or cancer surgery in which tissue damage occurs. Platelets and other clotting factors clump together in one location and form a clot. This clot is called a **thrombus**.

A thrombus can stay in one location and cause a blockage in blood flow, either venous or arterial. If **venous**, return of blood flow to the heart will be interrupted causing edema. If **arterial**, oxygenated blood will not flow to an extremity which causes duskiness and coolness of the limb.

A thrombus can break free and travel through the vascular system until it sticks in a smaller vessel. This is called an **embolus**. An example is a pulmonary embolism that blocks a vessel to the lungs and can be fatal.

Causes of Thrombotic Episodes

Cancer tumors can cause compression on vessels which can promote clumping of platelets and clotting factors. There are also certain types of tumors that secrete the proteins necessary for clotting, which can lead to thrombus formation. Abnormalities in blood counts with an elevation in platelets can promote clotting and thrombus formation, as well.

- Patients with an underlying **cardiac dysrhythmia**, especially atrial fibrillation, are more susceptible to developing blood clots. Patients with **vascular disease** are also more likely to suffer thrombus formation because of blood stasis.
- Patients may have a **decreased level of physical activity** because of pain or illness. This causes them to be at risk for developing blood clots, especially in the lower extremities. A deep vein thrombosis (DVT) can break free and travel through the system to the heart or lungs to become an embolism.
- Patients can also have a **congenital clotting disorder** that causes blood to clot easily. A condition called polycythemia vera causes an elevation in all blood cell types which can increase the risk for thrombus.

History and Physical Exam Findings in Patients Who Suffer a Thrombotic Event

When taking a **history** from a patient with suspected **thrombotic disease**, ask about any co-morbidity(s) that may be present and what treatments have been received for these illnesses. Assess the patient's activity level and whether they would be at risk for developing a DVT. Question the patient about habits such as smoking or drinking. Ask about pain the patient is experiencing and have the patient rate the severity of the pain. With pulmonary embolism, the patient may complain of acute onset of shortness of breath. This is a medical emergency and must be addressed immediately.

On **physical exam**, examine the patient's skin for any signs of bruising or stasis changes, especially in the lower extremities. A DVT can present as a hard, cordy feeling in the calf and the patient will have pain with firm dorsiflexion of the foot (Homan's sign). Assess the color and temperature of the extremities. With a pulmonary embolism, the patient will have diminished breath sounds and ineffective respirations.

Nonpharmacologic and Pharmacologic Treatments of Thrombotic Diseases

Nonpharmacologic treatments of thrombotic disease include measures to prevent any incidents from occurring. The patient should be encouraged to be as **physically active** as possible to prevent stasis of blood in the lower extremities. If the patient cannot get out of bed, exercises should be done with gentle limb movements while in bed. A Physical Therapy consult may be necessary to teach the patient exercises that can be done on their own. **Compression stockings** may be ordered to help with venous return in the lower extremities and decrease the risk of DVT formation. **Electronic devices** to compress the lower extremities may also be used to prevent DVT

Medical treatments can be used to prevent clot formation. These include aspirin therapy, Coumadin, Heparin, Lovenox, and Plavix. Many patients will go home on these medications, except for Heparin which is only given IV, to continue prophylactic treatment of thrombus formation. Lab tests with a PT and INR will need to be regularly monitored if the patient is taking Coumadin.

Hemorrhage, Hemostasis, and Coagulation

- **Hemorrhage** is uncontrolled bleeding whether from an injury within the body or on the outer surface of the body.
- **Hemostasis** is the action of bleeding being controlled and stopping due to the presence of clotting factors and platelet function.
- **Coagulation** is completely solidified blood which is caused by the action of fibrin and fibrinogen.

These processes are inter-related through a chain of events. *Hemorrhage* occurs because of some trauma to the outer body or an internal stimulus. This activates the body's clotting system with the migration of platelets and clotting factors to the site. A clot will form and stop the bleeding, if possible, through the action of *hemostasis*. *Coagulation* occurs when the blood thickens into a thickened clot using fibrinogen and other proteins. Both hemostasis and coagulation are necessary to control hemorrhage. If functioning properly, this cascade of events can prevent a patient from developing hypovolemic shock and even death from massive hemorrhage.

Hemorrhage Risk Factors

- **Cancers affecting the bone marrow** can cause a decrease in platelet production and decrease the clotting abilities of the body, which can lead to uncontrolled hemorrhage.
- **Tumors** are very friable and can bleed easily or cause bleeding if they damage other tissues. Brain tumors are susceptible to causing compression within the brain tissue and can possibly cause hemorrhage from the vessels located within the brain.
- **Chemotherapy** or other myelosuppressive treatments can lead to hemorrhage by decreasing the effectiveness of platelet cells.
- **Cancer surgery** places the patient at risk for excessive blood loss and hypovolemic shock.
- **Chronic steroid use** for treatment can decrease the effectiveness of platelet cells and slow down the clotting process.
- **Disease states affecting the liver** can cause a decrease in the production of clotting factors and proteins necessary for clotting, leading to an increased risk of hemorrhage.

Blood Transfusion Laboratory Testing

A **complete blood count (CBC)** with a hemoglobin and hematocrit is done first to determine the need for a blood transfusion. **Hemoglobin** is the primary level that is used to assess whether a patient needs to be transfused. When making the decision to transfuse, if the patient is symptomatic transfusion may occur anytime the hemoglobin drops less than 9. However, if the patient is asymptomatic, current guidelines recommend waiting until the hemoglobin is 7-8 g/dL. In the palliative care patient, transfusion is sometimes given to offer relief from advanced cancer symptoms in low but normal hemoglobin levels, but this must be decided on a case by case basis.

A **platelet count** is included in the CBC and is used to determine if a patient needs a platelet transfusion to promote blood clotting and avoid excessive bleeding. A transfusion is considered when the platelet count drops to less than 10,000, but may be considered at higher levels if the patient is bleeding or if they will be in a situation in which bleeding is a possibility.

Before blood can be transfused, a **blood typing** must be done to determine that patient's serotype. A type and screen is done if it is unknown whether blood products will be used, and a type and crossmatch is done for a certain number of units of blood when a transfusion if necessary.

Homologous Blood, Autologous Blood, and Directly Donated Blood

- **Homologous blood** – This is blood collected from one person and given to another. This is the most common type of blood collection. Local blood drives are conducted for this type of blood collection to be stored and used as needed by local hospitals.
- **Autologous blood** – A patient donates his or her own blood in preparation for surgery in which a blood transfusion will be necessary. This avoids the risk of contracting any blood borne illnesses from accepting homologous blood, though this risk is very slim anyway. Blood lost during surgery can also be collected through special equipment and recycled to be given back to the patient.
- **Directly donated blood** – A person donates blood to be used specifically for a certain patient who requires a transfusion. This is usually done by a friend or family member before surgery or in the case of a rare blood type. Some patients prefer to receive blood from a person they know rather than from a blood bank.

Endogenous vs. Exogenous Organisms

Endogenous organisms are those organisms which live naturally in our body. They function to keep other organisms in check and prevent infection by these organisms.

Exogenous organisms are those organisms which are found outside the body in the world around us.

Organisms can be transmitted to humans via 3 different routes:

1. *Direct contact* involves coming in contact directly with an organism, such as by coming in contact with an infected wound or contaminated blood or other bodily fluids. This includes contamination with bodily fluids during sexual activity.
2. *Indirect contact* is when an organism is contracted by contact with an inanimate object on which the organism is located. Examples include contaminated surfaces such as tables, door knobs, and drinking fountains.
3. *Airborne contact* is contact with an organism by respiratory droplets which are present in the air from coughing or sneezing. Certain diseases, such as tuberculosis, are transmitted via airborne respiratory droplets.

Risk Factors for Infection

- A cancer patient receiving chemotherapy will have a **decreased WBCs** which puts them at risk of acquiring an infection. Steroids are occasionally used to treat some forms of cancer and can also cause suppression of the immune system.
- The development of **skin breakdown** due to radiation therapy or bed rest and immobility can lead to localized infections.
- **Incision sites** from cancer surgery are also locations at which an infection can occur.
- Any **indwelling device**, such as a central line, PICC line, peripheral IV, Foley catheter, or port can be sites of an infection. Since these are implanted devices, an infection can be localized at the site or become systemic as organisms enter the circulatory system.
- **Co-morbidities** can put a patient at risk for developing infection. For example, peripheral vascular disease can cause a decrease in blood flow to the extremities and affect the body's ability to fight off infection in a limb. Other common co-morbidities include diabetes and lung disease.

Diagnosing an Infection

On **physical exam**, a patient with an infection will have a *fever*, usually greater than 100.4°. The patient may or may not be flushed, due to fever, and may have chills. Some infections can cause nausea and vomiting, and possibly pain at the site of the infection if localized. A *localized site of infection* will show edema, erythema, induration, warmth, and possibly purulent discharge. If severe, an infection can cause changes in mental status and delirium from fever.

Laboratory tests for assessing for infection include a CBC with an elevated WBC. If a respiratory infection is suspected, a chest x-ray will be performed. If an internal organ is the suspected site of infection, a CT scan can show a fluid collection or abscess near the organ. Blood cultures can be done to assess for growth of a specific bacterial organism causing sepsis. Urine cultures can also be performed to assess for bacterial growth in the urine. If an infection is localized, cultures may be done of any discharge present.

Antibiotic Therapy for an Infection

When bacterial growth is present on culture, a **susceptibility test** is done to test the organism against several antibiotics. This indicates which antibiotics are most likely to be effective in fighting this organism. If cultures do not show any growth, but it is evident an infection is present, a **broad-spectrum antibiotic** will be given for at least 1 week. A negative culture could also indicate infection with a virus and antivirals may need to be considered.

Another factor to consider is the possible resistance of an organism to certain antibiotics. This can vary geographically in which certain areas of the country have common organisms that have built resistance to antibiotics that were previously used to treat the infection.

With some IV antibiotics, such as vancomycin, a test called a peak and trough will be done to assess the amount of antibiotics in the patient's system right before administering the drug and again after administering. This allows adjustments to be made to reach therapeutic drug levels while preventing adverse side effects.

Dysphagia

Dysphagia is a dysfunction in swallowing which can sometimes be uncomfortable. Patients will often describe a feeling of having something stuck in their throat. This can lead to aspiration of materials if food or fluids pass through the airway.

- Risk factors of dysphagia can be due to **neurologic difficulties**. Several cranial nerves are responsible for the action of swallowing and impairment in these can lead to an inability or difficulty with swallowing. Cancer tumors that affect the mouth, esophagus, and stomach can cause mechanical difficulties in swallowing food and fluids.
- **Cancer surgery** for these cancers can cause pain and dysfunction with swallowing, as can radiation to the area. Some patients can develop a constriction in the esophagus due to scar tissue from radiation or surgery, which can cause food to become lodged.
- **Chemotherapy** can suppress the immune system, which can result in an oral *Candida* infection, which is painful and can impair swallowing. Some drugs with anticholinergic affects can cause a dry mouth and difficulty swallowing.

Dysphagia Treatments

The primary goal in **treatment of dysphagia** is to treat the cause.

- If there is a mechanical blockage of the esophagus due to a tumor, cancer surgery or radiation may be done.
- If stenosis of the esophagus is the cause of dysphagia, a dilatation procedure may be done to widen the esophagus.
- Another option when treating dysphagia is to provide food and nutrients via another route instead of orally, especially if there is no cure for the dysphagia or this cannot be remedied in a timely fashion. Total parenteral nutrition or tube feedings via a PEG tube may need to be considered. If the patient is having problems with liquids, thickeners can be added to ensure the patient is able to stay well hydrated without the risk of choking or aspirating on thin liquids.
- Speech therapy can assist the patient with relearning to swallow. They are trained to provide patients with special maneuvers and training to perform swallowing while minimizing the risk of aspirating.

Anorexia

Anorexia due to cancer is defined as a decrease in the desire to eat. It usually results in weight loss. This is different from anorexia nervosa in which a person has an altered sense of body image and consciously limits the amount of food they eat in an effort to lose weight.

- Physical changes due to **cancer** can be a cause of anorexia. This can be caused by a tumor compressing the stomach which can lead to a decreased ability to take in food. Cancers affecting the hypothalamus and satiety center can alter the sensation of hunger.
- **Cancer surgery** can alter appetite by causing pain or dysfunction of the oral cavity, esophagus, or GI tract. Brain surgeries near the hypothalamus may have an effect on the satiety center and lead to an alteration in the sensation of hunger.
- **Chemotherapy or radiation** can cause nausea and vomiting and may alter appetite.
- Other **medications** used for treatment can also cause side effects that may decrease a patient's desire to eat.

History and Physical Exam Findings in Anorexia Patients

When taking a **history** from the patient with anorexia, assess the cause of the anorexia. Ask the patient about pain with chewing or swallowing, find out if nausea is the cause of a decrease in appetite. Ask about current or past cancer treatments that may be hindering the patient. Also assess whether the patient had a problem with anorexia in the past and what treatments were used to help overcome this problem. Ask about their eating habits before the anorexia started and what types of foods they liked in the past.

On **physical exam**, assess the patient's overall nutritional loss. Evaluate hydration status and examine for muscle wasting or cachexia. Examine the oropharynx for any sores or signs of irritation. Regular weights should be taken at the same time of day, on the same scale, and with the patient wearing as little clothes as possible in order to assess a trend of weight loss. Also assess the patient for any psychological problems that may be affecting their ability to eat.

Anorexia Long-Term Effects

A decrease in appetite can cause the patient to decrease the amount of nutrients taken in, which causes an overall **decrease in nutritional status**. This can lead to a loss of muscle mass and weakness, which can affect the patient's ability to be physically active. The effects of **inactivity** include increased weakness, pressure ulcers, increased risk for infection, and impaired respiratory and/or cardiovascular status.

Along with muscle wasting and poor nutritional status, a patient can suffer from metabolic imbalances which can lead to renal dysfunction, cardiac effects, and altered metabolism and GI function.

Patients who do not have adequate nutritional intake may not respond as well to medical treatments because of decreased vascular function. They are also at increased risk of suffering from more side effects due to poor metabolism of medications. Cancer surgeries may result in increased recuperation time and increased risk of post-operative infection because of altered immune status and decreased muscle mass. The effects of decreased mobility also increase the risk of developing more post-operative complications.

Anorexia Treatments

Ask the patient what kinds of foods they enjoy and try to implement these into their diet, if not contraindicated. **Supplement** the diet with high calorie, high protein foods. Also offer snacks and small meals during the day to boost caloric intake. Try to avoid medical treatments or therapies at times when the patient may be able to eat, if possible. Avoid factors that tend to cause the patient to feel nauseous or decrease appetite, if possible.

Educate the patient and family members or caregivers on the foods that will best replenish nutritional stores in the body and develop some menu ideas that are appetizing to the patient. Obtain a **dietary consult** to provide counseling to the patient and family members or caregivers to ensure caloric needs are being met. Also offer any anti-nausea or pain medications if these are symptoms that interfere with a patient's ability to eat. Provide appetite stimulants as ordered. If metabolic imbalances occur, administer medications as ordered to help correct these.

Mucositis, Stomatitis, Esophagitis, and Gastroenteritis

- **Mucositis** is the development of irritation throughout the GI tract due to the presence of a noxious stimulus. Normally, the tissues would regenerate when destroyed, but this does not happen when the inflammation and irritation is due to cancer treatments.
- **Stomatitis** is the condition that results when the tissue damage occurs in the mouth.
- **Esophagitis** occurs when the irritation takes place in the esophagus.
- **Gastroenteritis** results when the damage occurs in the stomach and intestines.

Cancer treatments cause irregularities in cell reproduction. When tissue damage occurs in the mucous membranes, the tissues attempt to repair themselves by quickly reproducing more cells. Since the cancer treatments interfere with this process, the tissues are never able to replace the damaged cells with normally functioning cells. This results in ulceration and damage to the membranes. The time it takes for mucositis to occur varies on the location of the damage and the treatments received. Some sections of the GI tract take longer than others to reproduce cells and repair damage.

Risk Factors for Mucositis

Cancers that affect the tissues of the GI tract can cause mucositis by physically damaging healthy tissues. Normally healthy mucous membrane cells can be replaced by cancer cells and lead to reproduction of more cancer cells.

Cancer treatments can cause mucositis and this can be quite severe and intolerable:

- *Chemotherapy drugs* can directly damage membrane cells when they come into contact with them. They can also cause damage indirectly. The decrease in WBCs caused by chemotherapy can lead to infections in the GI tract. These infections can cause inflammation and damage to the mucous membranes. This can develop into a chronic condition.
- *Radiation therapy* directly damages mucous membrane cells, which impair their ability to reproduce and repair. This is dose-dependent with more damage occurring with larger doses of radiation.
- **Cancer surgeries** can cause permanent damage leading to mucositis, also. Scar tissue can develop after surgery causing replacing of normally healthy tissue with scar tissue.

Mucositis Treatments

First find out the **cause** of the mucositis and what portion(s) of the GI tract is involved. Attempting to treat the cause may not always be possible if the cancer treatment is necessary.

Relieving the symptoms is the goal to prevent a change in the patient's nutritional status.

- **Analgesics** can be given to help reduce the irritation. Keep in mind that the patient may not tolerate analgesics when given orally.
- **Topical anesthetics** may be necessary to help reduce the pain, especially when the oral mucosa is affected by mucositis.

- **Medications** are also available to help coat the GI tract and prevent further damage. If infection occurs due to ulcerations in the mucous membranes, appropriate **antibiotics** should be given. When mucositis affects the intestinal tract, medications to treat diarrhea may also need to be given. **Vitamins** can be given to help increase energy and aid the immune system. **Protein supplements** may also be helpful in restoring depleted protein stores and aid in tissue repair.

Nonpharmacologic Treatments of Mucositis

- Try to **avoid additional irritation** to the area of mucositis. If the oral cavity is involved, offer foods that are soothing and smooth that do not require a lot of chewing to swallow. Avoid spicy foods or drinks that further irritate the area of mucositis.
- **Educate** the patient on the **causes and risk factors** for mucositis to help control or prevent symptoms. Include education on the importance of appropriate oral care and perineal care to prevent further irritation, infections, and damage.
- Encourage **adequate fluid intake** to prevent dehydration. Cool liquids may be soothing to the oral mucosa, also.
- **Assess** what **treatments** seem to be causing the mucositis and provide symptomatic treatment when these are going to be given, if possible. This may help to decrease the severity of tissue damage.
- **Educate** the patient on the **signs and symptoms** of infection. Ensuring that proper oral and perineal care is performed will help to reduce the risk of infection.

Xerostomia

Xerostomia is a decrease in moisture in the mouth due to a change in saliva production. Risk factors include:

- **Cancers** involving the salivary glands can lead to a decrease in their function and a decrease in saliva production. Other disease states and infections can also cause xerostomia to develop.
- **Cancer surgeries** can cause damage to the salivary glands or may result in complete excision of the glands. Cancer treatment with radiation can cause permanent cellular and tissue changes within the glands which affects the production of saliva. Radiation can also cause damage to the oral mucous membranes which affects the ability of saliva to effectively moisturize the mouth.
- Many **medications** also cause a dry mouth sensation, such as antidepressants, some analgesics, and any medications with anticholinergic effects.

Impairments in saliva production may be temporary or permanent. Of course, removal of the glands will result in permanent loss of saliva production, but if caused by drug treatments, the glands may rebound and function properly after treatments are completed.

Nonpharmacologic Treatment of Xerostomia:

- Offer items that will **stimulate saliva production**, such as hard candies. Citrus-flavored or sour candies are more likely to stimulate the salivary glands. Also offer frequent sips of water, if not contraindicated.
- Increase **moisture content** in foods by adding water and liquids to them.
- Offer **frequent snacks** that are high in fluid content.
- **Prevent mucosa from drying** out and increasing xerostomia.

- Educate the patient in **adequate oral hygiene** or perform regular oral hygiene to prevent infection and excessive dryness in the mouth.
- Advise the patient to **keep the lips well moisturized** to prevent drying, chapping, and cracking. The oral mucosa can also be lubricated with non-toxic oils before eating.
- **Assess which foods and fluids the patient prefers** and attempt to incorporate these into the diet, if not contraindicated.
- Encourage the patient to **report any change** in symptoms, especially response to any treatments that are given that may help or worsen the symptoms of xerostomia.

Nausea

Pathophysiology

Nausea is the sensation of GI upset that includes stomach pain and a feeling that vomiting may occur. It does not always result in vomiting, though, and can be triggered by multiple factors that may be actual or perceived triggers.

Nausea is caused by stimuli applied to the **vomiting center** in the brain. Specialized receptor cells are located outside the blood-brain barrier and they receive stimulation from substances traveling through the bloodstream that can cause nausea and vomiting, such as medications. Once stimulated, these receptor cells send a signal to the vomiting center in the brain. If the signal is strong enough, vomiting will occur. If not, the patient will only experience nausea.

The **stimuli** necessary to cause stimulation of the vomiting center can vary from medication, certain foods or smells, or by perceived stimuli that the patient thinks about. This can be an impending treatment or other event that has caused nausea in the past.

Risk Factors

The risk factors for nausea:

- **Tumors** in the brain that involve the vomiting center can cause a patient to experience regular nausea and require chronic anti-nausea medication use. Tumors that occur in the GI tract and cause obstruction or prevent proper digestion can also stimulate nausea. Though rare, cancers involving the semicircular canals within the inner ear can cause chronic vertigo, which can lead to nausea.
- **Metabolic imbalances** can cause nausea, as can infections or other illnesses that accompany a patient's cancer.
- **Cancer treatments** can lead to nausea, and the most likely of these is chemotherapy. It is standard to administer anti-nausea medications regularly to patients who are receiving **chemotherapy**. **Radiation** can cause nausea, as can oral medications. Other non-cancer medications can also cause nausea and this may be exaggerated when taken along with cancer medications.
- A patient's **anxiety level** may exacerbate nausea and make it worse because of stimulation to the vomiting center. This anxiety can be provoked just by the fear of developing nausea or may be due to a past negative experience.
- Always rule out **pregnancy** as a cause of nausea, as pregnancy may change cancer treatment decisions and options for the patient.

> **Review Video:** Nonpharmacological Interventions
> Visit mometrix.com/academy and enter code: 675095

Medical and Nonpharmacologic Treatments of Nausea

Medical treatment of nausea is mainly through **antiemetic medications**. These include ondansetron (Zofran), metoclopramide (Reglan), and prochlorperazine (Compazine). Phenergan is another popular medication used for treatment of nausea. If the patient is suffering from anxiety that is causing nausea, antianxiety medications may be used to help reduce the anxiety. Though controversial and not legal in all states, using cannabis (marijuana) to treat cancer nausea can be very helpful. This can also help stimulate the appetite.

Nonpharmacologic treatments can include removing the patient from the stimulus that is causing the nausea, if possible, and various alternative treatments. Imagery and relaxation can help the patient to focus on any time or place to block the unpleasant sensation of nausea. Massage can help with relaxation, foot massage especially, or reflexology, can be helpful in relieving nausea. Some patients respond well to hypnosis or deep breathing exercises. Acupuncture can also be used to block the sensations of nausea.

Vomiting

Vomiting is the powerful ejection of food and liquid that has not been fully digested within the stomach or from the proximal end of the small intestine. It is usually preceded by nausea.

The **vomiting center** is located within the brain. When certain processes occur within the body, a signal is sent through nerve fibers to the brain to stimulate the vomiting center. Signals are also sent to the **vagus nerve** to cause strong contraction of the diaphragm which assists in expelling the stomach contents. This stimulus can be an actual event such as a medication that has been taken, a certain food that has been eaten, or something that has been drunk. This stimulus can also be a perceived event such as a memory of a previous stimulus that caused vomiting or anticipation of an event that may cause vomiting. Psychological changes such as anxiety can also lead to vomiting.

> **Review Video: Nausea and Vomiting**
> Visit mometrix.com/academy and enter code: 631968

Constipation

Constipation is a decrease in the frequency of bowel movements accompanied by pain and straining with trying to defecate. Stool is not passed easily to the rectum which causes more water to be absorbed by the intestines. This results in very hard stool that is hard for the patient to pass. This can lead to anal fissures and vagal reactions with light-headedness or losing consciousness.

- *Primary constipation* results from external causes such as immobility, not following a regular routine, or changes in diet. A decrease in fiber or water intake can result in this type of constipation.
- *Secondary constipation* occurs due to a disease process. This can result from a blockage within the bowels, neurologic dysfunction, or electrolyte imbalances. Surgery can cause scar tissue to form in the wall of the intestines, which may result in strictures that prevent stool to move through easily.
- *Iatrogenic constipation* is a result of certain medications. Narcotic analgesics and some chemotherapy medications, as well as other drugs, can result in this form of constipation.

<u>Risk Factors</u>

Risk factors for bowel obstruction include:

- **Cancer tumors** that cause compression of the bowel can result in a bowel obstruction and blockage of the passage of stool. Tumors that cause impingement on the spinal cord through the lower thoracic and upper lumbar spine can cause neurologic dysfunction in bowel control.
- Constipation can result from **electrolyte imbalances** involving calcium or potassium.
- Overall **fatigue** and malaise can decrease activity, which can decrease the frequency of bowel movements.
- Uncontrolled **nausea** and vomiting can decrease a patient's appetite and lead to decreased bulk in the diet, which will affect defecation. Treating nausea with phenothiazines or other anti-emetic medications that have anticholinergic effects can cause constipation.
- **Cancer surgery** can decrease motility of the GI tract and cause constipation.
- Excessive **pain** can cause a patient to be apprehensive about having a bowel movement.
- **Medications**, especially opiate analgesics, can cause constipation. Some chemotherapy medications can cause neurologic side effects that may affect defecation.

<u>History and Physical Exam Findings in Patients with Constipation</u>

When taking a **history** from a patient with **constipation**, assess their normal bowel habits and how frequently they usually have bowel movements. Assess their pain level associated with the constipation and the presence of any cramping. Evaluate the patient's diet and ask about any recent changes in their eating habits. Ask about any changes in size, shape, or consistency of stool. Assess for any side effects of constipation such as hemorrhoids, both internal and external, and any cracking or fissures.

On **physical exam**, listen to bowel sounds and assess for the presence of sounds and any abnormalities. Feel the abdomen for any hardness and assess for tenderness. A rectal exam should be done to assess for hemorrhoids, collection of stool, adequate rectal tone, or fissures. Assess the patient for any alteration in their nutritional status as evidenced by muscle wasting or recent weight loss. Observe the patient for any objective signs of pain.

<u>Treatments</u>

Treatments of constipation:

- A **non-pharmacologic treatment for constipation** is to encourage adequate fluid and fiber intake, if not contraindicated. A patient should also be as active as possible to promote GI motility and prevent constipation.
- **Pharmacologic treatment for constipation** includes various forms of **laxatives**. These can act as a stimulant to promote tightening of the bowel. They also can function to decrease the amount of water in stool, which causes firmer stools. Other laxatives can function to moisten feces to promote easy passage of the stool. Laxatives are available in pill, liquid, and suppository form.
- **Stool softeners** can be given on a regular basis to assist with bowel movements. These help to keep bowel movements regular without the stimulant effect of a laxative.
- **Enemas** may be used when evacuation of the bowel is necessary. These are contraindicated when a bowel obstruction is present. Enemas are not used regularly now because of more laxative and stool softener agents being available.

Diarrhea

Types of diarrhea include:

- **Osmotic diarrhea:** Occurs when there is excess water in the stool. This is usually due to matter present in the intestines that cannot be absorbed. This causes water to remain in the intestine instead of being absorbed. This type of diarrhea can be caused by food allergies, such as an allergy to lactose in dairy products.
- **Secretory diarrhea:** Occurs when some form of an irritant causes the intestine to emit liquid. Electrolytes can also be secreted along with the fluid. This type of constipation can be caused by infections, such as an *E. coli* or *C. difficile* infection.
- **Hypermotility diarrhea:** Due to excitability of the intestine causing matter to move through very quickly. This decreases the time that solid waste is within the intestine, thus decreasing the amount of fluid absorbed from the stool. This can be caused by inflammation within the intestine and various drugs that irritate the intestinal wall.

Risk Factors

- **Cancers** of the intestine can lead to diarrhea by causing blockages, which lead to only fluid being able to pass through.
- **Cancer surgeries** can cause irritation and inflammation of the bowel leading to diarrhea.
- **Cancer treatment** with medications that irritate the GI tract can lead to diarrhea. *Radiation therapy* to the abdomen can cause irritation of the intestine and bowel causing inflammation and an increased risk for diarrhea. *Chemotherapy* can cause suppression of the immune system, leading to an increased risk for infections.
- **Antibiotics and antivirals** used to treat these infections can be very irritating to the GI tract, causing nausea, vomiting, and diarrhea.
- Irritability of the bowel can also be caused by **psychological factors**. Increased *stress and worry* can cause intestinal cramping and hypermotility. *Depression and anxiety* can cause a decrease in appetite, leading to poor health habits, including a change in diet. This can put a strain on the intestines and cause diarrhea.

History and Physical Exam Findings in Patients with Diarrhea

When taking a **history** from a patient with **diarrhea**, obtain a thorough explanation of the patient's past bowel habits. This includes frequency, activities that have triggered bowel movements, and any past treatments for constipation or diarrhea. Evaluate their current bowel pattern including frequency of the diarrhea, consistency, color, and any accompanying pain. Also question the patient about nutritional habits and diet preferences, as well as any recent changes. Ask about any medications they are taking as well as any co-morbidities present.

On **physical exam**, assess the patient's nutritional status and monitor for signs of dehydration. This includes examining mucus membranes for dryness and testing skin tenting. Heart rate may be elevated with dehydration and, if severe, patients may have changes in mental status. Assess for any electrolyte imbalances with signs and symptoms of these depending on which electrolyte is affected. Examine the skin in the perineum for signs of inflammation or breakdown. Listen to bowel sounds to assess for hyperactivity. Also palpate the abdomen to assess for tenderness.

Treatments

Treat the **cause** of the diarrhea first, if possible. If *food allergies* are present, avoid those foods in the patient. If certain *medications* cause the intestinal irritation and diarrhea, ask the physician if an alternative medication can be used. Start the patient on a bland diet with plenty of fluids to prevent dehydration. Administer IV medications as ordered. If *stress* is causing irritability in the bowels, try to provide a calming environment for the patient to decrease stress. Answer any questions the patient may have to help keep them informed and avoid stress related to their situation.

Medical treatments are aimed at slowing down the GI motility. Loperamide (Imodium) can help to decrease the passage of stool through the intestines and increase the absorption of water. Medications can also be given to calm down inflammation and irritation in the bowel. If an infectious process is the cause of the irritability, treat with the appropriate antibiotic. Medications may need to be added to increase bulk in the stool.

Ascites

Ascites is a collection of **fluid within the abdomen**. This fluid is often not taken up by the circulatory system.

- Most instances of ascites are not due to cancer, but rather occur because of primary *liver disease*, such as cirrhosis. Liver disease can lead to a buildup of fluid in the abdominal cavity. This can occur when liver cancer causes liver failure.
- Ascites can occur from *tumors* that leak fluid into the abdominal cavity and may prevent the fluid from being reabsorbed into the circulatory system. This fluid can be a protein-rich fluid called exudate or blood from the tumor.
- *Lymph fluid* can also accumulate due to cancers affecting the lymph system.
- *Abscesses or infections* in the GI tract may cause pus to accumulate in the abdomen.
- *Pelvic cancers* can also cause ascites to develop.
- *Treatments*, such as radiation, can cause vascular and lymphatic changes that result in abnormalities of fluid absorption and the accumulation of fluid in the abdomen.

History and Physical Exam Findings in Patients with Ascites

When taking a **history** from a patient with **ascites**, ask about other illnesses the patient may suffer from, especially chronic liver disease. Question the time frame in which the ascites occurred and what has been done in the past to relieve this. Assess for any other symptoms the patient may have indicating an increase in fluid overload. Ask about any swelling or difficulty breathing that has occurred recently. Ask about pain and any triggering events that may increase pain.

On **physical exam**, abdominal girth should be measured and recorded over time to assess for increases or decreases in fluid accumulation. Pitting edema may be present over the abdomen and the patient should be assessed for the presence of a fluid wave. Laboratory tests should be performed to assess protein levels and the fluid collected via paracentesis should be tested for the presence of cancer cells. Radiographic studies are helpful in locating the source of the fluid. Ultrasound and CT scan can further evaluate the abdominal and pelvic cavities.

Treatment

Treatments for ascites include:

- *Fluid restrictions* to help to decrease fluid retention and further buildup of fluid within the abdomen.
- *Sodium restrictions* to also help by preventing water retention.

- **Paracentesis** can be performed. This involves inserting a long needle through the abdominal wall into the abdominal cavity and withdrawing the fluid. This procedure may need to be repeated several times over the course of treatment if the ascites continues to occur. There is a risk of infection with this procedure and other possible complications, including organ puncture.
- A **shunt** can be used to drain the fluid from the abdomen into the blood stream. If severe, the fluid drained into the circulatory system may lead to fluid overload. The patient needs to be closely monitored for signs of edema or increase in respiratory secretions.
- A **drain** can be placed to remove the fluid from the abdominal cavity, but this is a permanent access through which organisms can enter the abdominal cavity and could possibly cause an infection.

Types of Intestinal Mechanical Obstruction

Mechanical obstruction is the most common type of bowel obstruction. It has 3 main causes: influencing factors outside the bowel, inside the bowel, or physical blockage within the bowel.

- Causes of a bowel obstruction that occur **outside of the bowel** include adhesions or hernias.
- **Within the bowel**, obstruction can occur due to tumors or conditions in which the bowel wall is inflamed or is receiving a decreased amount of oxygen.
- **Blockages** within the bowel can also lead to obstruction. The blockage can be caused by objects which are ingested or by stool. There are 3 main types of bowel obstruction:
  - A **simple obstruction** is a noncomplicated bowel obstruction in which blood supply remains intact.
  - A **closed obstruction** occurs when there is more than one area of blockage.
  - A **strangulated obstruction** occurs when the blood supply becomes compromised and is considered a medical emergency requiring urgent surgery.

Nonmechanical Intestinal Obstruction Causes

A **nonmechanical intestinal obstruction** is not due to an actual physical blockage. Rather, waste products cannot move through the intestines because of neurologic deficits or because of a decreased blood supply. This can have causes arising from within the abdomen or outside the abdomen.

- Events **within the abdomen** that can cause an obstruction include intestinal movement during surgery, irritation of structures within the abdomen, or decreased blood flow to the bowel.
- Causes occurring **outside of the abdomen** can include injuries that prevent a patient from bearing down to evacuate the bowels, use of medications with anticholinergic side effects, narcotic analgesics which cause constipation, and electrolyte imbalances. The patient's inability to drink fluids can also cause a bowel obstruction if constipation becomes severe enough. This causes the stool to be too hard and the patient is not able to pass it. Immobility can also decrease motility of the GI tract and slow down peristaltic movement. This can result in constipation and may lead to a bowel obstruction.

<u>Risk Factors</u>

Risk factors for intestinal obstruction include:

- **Cancer tumors** that compress the intestines can cause an obstruction. Cancer that affects the spinal cord in the lower thoracic and upper lumbar areas can cause a nonmechanical obstruction. Any damage to this area of the spinal cord during surgery can also cause the patient to be more susceptible to developing a bowel obstruction.
- **Cancer surgeries** can cause adhesions and may lead to a bowel obstruction due to stricture of the intestinal lumen. Surgery in which the intestines are handled frequently can also cause the bowel to become less active, leading to an obstruction.
- **Radiation therapy** to the abdomen can cause damage to the intestinal wall, along with weakening of the smooth muscle. This can lead to a decrease in peristalsis, causing formation of a bowel obstruction.
- The **formation** of diverticulum, or outpouches, in the intestinal wall can cause an obstruction to form.
- **Additional disease processes** that may promote development of a bowel obstruction include inflammatory bowel disease, a hernia, and ulcerative colitis.

<u>History and Physical Exam Findings in Patients With Intestinal Obstruction</u>

When taking a **history** from a patient with a **bowel obstruction**, try to assess the time frame in which their symptoms occurred. Ask how long abdominal pain has been present, when the last bowel movement was and the characteristics of the bowel movement. Depending on the location of the obstruction, the patient may experience leakage of watery stool or may even develop vomiting of fecal material if the blockage is high in the small intestine. Ask if a fever or chills have been present. Question the patient about co-morbidities and any past or present treatments they have received.

On **physical exam**, vital signs should be assessed for presence of a fever or an increase in heart rate which could indicate an infection or dehydration. An abdominal exam should include auscultating for bowel sounds and recording their frequency and tone (high pitched, rumbling, etc.) Palpate the abdomen for any hardness or tenderness. Include a rectal exam to see if there is any hard stool or blood present on exam.

<u>Treatments</u>

Patients who are diagnosed with an intestinal obstruction are placed on **NPO status**. Usually a **nasogastric tube** will be inserted and set to low suction. This may be done for a few days while waiting for the obstruction to resolve by itself. During this time, it is important to assess the patient's nutritional status. **Parenteral feedings** will need to be used to provide the patient with nutrients necessary to meet the body's needs. **Hydration status** should also be regularly examined as well as electrolyte levels to ensure there are no abnormalities. **Surgery** may be required to either resect the section of bowel that contains the obstruction or to treat the cause of the obstruction if it is a tumor causing compression or adhesions. The patient may require a **colostomy** following surgery which may be temporary or permanent depending on the severity of the obstruction and the amount of bowel involved.

<u>Fecal Impaction</u>

Fecal impaction is the state in which feces is not passed for some time and forms a hard impassable mass which requires **intervention** in order to clear the tract. Fecal impaction is more common in the elderly due to slowing of the GI tract.

During **assessment**, evaluate bowel sounds, and rule out metabolic changes, inadequate food intake, narcotics, decreased exercise, surgery, and any medication to make a tentative diagnosis regarding the constipation.

Urinary Incontinence

Types of Urinary Incontinence

- **Stress incontinence** is leaking of urine when any activities are performed that involve a bearing down function. This includes laughing, sneezing, and coughing. Talking or yelling loudly can also cause this. Patients will often describe this as a dribbling or leaking sensation whenever they perform these actions.
- **Urge incontinence** is leaking of urine very suddenly in response to a sensation of needing to urinate. Patients describe it as not being able to make it to the bathroom.
- **Reflex incontinence** is leaking of urine without any feelings of having to urinate. The patient may often not realize this is occurring until they notice the wetness on their clothes.
- **Functional incontinence** is when a patient voids because they are not physically able to reach the bathroom before having to urinate.
- **Total incontinence** is constant leaking of urine because there is no sensation of having to urinate. It is a complete lack of control of the function of urinating.

Risk Factors

- **Cancers** that primarily affect the urinary system and rectum can cause incontinence. These may involve dysfunction of the sphincters or muscle tissue of the bladder or rectal walls. Cancers affecting the neurologic system can cause nerve compression and prevent the nervous stimulation necessary to promote urinary or fecal control.
- **Cancer surgery** can result in incontinence. Removal of bladder tumors can result in damage to the bladder wall and muscle tissue, resulting in involuntary spasms or loss of control. Prostatectomy can result in incontinence by decreasing urge.
- **Radiation treatments** can cause tissue and muscle damage resulting in incontinence. While killing cancer cells, the destruction of healthy cells can occur.
- **Weakness and decreased mobility** can lead to functional incontinence when the patient is unable to move quickly enough to get to the bathroom before voiding.
- **Change in mental status** can also cloud judgment and decrease the patient's sensation to void.

Mechanism of Action Behind Types of Urinary and Fecal Incontinence

Urinary incontinence occurs because of problems with holding urine within the bladder or because of problems with emptying the bladder. It can also occur from a combination of the two mechanisms.

- Problems with *holding* urine in the bladder can be due to malfunction of the bladder neck and muscle control. Bladder spasms may contribute to the inability of holding urine within the bladder by forcing the urine out involuntarily. Cancers of the bladder wall may contribute to spasms and irritability within the bladder.
- Problems with *voiding* can include obstructions of the bladder or urethra which prevent urine from being able to pass. There can also be problems with muscle contraction in the bladder and weakness which prevents urine from being forced out of the bladder.

Fecal incontinence can occur because of a loss of control of the anal sphincters. This can be due to tissue damage or neurologic damage. Patients may also develop a loss of sensation within the rectum which prevents them from knowing when they need to defecate.

History and Physical Exam Findings in Patients with Incontinence

When obtaining a **history** from a patient with incontinence, ask questions pertaining to when this started and if any treatments coincide with the beginning of the incontinence. Question the patient to determine the type of incontinence they are experiencing, i.e., urge, stress, functional. Ask about any past or present treatments that the patient has undergone that may be contributing to the incontinence.

On **physical exam**, an abdominal exam should be performed to palpate the bladder, if possible. The bladder may be full of urine when there is a problem with emptying and feel empty if the patient has continual leakage of urine. Examine the patient's skin for skin breakdown that may occur due to urine or feces being in contact with the skin. Assess the patient's mental status for any decrease in awareness and possible dementia. Physical activity level should also be assessed to determine if physical impairments or pain are preventing the patient from getting to the bathroom before voiding.

Renal Dysfunction

Physiology

The **kidneys** are responsible for filtering the blood. They are comprised of a series of tubules that retain substances that are needed by the body and excreting others that are not needed. Cancer can invade the kidney tissue and cause malfunction in the filtering system which would result in the reabsorption or excretion of improper amounts of fluid or electrolytes. The kidneys play a huge role in the human body in maintaining the fluid and electrolyte balance, so any damage to the kidneys can result in life-threatening results.

Any cancer affecting the kidneys can cause dysfunction within the organs. The dysfunction may result in the resorption of too much fluid, leaving the body in fluid overload with diluted electrolyte levels. Or the kidneys may not be able to function appropriately in excreting electrolytes, causing the urine to be diluted with an excess of certain electrolytes within the blood stream. This can result in electrolyte levels that are too high.

Risk Factors
- **Cancer** that affects the kidneys may cause dysfunction within the organs. This can be due to a decrease in blood flow to the kidneys, cancer invasion within the organs, or cancer affecting a portion of the urinary system distal to the kidneys which causes a reflux of waste products back into the kidneys.
- **Co-morbidities** may contribute to renal dysfunction. Diabetics are at risk for renal dysfunction because of microvascular affects along with poorly-controlled glucose levels. Recurrent urinary tract infections with renal involvement can also progress to renal dysfunction. Any conditions or urinary diversions that result in reflux of the urine back to the kidneys can result in altered filtering performance. Recurrent renal stones can also cause scarring in the kidney.
- **Cancer surgery** can cause scarring, which may affect urine flow, or nerve damage, which can lead to retention and reflux of urine into the kidneys. *Radiation* therapy can cause scarring and damage from the urethra to the kidneys. *Chemotherapeutic medications* can be toxic to the kidneys when passing through the organs.

- 136 -

History and Physical Exam Findings in Patients with Renal Dysfunction

When taking a **history** from a patient with impaired renal function, ask about current and past medications that have been prescribed. Review the type of cancer the patient has and if there is any direct renal involvement. Assess for any co-morbidities that may affect renal function such as diabetes or past history of kidney stones. When discussing past treatments, find out where radiation was done and which chemotherapeutic medications were given. Also ask about any surgical procedures that have been done in the past.

On **physical exam**, do a thorough skin exam to assess the patient for dryness and tenting of the skin, which can both be signs of dehydration. Also examine the extremities for any signs of edema. Listen to the heart and evaluate for any irregularities in heart sounds. Also assess the lungs for any sounds of fluid accumulation. An abdominal exam should be done to check for any organ enlargement or bladder fullness.

Treatments

Nonpharmacologic treatments include accurate recording of urine output. The amount of fluid intake should also be recorded, including IV fluid, parenteral nutrition, and oral fluids. Salty foods should be avoided if a fluid volume overload problem is present. Examine the intake and output records for any changes in pattern. Daily weights should also be performed to assess for sudden gains due to fluid accumulation. Laboratory tests should be closely monitored for changes in renal function and electrolyte abnormalities. Alert the physician to any sudden changes in lab findings. Encourage the patient to be as physically active as possible. Instruct the patient in exercises that can be performed in bed if they are not able to get out of bed. Obtain a physical therapy consult if warranted.

Medical treatments are aimed at treating the sequelae of renal impairment. This includes correcting any electrolyte imbalances that occur to prevent potentially life-threatening side effects. Any medications that are to be given should be reviewed for any possible nephrotoxic side effects.

Skin

Role of the Skin in Protecting the Body

The **skin** is the body's primary defense for protection against outer stimuli. The skin is made up of the **epidermis**, **dermis**, and **subcutaneous tissue**. Each layer plays a vital role in protecting the body by serving as a barrier, serving as a carrier of blood vessels and nerves, or providing fatty tissue to protect the body and maintain body temperature.

Excessive moisture can cause a breakdown in the outermost layer of skin, which can provide a portal through which bacteria enter the body and cause infection. The fatty tissue provides a cushion to protect body tissues and organs. It also insulates the body and prevents heat loss. The skin also absorbs nutrients to provide nourishment to the underlying tissues. Some vitamins are also produced within the skin, such as vitamin D due to exposure to sunlight. The skin also serves to cool the body through perspiration and by emanating heat.

History and Physical Exam Findings in Patients with Altered Skin Integrity

When taking a **history** from a patient with a risk for altered skin integrity, be sure to ask about current and past treatments received. Also assess for any complications or side effects from previous treatments. Current medications should be examined for any potential skin effects. Nutritional status should be examined for any muscle wasting or altered fluid or food intake which may deprive the skin of the nutrients necessary to function properly.

- 137 -

On **physical exam**, do a very thorough skin exam and assess for areas of skin breakdown that are already present and those areas that may be at risk. Check for redness or swelling at any pressure points and provide appropriate cushioning to decrease pressure on these areas. Check mental status and the patient's ability to understand the importance of frequent turning in bed or frequent movement to prevent pressure ulcers. Also assess physical activity level; for instance, is the patient able to move on their own or do they require assistance with moving in bed or walking?

Risk Factors for an Alteration in Skin Integrity

- **Primary skin cancer** can cause an alteration in the functions of the skin. It can also lead to destruction of skin cells and tissue.
- A **decrease in platelets** can cause bleeding from blood vessels, which can cause compression of vital structures within the skin and interrupt their function.
- **Radiation treatment** can damage skin cells and cause injury, impairing function.
- Treatment with **steroids** can also impair skin integrity and lead to easy tearing of the skin and bruising.
- Patients frequently receive **cancer treatments via IV.** These medications can be caustic to the skin and lead to inflammation and irritation.
- **Cancer surgery** causes injury to the skin and underlying tissues and may lead to infection at the surgical site. This can cause death or destruction of skin tissue.
- **Impaired mobility** due to illness can cause decubitus ulcers and further skin breakdown.
- **Severe illness** can also cause impaired nutritional status, which can deprive the skin of the fluids and nutrients necessary to function properly.

Pruritus

Physiology

The physiology of **pruritus**, or itching, is similar to that of pain. Some type of **stimulus** is applied, either external or internal in nature. This causes the affected tissues to release histamine from immune cells which also activates the inflammatory process and causes prostaglandins, substance P, and other factors to be released. This causes the transmission of a signal into the spinal cord and then to the brain. The brain responds by releasing naturally produced **opioid-like substances**. The release of these opioid-like substances is responsible for mediating the pruritic response and is the body's natural way of trying to fend off pruritus.

External factors that can cause a pruritic response include radiation, poison ivy, or soaps and detergents. Any item that can stimulate histamine release and the cascade of reactions that leads to an allergic or inflammatory response can cause pruritus. **Internal factors** include medications that cause an allergic reaction manifested in the skin, similar to hives.

Risk Factors

Risk factors for pruritus can be disease-related, treatment-related, or lifestyle-related.

- **Disease-related factors** include prostate cancer, which can cause itching in the genital area, liver cancer that may cause jaundice and severe pruritus all over, and malignant melanoma, which may cause itching at the site of the malignant lesion. Diabetics may also describe an itching sensation in extremities that are affected by diabetic peripheral neuropathy.

- **Treatment-related factors** include any allergic reaction that may occur from medications. This is called a wheal and flare reaction, or hives. Several chemotherapeutic drugs can potentially cause pruritic reactions. Radiation can cause pruritus and skin irritation at the site that is being radiated. Patients who undergo surgery may complain of itching at the surgical incision site.
- **Lifestyle-related factors** include somatic responses to anxiety and depression. If a patient is suffering from profound fatigue, there may be difficulty with simple ADLs and poor hygiene can contribute to pruritus.

History and Physical Exam Findings in Patients with Pruritus

When obtaining a **history** from a patient with pruritus, it is important to ask about anything the patient may be taking or using that is new to them. For example, new medications, personal care items, soaps or detergents. Co-morbidities also need to be considered as a possible source of the pruritus. Also try to find some possible pattern that may be present with the pruritus; is it only present at night, when they are alone, in a certain place, etc.

On **exam**, the patient's skin will often be reddened with or without a rash appearance, possibly with excoriated areas. Assess for the presence of any secondary skin infections which can occur with intense itching causing the skin to break or bleed. Assess the sclera of the eyes for signs of jaundice; in dark-skinned patients, compressing the end of the nose can show yellow discoloration. Lab tests may show a rise in eosinophils on CBC with an allergic reaction, abnormal liver function tests with jaundice, or abnormal glucose levels in diabetic patients.

Treatments

Anti-histamines, such as Benadryl, are the preferred drugs to use to relieve pruritus. However, they can cause sedation, dry mouth, and constipation and care should be used when administering them to elderly patients or patients who are already somewhat sedated due to fatigue or medication side effects. If the pruritus is not widespread and is confined to only one area of the body, **topical steroids** may be used. These help to decrease irritation and inflammation and can be used in conjunction with anti-histamines. A **cool bath** may help to soothe the burning sensation associated with pruritus and help to alleviate the stinging from excoriated skin. Many over-the-counter **oatmeal bath agents**, such as Aveeno, are available to help soothe irritation. The patient should avoid products that have strong perfumes or dyes, which may only increase irritation of the skin. **Sunshine therapy** may also help to reduce the irritation. Low dose **ultraviolet light** is especially helpful with pruritus due to jaundice.

Dyspnea

Dyspnea is the feeling of not being able to breathe or a sensation that not enough air is being drawn in which each breath.

- An obvious disease-related risk factor for dyspnea is any illness that prevents the **respiratory system** from functioning properly. For example, a tumor that compresses the lungs or the airway may cause dyspnea.
- **Co-morbidities** that frequently accompany cancer can affect a patient's ability to breathe effectively. For example, anemia can cause a patient to have an increased respiratory rate to compensate for the decreased oxygen available to the body's tissues.
- **Pain** that may be present from the cancer itself or due to cancer surgery can prevent full expansion of the lungs with deep breathing. A patient may be afraid to take deep breaths because of the pain that accompanies deep inspiration.

- **Anxiety** can also affect the respiratory rate by causing a patient to increase their breathing and start to hyperventilation. This actually leads to a decrease in the amount of oxygen that is drawn in.

History and Physical Exam Findings in Patients with Dyspnea

Dyspnea is subjective and many of the descriptions a patient uses to explain the way they feel can point to a cause. Feelings of a heavy weight on the chest, of pain, of panicking can all help to determine a cause of the dyspnea. History of exposure to pollutants, cigarette smoke, or allergens is necessary when taking a history. If no specific trigger can be found, evaluate what the patient was doing when the dyspneic episode occurred including if they were sitting still, moving around, or sleeping. Also assess what they have done or what medications have been taken to help relieve the symptoms.

On **exam**, obvious difficulty breathing with sitting upright, leaning forward, possibly even panting are all objective signs of dyspnea. When severe, a bluish discoloration around the lips or in the fingertips and toes (cyanosis) may be present. Many patients may have difficulty completing even short sentences without stopping to take a breath.

Risk Factors of Dyspnea Due to Treatment

- One of the most common treatment-related risk factors of dyspnea is **pain**. This can be due to cancer surgery, compression of an organ or nerve by a tumor, or from metastasis of a cancer. Bony metastasis of cancer to the ribs can prevent full expansion of the lungs while breathing.
- Another treatment-related risk factor is an accumulation of **fluid** in the lungs due to a tumor bleeding or due to decreased effectiveness in cardiac function with resultant right-sided heart failure and development of pulmonary edema.
- **Radiation** can cause tissue damage and scarring in the lungs when treatment is focused there, which can cause a decrease in lung expansion and pain with deep breathing.
- **Medications** used to treat cancer can also cause difficulty breathing. Pain medications and anti-anxiety medications (benzodiazepines) can cause respiratory depression and a decreased level of consciousness.
- **Allergic reactions** with respiratory effects can also affect a patient's ability to breathe effectively.

Dyspnea Diagnostic Test Findings

- Pulse oximetry will be decreased, usually below 90%.
- Arterial blood gases can be done to evaluate the serum oxygen level. This may be decreased with an increase in carbon dioxide. Arterial blood gases can also be used to diagnose respiratory acidosis or alkalosis.
- If accompanied with a productive cough, a sputum culture may be obtained for culture and sensitivity testing.
- Chest x-ray can also be done to determine if there is fluid accumulated within the lungs and pleural space.
- If a tumor is suspected, a CT scan may be done for further evaluation.
- Lab tests may be done including chemistry profile, a CBC (especially if an infection is suspected), and thyroid studies.
- If it is determined that a mass is present, a tissue biopsy will be done to determine if it is malignant or not. This is usually done through bronchoscopy or a more invasive thoracotomy for removal of a tumor.

Medical Management of Dyspnea

Maintaining the **airway** is the first priority when managing the patient suffering from dyspnea. Giving supplemental oxygen via nasal cannula or via mask if necessary can help to reduce the patient's feeling of oxygen starvation. Various medications can be given depending on the cause of the dyspnea.

- If due to ***pulmonary edema*** or a fluid overload, administering diuretics can help reduce fluid volume overload. Furosemide (Lasix) is frequently given IV but can cause a decrease in potassium so supplementation is frequently required.
- If dyspnea is due to an increase in ***pulmonary secretions***, nebulizer treatments are frequently administered to cause bronchodilation. These can also cause hypertension and increased heart rate.
- If the dyspnea is due to compression of the lungs or airways by a ***tumor***, consideration may be given to removing the tumor. If a tumor is large, a series of radiation treatments may be given to help shrink the tumor's size before surgical removal.

History and Physical Exam Findings in Patients with Altered Ventilation

Patients who are having difficulty breathing will frequently have **bronchospasm** which causes a persistent cough. They will also experience difficulty breathing with activities. If severe, dyspnea may be present at rest, also. Ask the patient about specific symptoms such as cough, shortness of breath, sputum production with cough, dizziness, and chest pain.

Assess co-morbidities and any treatments they have performed to help treat their breathing difficulties. Ask about the patient's ability to perform basic self-care activities. Also ask about difficulty sleeping because of shortness of breath and if they are able to lie down without breathing becoming more labored.

On **physical exam**, assess the patient's overall difficulty breathing. Many patients will lean forward to breathe easier and may brace their arms on their legs when sitting. Check for any circumoral or nail bed cyanosis. Assess vital signs for elevation in respiratory rate. Listen to the lungs for any wheezing or crackles. Look at the chest wall and back to determine if respiratory effort is equal bilaterally.

Impairments in Ventilation Risk Factors

- **Cancer** involving the lung tissue, pleural cavity, chest wall, or airways will impair a patient's ability to breath. Cancers that involve the neck and a tumor compressing the airway may also affect a patient's ability to take in oxygen. Brain cancers that affect the respiratory center in the brainstem can interfere with regular breathing as can tumors compressing the phrenic nerve, which controls the diaphragm.
- **Radiation treatments** can damage airway and lung tissues, which can decrease the effectiveness of breathing as well as impair the exchange of oxygen within the lungs. Some **chemotherapy medications** are more likely to cause a hypersensitivity response in patients, which can cause swelling of the airways and decreased ability to breath.
- **Surgical removal** of a portion of the lung or chest wall can inhibit breathing.
- Underlying **respiratory or cardiac disease** can also contribute to impairing a patient's respiratory effort.
- The presence of **anxiety** with panic attacks can cause a patient to hyperventilate which causes ineffective breathing.

Pleural Effusion

Causes of Benign and Malignant Effusions

A **pleural effusion** is an accumulation of fluid within the pleural cavity. Patients who have had a pleural effusion in the past are susceptible to developing subsequent, repeated pleural effusions.

Any process that has the potential to cause fluid to leak into the pleural space can cause a pleural effusion.

- When the **heart** does not work effectively as a pump, as with right-sided congestive heart failure, blood can back up into the lungs and cause a pleural effusion.
- **Tissue damage and cell death** within the pleural cavity can cause fluid to leak out of the cells and accumulate within the lungs.
- Some **infections**, like pneumonia, can cause the lungs to secrete more mucus and other secretions. This can also cause a consolidation of fluid within the lungs. Pus-like fluid and mucus can accumulate within the lungs and cause a pleural effusion.
- Some **tumors within the lungs** can bleed and cause fluid to accumulate within the lungs.

Treatments

The **cause** of the pleural effusion should be treated, if possible. If the patient is suffering from congestive heart failure, **diuretics** should be given and cardiac function should be maximized. If infection is the cause, appropriate **antibiotics** should be given. If the infection appears to be resistant to treatment, a culture and sensitivity of the patient's sputum should be performed.

If these measures do not help to treat the pleural effusion, a **thoracentesis** may be done, in which a needle is inserted into the pleural cavity and fluid is withdrawn from the space. Thoracentesis can help by making the patient more comfortable and relieving severe shortness of breath. Unfortunately, patients who develop a pleural effusion that requires thoracentesis may require this procedure to be done repeatedly as the pleural effusions is likely to reoccur. A chest tube may also be inserted to help drain fluid from the pleural cavity. This is set to suction to promote drainage.

Peripheral Neuropathy

Pathophysiology
- Any cancers that affect the nervous system can lead to **peripheral neuropathy**.
- **Nerve compression** due to a tumor encapsulating a nerve or on a surrounding structure and causing pressure on a nerve can lead to nerve pain.
- Any **tumors more proximal on a nerve** can interrupt the signal traveling down a nerve and lead to peripheral pain also.
- **Treatments** can cause damage or destruction to nerves and lead to nerve pain.
- **Alterations** can occur in neurotransmitters at the synaptic junction where nerve impulses travel. This can cause an alteration in sensory perception and ultimately pain.
- **Decreased nutrients to nerve cells** can alter their function and result in pain or dysfunction also.
- Some nerves have a myelin sheath surrounding them, which aids in protection and transmission of nerve signals. **Cancers** and other diseases affecting the myelin sheath can cause distortion of the nerve signal and lead to peripheral nerve pain.

<u>Risk Factors</u>

- Any **cancers** affecting the nervous system can lead to nerve pain. For patients who had peripheral neuropathy before the cancer diagnosis, this can be quite severe. This can be due to diabetes, vascular disease, and other causes.
- **Edema** in joint spaces can cause excessive pressure to be applied to the nerves and result in pain.
- **Chemotherapeutic medications**, and other medications, can cause nerve damage and result in nerve pain.
- **Radiation** can also cause nerve irritation and damage which leads to chronic pain.
- Underlying **depression** or anxiety can exacerbate pain sensations and cause the pain to be perceived as being more severe.
- The stress on the **immune system** that occurs with cancer can lead to the development of shingles, or a herpes zoster infection. Occasionally a permanent nerve pain can develop after the shingles rash has resolved, called postherpetic neuralgia. This can be quite severe and will be located at the site of the shingles infection.

<u>History and Physical Exam Findings in Patients with Neuropathy</u>

It is important to question the patient about any pre-existing conditions that may be present, especially diabetes, thyroid disorders, or vitamin B_{12} deficiency. Any treatments that the patient is undergoing or has received are also important, such as chemotherapy or radiation. Assess the patient's symptoms such as burning, tingling, or decreased sensation and assess triggering factors, if any. Also question the patient about any change in motor skills or balance.

On **physical exam**, do an overall exam on the patient and observe their gait, balance, and any objective signs of pain. Assess motor function and strength in all four extremities to ensure that strength is appropriate for age and build. Test the patient for any sensory deficits by using a monofilament for light touch and a safety pin for sharp sensation testing. Examine the skin for any color changes or changes in hair distribution. Deep tendon reflexes should be assessed in all four extremities also. Chemotherapy-induced peripheral neuropathy (CIPN) is a common side effect that often causes both physical and emotional symptoms. Healthcare providers must be diligent and proactive in their assessment of CIPN. Patients receiving chemotherapy should be assessed for CIPN at every visit. Upper extremity symptoms can be present, although not as common as deficits in the lower extremities. Physical and occupational therapies should be included in the treatment plan for those patients experiencing neuropathy causing physical limitations.

Nutritional Assessment

<u>Reasons for Nutritional Assessment</u>

Nutritional assessment is done to evaluate several factors:

1. To screen for **potential problems** with nutrition.
2. To recognize patients with existing nutritional deficits.
3. To look at the **nutritional necessities** for the patient.
4. To see the **body's reaction** to diet already given.

Physical factors influencing nutrition begin with the ingestion of food. Ingestion begins with appetite (which may be nonexistent), chewing of the food, swallowing of the food (both may be altered by the cancer process or the type cancer) and the effects of digestion of the food (altered by cancer or its produced substances or by the therapy) also. Obviously, to combat the cancer a normally functioning and uncompromised digestive system needs to be present. A normally cycling blood glucose level must be maintained. Anything that affects blood glucose level also directly affects nutritional status.

<u>Assessing Nutritional Status</u>

On **physical exam** the patient's overall *hydration* and *body mass* **status** should be evaluated. This includes evaluation for signs of dehydration which can cause dry mouth, tenting of the skin, and changes in mental status. Body weight should be assessed regularly for excessive weight gain or weight loss. Fat measurements should also be done using calipers. Also assess the patient for any loss of muscle mass.

Laboratory data is used to assure that proper nutritional needs are being met without causing any type of metabolic imbalance. Albumin and total protein levels are used to assure that TPN is meeting the protein needs of the patient to prevent loss of muscle mass. Glucose levels are monitored regularly for hyper- or hypoglycemia. Insulin may be given with the TPN if hyperglycemia is a chronic problem. Other lab tests include a chemistry panel to assess electrolytes and renal/liver status, and CBC and iron levels to assess for anemia.

Taste Alteration, Hypogeusia, Dysgeusia, and Ageusia

- **Taste alteration** is a modification in the way a person perceives taste or may involve a complete deficit of taste sensation. This can be due to treatments with radiation or medications, or may be due to surgical changes involving the mouth and taste buds.
- **Hypogeusia** describes a diminished sense of taste. This may be only temporary and normal taste sensation may return after treatments, or other causes, are completed.
- **Dysgeusia** is an alteration in the way a person interprets taste. This may involve a certain food or flavor that was pleasant to the person, but is now sensed to be distasteful. Some medications can cause a metallic taste in the patient's mouth, which may alter the taste of foods and drinks.
- **Ageusia** is the complete loss of taste perception. This can be due to damage to the taste buds on the tongue because of surgical removal of the tongue because of malignancy or because of radiation treatments that cause permanent damage to the taste buds.

Alteration in Taste Sensation Risk Factors

- **Cancer tumors** can cause alterations in taste, especially when the mouth and throat are involved. Tumors in the mouth can affect the taste buds and cause them to not function correctly or not function at all. Cancers that cause an infection can also affect the sense of taste.
- **Cancer surgery** can alter the sensation of taste by removal of taste buds. Also, any surgery involving removal of the salivary glands can lead to an alteration in the perception of taste.
- **Radiation** to the mouth and throat can cause tissue damage and possibly alteration in the taste buds which will affect taste sensations.
- **Chemotherapy** can also cause changes in taste perception, most frequently causing a metal taste in the patient's mouth which interferes with eating. Chemotherapy may also cause nausea and vomiting which may affect how the patient perceives certain foods. If a patient has had some nausea and vomiting with certain foods, they may perceive a change in the way they taste because of the unpleasant experience.

Preventing or Decreasing an Alteration in Taste

Question the patient regarding which foods they enjoyed eating before the alteration in taste occurred. Try to supply these foods, if possible and if not contraindicated. Also try flavoring foods differently to obtain a desirable flavor for the patient. Obtain a **dietary consult** to assist the patient in choosing foods that will be palatable while still meeting all the necessary nutritional requirements.

Try to prevent any **stimulus** in the patient's environment that may exaggerate this alteration in taste. Remove any triggers that may be present that have caused the patient to experience changes in taste. Try to time medical treatments away from regular eating times to help with any perceived changes the patient may experience.

If a decrease in salivation is the cause of the patient's alteration in taste, try **promoting saliva excretion**. Offer frequent sips of water or hard candies for the patient to use to help with saliva production.

Hypercalcemia and Hypocalcemia

Pathophysiology

Hypercalcemia is an increased level of calcium in the serum, **>10.5 mg/dL.** Calcium levels within the bloodstream are controlled by many factors, one of which is parathyroid hormone. This causes calcium to be reabsorbed by the bones if the level is too high or causes it to escape the bones and enter the circulating bloodstream if levels are too low. Any tumors affecting this process can alter calcium levels and cause an elevated calcium level. Calcium is excreted by the renal system and any alteration in kidney function could result in hypercalcemia.

Hypocalcemia *(serum calcium of < 8.5 mg/dL)* can be caused by under-secretion of parathyroid hormone, resulting in more calcium remaining in the bones and less being circulated into the bloodstream. Calcium requires vitamin D to be present in order to be absorbed in the GI tract. A vitamin D deficiency can lead to hypocalcemia. This can also result from an alteration in renal function. There are certain cancer medications that can also cause a decrease in calcium levels.

Symptoms

Calcium is necessary for normal function of nerves and muscles. Any alteration in the calcium levels will affect these actions in the body. If the calcium level is too high, as with **hypercalcemia**, you can see an increase in heart rate. The patient will have changes in mental status with lethargy and somnolence being present. There may be a decrease in the peripheral reflexes because of malfunction in nerve transmissions. The patient may also develop a decrease in kidney function which can result in decreased urinary output.

With **hypocalcemia** there is excitability of the nervous system. The patient may exhibit spasm of the facial muscles (a positive Chvostek's sign). Mental status will be altered and the patient may even experience hallucinations. The heart rate may become irregular and changes may be present on EKG. Muscle spasms can also occur, even in the smooth muscle such as the bronchial passages, which could lead to respiratory arrest.

Treatments

Treating **hypercalcemia** is accomplished through administering IV fluids and giving medications such as steroids and gallium. Close monitoring should be done to assess renal function and any EKG changes that may be present. The patient should be encouraged to increase activity levels and perform light exercise as tolerated. This helps to build bone density and prevent weakening of the bones due to a decrease in calcium content.

Hypocalcemia can be treated with calcium replacement if calcium levels have dropped dangerously low. The patient must be closely monitored for mental status changes, EKG changes, and any changes in motor activity. Serum calcium values should be monitored regularly to assess for resolution of the condition and to detect if the calcium levels are decreasing further. Seizures precautions may be necessary if the patient is developing alterations in motor activity. Once calcium levels have begun correcting themselves and are beginning to return to normal, the patient may need to take oral calcium supplements to maintain normal serum calcium levels.

Hypermagnesemia and Hypomagnesemia

Magnesium is responsible for maintaining electrolyte concentrations within cells. If there is an alteration in magnesium, there may also be alterations in other electrolytes, such as potassium and sodium.

Hypermagnesemia is defined as a *serum magnesium level >2.5 mg/dL*. Magnesium is obtained from foods as they pass through the GI tract, but it is excreted in the urine. Renal dysfunction that results in a decrease in urine output can result in increased magnesium levels.

Hypomagnesemia is defined as a *serum magnesium level <1.8 mg/dL*. Magnesium is stored in the liver. Liver failure can cause the magnesium stores to be depleted and result in a lowered magnesium level. Some medications, like certain antibiotics and diuretics, can cause a decrease in magnesium levels. Since magnesium is responsible for maintaining electrolyte levels within the cells, changes in magnesium levels can also result in decrease in potassium and sodium levels. Magnesium has an adverse relationship with calcium levels, so if there is an increase in calcium, there will be a concomitant decrease in magnesium.

Symptoms

The symptoms for hypermagnesemia and hypomagnesemia are very similar to each other. Both conditions can cause changes in the **neurologic system** with changes in **mental status** and **somnolence**. There can also be decreased nervous system activity as evidenced by decreased reflexes. With hypomagnesemia, the nervous system symptoms can become severe enough that seizure activity can be present. There can be a vasodilation effect that causes erythema and hypotension. Respiratory changes may be evident with a decrease in respiratory rate and increased difficulty with taking effective breaths. With hypomagnesemia, there may also be signs of decreased potassium and sodium levels. These include nausea and vomiting, muscle cramps, seizures, tingling of the extremities, and EKG changes with cardiac dysrhythmias.

If hypomagnesemia is present and is due to an increase in calcium levels, symptoms of hypercalcemia may be present. These include mental status changes, increased heart rate, decrease in reflexes, and renal dysfunction.

Treatments

To treat **hypermagnesemia**, diuretics are often given to increase excretion of magnesium through the urine. This can also cause an increase in potassium excretion, though, so laboratory tests should be frequently monitored to achieve the desired effect without causing too large a decrease in magnesium or potassium. Sodium levels should also be monitored to ensure levels do not become too low with increased magnesium excretion.

To treat **hypomagnesemia**, magnesium sulfate can be given. There are also medications that help to decrease the amount of magnesium that is excreted through the renal and urinary systems. Again, laboratory tests should be closely monitored to ensure the desired effect is achieved without increasing magnesium levels dangerously. Potassium and sodium levels should also be closely monitored to ensure these remain within normal limits. If a patient has primary hypercalcemia, magnesium levels should be monitored while the disorder is being treated to prevent a dangerous increase in magnesium levels.

Hypernatremia and Hyponatremia

<u>Pathophysiology</u>

Sodium is the main electrolyte present in plasma. Its serum levels are monitored by receptors in the body that stimulate changes in the body's water content. Management of sodium levels is accomplished by changes in absorption and excretion in the renal system. Hormonal control of sodium is accomplished through ADH, or antidiuretic hormone, secreted by the adrenal glands.

Hypernatremia *(serum sodium > 145 mg/dL)* can be caused by a decrease in fluid intake or dehydration. Diabetes insipidus can result in changes in ADH levels which can alter sodium regulation. Renal dysfunction can alter the excretion of sodium and result in higher levels within the blood stream. An increase in magnesium can also cause an increase in sodium levels.

Hyponatremia *(serum sodium < 135 mg/dL)* is due to changes in ADH, as seen with SIADH (syndrome of inappropriate ADH) and suddenly stopping steroid treatment without tapering the medication. A decrease in magnesium levels can also cause a decrease in sodium levels.

<u>Symptoms</u>

The symptoms of whatever is causing the electrolyte imbalance will be the symptoms seen with **hypernatremia**. If renal dysfunction is contributing to increased water wasting, increased urinary output will be present. If dehydration is the cause, excessive sweating and a dryness of the oral mucosa can be present. The patient may also have had some nausea and vomiting with a decrease in oral fluid intake if that is the cause of the dehydration. Nervous system effects include changes in mental status with irritability, somnolence, and, if severe, seizures. There may also be decreases in the deep tendon reflexes.

Symptoms of **hyponatremia** can vary from mild, nonspecific symptoms to severe symptoms with seizures and coma depending on the severity of the illness. Mild hyponatremia will result in nausea and vomiting and other vague flu-like symptoms. Moderate hyponatremia causes muscular effects of weakness and muscle pain. Severe hyponatremia causes changes in mental status with lethargy and psychosis. If severe, seizures can occur that may lead to coma and possibly even death.

<u>Treatments</u>

Treatment of sodium imbalances should focus on treating whatever is causing the change in sodium levels. If sodium levels are **increased**, treat the patient for dehydration if this is the cause. Provide IV fluids to correct the imbalance if the renal system will allow this. If caused by increases in magnesium levels, then the hypermagnesemia should be treated.

Decreases in the sodium level may be dilutional effects from over-hydration. Fluid restrictions can be implemented to return the sodium levels to normal. If severe, IV fluids with high sodium content can be administered along with a diuretic to increase fluid output. If an abnormality in the amount of ADH is present, as with SIADH, an antibiotic can be given to correct this. If the SIADH is due to malignancy, treatment of the cancer can help to correct the condition and normalize sodium levels.

- 147 -

Significant diuresis may need to be accomplished if fluid overload is causing a dilutional hyponatremia.

Hyperkalemia and Hypokalemia

Pathophysiology

Potassium is different in that the body has no way to prevent excretion of potassium in order to maintain normal potassium levels. Potassium is the main electrolyte present within blood cells. It has an adverse relationship with sodium so that an increase in potassium causes a decrease in sodium.

Hyperkalemia is defined as a ***serum potassium level > 5.5 mg/dL***. Potassium is excreted through urine so any dysfunction of the renal system that results in a decrease in urine output can result in increased serum potassium levels. Because potassium is the main electrolyte in blood cells, any process that causes blood cell destruction, such as hemolytic anemia, can cause a rise in potassium levels. Various medications can lead to hyperkalemia.

Hypokalemia is defined as a ***serum potassium level < 3.5 mg/dL***. Increased excretion of potassium, such as with diuretics or through diarrhea and vomiting, can cause decreased levels of potassium. Various antibiotics can also cause hypokalemia.

Symptoms

Both hyperkalemia and hypokalemia can cause the same neuromuscular symptoms of weakness, lethargy, diminished reflexes, and tingling of the extremities. **Hyperkalemia** also causes decreased heart rate and cardiac dysrhythmias. EKG changes can be evident with a wide QRS complex and elevated T waves. GI symptoms can be present with nausea, vomiting, and diarrhea. Because sodium and potassium have an adverse relationship, a decrease in sodium can cause hyperkalemia and result in mild to severe symptoms ranging from nausea and vomiting to coma and death.

Hypokalemia can also have cardiac effects with cardiac dysrhythmias and an increased heart rate. Decreased blood pressure may also be present along with mental status changes. If potassium levels drop severely low, fatal cardiac dysrhythmias can occur with cardiac arrest. EKG changes include flattened T waves and ST depression, similar to cardiac ischemia. An increase in sodium levels can cause hypokalemia and increased mental status changes, somnolence, and possibly seizures.

Treatments

Treatment of **hyperkalemia** is achieved by increasing the excretion of potassium. This can be done with diuretics that increase potassium excretion through urine. Kayexalate binds with potassium to increase secretion and can be given rectally by enema. This will cause increased excretion of potassium through the GI tract. IV fluids high in glucose concentration can cause potassium to move from the extracellular to the intracellular space. Laboratory tests should be closely monitored to assess effectiveness of the treatment and prevent abnormalities in other electrolyte levels during treatment. Hypokalemia can also develop if treatment is too aggressive, so potassium levels should be closely monitored.

Hypokalemia can be treated with IV solutions with added potassium chloride. This may be caustic to the veins so monitor for irritation at the IV site and for infiltration of the IV fluid. Potassium-rich foods can also be given to increase intake of potassium. Closely monitor for signs and symptoms of hyperkalemia, especially cardiac effects. Other electrolyte levels, especially sodium, should be closely monitored for abnormalities.

- 148 -

Weight Change

Cancer-Related Weight Gain

Weight gain can result from **fluid accumulation**. There can also be **electrolyte imbalances** that result in fluid retention and increased weight. **Decreased renal function** can also cause fluid retention as urine excretion is decreased, resulting in increased weight. **Tumors** that secrete hormones can cause fluctuations in weight. Treatment with **steroids** can stimulate appetite and cause an increase in weight. Several **chemotherapy medications** can also contribute to weight gain. Treatments that impair **physical activity**, such as surgery, can result in weight gain because of decreased exercise. As cancer progresses, it may be harder for a patient to perform regular exercise, resulting in weight gain.

Psychological changes in a patient can contribute to weight gain. Many people respond to feelings of depression by increasing food intake as a means of comfort. This, accompanied with decreased physical activity, can result in weight gain. Feelings of anxiety may also cause a patient to decrease physical activity.

Cancer-Related Weight Loss

The cancer-related causes of weight loss:

- **Cancer** affecting the GI tract can result in weight loss. This may compress organs and inhibit patients from eating as much food as they normally would.
- **Cancer surgeries** can result in pain and decreased ability to eat, which could result in weight loss. A patient may also have decreased absorption of nutrients following gastric surgery to remove a tumor. If unable to eat food because of dysphagia or absorption issues, total parenteral nutrition may need to be used but there is a risk of decreased nutritional needs being met.
- **Cancer treatment** with chemotherapy and radiation can result in nausea and vomiting with a decrease in appetite, which can result in decreased intake and weight loss. Cachexia can also result with severe muscle wasting.
- The presence of **concomitant illness and infections** can result in decreased appetite and weight loss. Some medications can result in feelings of nausea and decreased appetite.

Dietary consultation should be obtained to evaluate causes of weight loss and formulate a treatment plan.

History and Physical Exam Findings in Patients with Weight Changes

On **history**, assess the patient's food preferences and accommodate these, if possible. Question the patient about certain triggering events that may cause nausea, vomiting, and food aversions. Ask the patient about the trend in weight loss and how quickly this has occurred. Ask about any changes that have occurred that seemed to lead to the weight loss and cachexia. Assess which treatments the patient is currently undergoing or has undergone in the past. Evaluate for any co-morbidities that may be contributing to weight loss.

On **physical exam**, regular weights should be assessed to determine if the weight loss is ongoing and if there is any response to treatment designed to promote weight gain. Evaluate the patient's mobility and if they are able to move independently since developing muscle loss. Evaluate for dehydration and treat accordingly.

Laboratory tests should be regularly monitored for any electrolyte abnormalities and any liver or renal dysfunction. Check serum albumin and total protein levels to assess for muscle wasting.

- 149 -

Cachexia

Cachexia is the condition in which excessive weight loss with depletion of muscle mass occurs due to decreased intake of nutrients necessary for the body to function appropriately.

- *Primary cachexia* occurs as a result of several factors occurring at once. The patient may experience anorexia with decreased appetite. This can lead to electrolyte and metabolic abnormalities that cause the release of several inflammatory cells by the immune system. The metabolic abnormalities include changes in the way glucose is metabolized and changes in the metabolic rate. This causes weight loss and can lead to cachexia.
- *Secondary cachexia* occurs as a result of other factors. This includes nausea and vomiting from treatments that lead to weight loss and depletion of muscle mass. Malabsorption syndromes can occur as a result of tumors or after cancer surgery in which the surface area of the GI tract through which nutrients are absorbed is decreased, resulting in a decreased amount of nourishment.

Treatment

Treating the underlying **cause** should be the focus of treatment. If medications or treatments are leading to nausea and vomiting and aversions to foods, try not to time these around meal times, if possible. Offer **foods** that the patient finds pleasurable to increase intake and promote weight gain. If the patient is not able to eat, total parenteral nutrition (TPN) or tube feedings via a PEG tube may be necessary to reverse poor nutritional status and cachexia.

Medications can be used to stimulate appetite. These include steroids, if not contraindicated, and Reglan which will promote gastric emptying and decrease the sensation of feeling full.

Though controversial and not legal in some states, **cannabis** (marijuana) can stimulate appetite and decrease nausea. This is used by some cancer patients to help promote eating and weight gain.

Any metabolic abnormalities should be treated. Renal status should be closely monitored to assess for any dysfunction.

Effects That Cancer Treatments Have on Nutritional Status Patients

- **Chemotherapy** can cause a decrease in appetite with nausea and vomiting which will have an impact on a patient's nutritional status. Weakness and fatigue from anemia due to chemotherapy can cause the patient to have so little energy that they are just physically not able to eat.
- **Radiation** can cause pain if focused near the neck or throat. It can also alter the taste buds and cause food to taste differently, which may affect appetite.
- **Surgery** can affect nutritional status by possibly removing a portion of or all of an organ, causing an alteration in the digestive tract. There can also be a problem with dumping syndrome, which occurs when food "dumps" from the stomach and through the GI tract immediately after eating. This causes diarrhea and cramping. Surgeries performed on the mouth, jaw, or throat can impair the physical act of eating and chewing, which will affect nutritional status.

Pathophysiology of the Effects of Cancer on Nutrition and Metabolism

Cancer cells need energy to function and they will fight with normal cells for **nutrients** needed to thrive. Tumor cells will alter the **metabolism** of glucose to produce the types of nutrients that are necessary for energy for cancer cells. There is also an increase in glucose metabolism in order to support the tumor. The tumor cells cause the body to not respond to glucose like it should so that less is used by the body's normal cells, leaving more for the cancer cells.

There is an increase in the **breakdown of protein** in the body's muscle tissue in order to provide more nutrition to cancer cells. This results in muscle wasting and profound weight loss.

Cancer also causes a **decrease in appetite**, which can lead to more weight loss and failure to provide the body with the nutrients necessary to function appropriately.

Large tumors can cause **pressure on organs**, leading to **pain** which can decrease appetite or lead to inability of the body to breakdown food because of organ malfunction.

Enteral Feeding

Enteral feeding is done when food is given to a patient via the digestive system but not delivered through the mouth. This can be accomplished through a ***PEG tube*** in the abdomen or through a ***nasogastric (NG) tube***. Enteral feeding is considered when a patient can no longer feed themselves and it is expected that this route of delivery will be necessary for an extended period of time.

Formulas used in enteral feedings are specially designed based on the patient's nutritional needs. These can be high in protein or low in protein, or based on a diabetic diet. Some formulas are designed for specific illnesses, for example, a special respiratory diet or a diet specifically designed for those patients with renal failure. The patient's ability to digest foods needs to be considered when choosing the best formula for enteral feedings. Formulas are available for a digestive tract that is functioning normally and for a digestive system that has a malfunction in absorbing nutrients.

Possible Adverse Effects of Enteral Feeding

An enteral feeding tube can be placed in the **wrong location**, particularly with a nasogastric tube. It is possible that an NG tube can enter the airway instead of the esophagus. After initially inserting the tube placement, location is confirmed by aspirating contents from the NG tube and testing for pH. An x-ray can also be performed to verify placement, and is the most definitive method of confirmation. Of note, former methods of confirming placement, including auscultation during air bolus over the epigastrium or flushing with 30 mL of normal saline, are not acceptable ways to confirm placement of an NGT. Always confirm the placement of a tube that will be used to give medications or feeding with radiographical evidence.

Aspiration is also a concern with enteral feeding. Always be sure the patient is not lying flat during and immediately after feedings to prevent regurgitation and subsequent aspiration of the formula.

With a PEG tube, there is the **risk of infection** at the tube site. Care should be taken to keep the site clean and free of any leaking gastric contents.

An enteral feeding tube can become **blocked** with thickened formula and may be severe enough to require changing of the tube. The tube should be flushed well before and after giving meds or formula through it to prevent clogging.

Parenteral Feeding

Parenteral nutrition is administered through an IV line and is for short-term use, usually less than 30 days. This is usually infused through a central line or PICC line. The specific type of fluid used, called **TPN (total parenteral nutrition)**, is designed to meet the nutritional needs of the patient. The amount of glucose, protein, and fat can be adjusted through different types of formula.

Possible Adverse Effects of Parenteral Feeding

The **possible adverse effects** related to parenteral nutrition are problems that can arise due to the central line or PICC line placement. These include the risk of pneumothorax with a central line, an infection at the site of the line placement, or blockage occurring in the line. Blood sugars can also vary with TPN and levels need to be monitored regularly while a patient is receiving parenteral nutrition. It is not unusual for a patient to receive insulin, usually directly infused through the line, to help with glucose metabolism while TPN is being used.

Change in Mental Status

- Any **cancer affecting the brain** can cause changes in mental status and mood. This can be a metastatic lesion from another primary cancer source or a primary brain cancer, such as a glioblastoma multiforme.
- Patients with **traumatic brain injuries or dementia** will also exhibit mental status changes. As can those with a past history of **cerebrovascular accidents** or TIAs.
- **Sepsis** can affect a patient's mental capacity as can infections affecting the central nervous system, such as meningitis.
- **Renal failure** and severe liver failure can also cause changes in mental status due to alterations in metabolism.
- **Medical treatments** can cause changes in mental status, such as chemotherapy and radiation. These changes may be permanent or temporary. Pain medications can cause transient changes in mental status as a potential side effect.
- Any **fluid or electrolyte imbalances**, especially with decreases in sodium or potassium, can lead to mental status changes.
- **Alcohol or drug use** for self-medication can cause transient or permanent changes in a patient's mental capacities.

History and Physical Exam Findings in Patients with an Alteration in Mental Status

A thorough **history** should include questions regarding current medical conditions and past and present treatments. Family members or friends/significant others may need to be questioned if the patient is not able to answer questions on his own. Assess if the patient uses alcohol or drugs on a regular basis. Ask family members whether the patient suffers mental changes at different times of the day, such as with sun downing. Assess the patient's pain level, using a 0-10 scale, to determine if excessive pain could be causing changes in their mental status.

On **physical exam**, assess the patient's mental status using cognitive testing such as 3-word recall, naming objects, and orientation to date, time, and place. Be sure to include questions that test not only the present, but long-term memory also. Correct answers to these questions may need to be acquired from family members who are present. Laboratory tests should be assessed for any signs of infection with an elevated WBC, any changes in endocrine dysfunction, and any electrolyte imbalances.

Fatigue

Fatigue is an overwhelming state of exhaustion and a decrease in physical and mental tolerance that is not relieved by rest. Fatigue is common in cancer patients and is not fully understood. It is usually a chronic condition.

<u>Physiologic Causes</u>

Fatigue may result from:

- **Cachexia** (profound weight loss and wasting of the body muscle). This leads to a decrease in strength and energy, which makes it difficult to perform even simple everyday activities.
- **Anemia** is a common cause of fatigue and is one of the side effects of chemotherapy. Blood cell production is stimulated by a substance called erythropoietin, which is decreased in anemia. Erythropoietin has been found to have neuroprotective qualities that can have positive mental effects. Decreased amounts of erythropoietin have been found to contribute to impaired cognitive abilities.
- **Infection** and **depression** can also contribute to fatigue.
- **Pain** is another factor that can contribute to an overall sense of fatigue and lack of energy.

<u>Risk Factors</u>

Risk factors for fatigue can be categorized as disease-related, treatment-related, or lifestyle-related.

1. **Disease-related fatigue** is the most common symptom present in cancer patients. Fatigue can occur in any stage of the illness and can be exacerbated by other conditions that occur such as electrolyte imbalances, anemia, dehydration, and pain.
2. **Treatment-related fatigue** is very common with chemotherapy, and in fact, it is the most common side effect of chemotherapy. It usually peaks within the first few days of treatment and will recur with each cycle of chemotherapy. This fatigue is most likely due to chemotherapy-induced anemia and nausea. Immunotherapy with such drugs as Interferon or Interleukin-2 will rarely cause fatigue. Radiation leads to fatigue in nearly all patients and is progressively cumulative throughout therapy. Surgery can cause fatigue due to pain, alteration in nutritional status, and apprehension regarding diagnosis.
3. **Lifestyle-related fatigue** can be due to anxiety, depression, financial pressures due to illness, and inactivity.

<u>Physical Exam and Diagnostic Test Findings in Fatigued Patients</u>

On exam, a patient who is suffering from fatigue would appear tired. They may have difficulty concentrating during a conversation, dark circles may appear under the eyes, and even basic hygiene may suffer if a patient has difficulty completing ADLs due to fatigue. It is important to assess the patient's mental status with special attention to possible depression. Evaluate **cognition** using three-word recall, counting backwards, level of orientation (name, date, place, time), and short-term and long-term memory. **Lab findings** that may appear abnormal will be reflective of the cause of the fatigue. For example, a decrease in red blood cell count (RBC), hemoglobin (Hgb), and hematocrit (Hct) are all indicative of anemia which is a likely cause of the fatigue. Pulse oximetry or arterial blood gases (ABGs) may show a decrease in oxygen or an increase in carbon dioxide (CO_2). **Chemistry studies** may reveal hypoglycemia, hyponatremia, and hypercalcemia. **Thyroid studies** should also be done to see if hypothyroidism could be a cause of the fatigue.

<u>Managing Fatigue</u>

To aid in **minimizing fatigue**, the oncology nurse can:

1. Institute regular bedtimes.
2. Monitor weight.
3. Provide frequent small meals to improve nutrition.
4. Control other symptoms that enhance or contribute to fatigue.

5. Schedule more time with family members.
6. Encourage meditation/prayer.
7. Schedule exercise periods.
8. Utilize distraction tactics, even for short periods of time.

Anemia Treatment Medications

- **Red blood cell (RBC) growth factors**, such as Epogen or Procrit, can be given to promote production of blood cells within the bone marrow. Side effects include pain at the injection site, headache, hypertension, edema, and paresthesia.
- **Aranesp** is another medication that stimulates the bone marrow to produce more RBCs. It is given less frequently than Epogen or Procrit because it has a longer half-life. Side effects include fatigue, hypertension, edema, nausea, and diarrhea.
- **Stimulants**, such as Ritalin and Provigil, may help to reduce the symptoms of fatigue, but do not treat the actual cause of the disorder.
- **Herbal remedies** along with vitamins are frequently used to treat fatigue. B-complex vitamins, iron, and amino acids can be helpful in treating the symptoms. With fatigue due to anemia, a blood transfusion may be considered if the anemia becomes severe. Continual monitoring of the RBC along with hemoglobin and hematocrit needs to be done to assess if a transfusion is warranted.

Nonpharmacologic Ways to Treat Fatigue

Administering **oxygen** provides oxygen-starved cells with the oxygen necessary for them to function properly. Hemoglobin is responsible for transporting oxygen throughout the body to the tissues. The **hemoglobin count** is decreased with anemia, meaning there is less oxygen being transported to the tissues. Administering oxygen helps to maximize the amount of oxygen being transported by the hemoglobin. Proper **diet** along with an appropriate balance of exercise and rest is very important in treating fatigue. A diet high in nutritional foods, especially those high in iron, will provide the necessary energy the body needs. Some light form of **exercise** is necessary, depending on the condition of the patient, in order to maintain adequate blood circulation, maintain metabolic levels, and to stretch muscles. **Rest** helps to rejuvenate the body and allow it time to heal and restore energy levels. **Emotional support** also helps to relieve fatigue by reducing stress and anxiety. A strong support team can help with mental well-being as well as provide the physical and mental assistance needed.

> **Review Video: Fatigue Severity Scale**
> Visit mometrix.com/academy and enter code: 451022

Sleep

Stages of Sleep

There are **two main stages of sleep**. Non-rapid eye movement, or non-REM sleep, and rapid eye movement, or REM sleep.

1. **Non-REM sleep** is further divided into four sub-categories. *Stage 1* is the phase between being awake and being asleep. It is not a restful period of sleep and does not usually last very long. Stage 2 of non-REM sleep is true, deep sleep. Stages 3 and 4 is the phase of sleep in which delta waves, or slow waves, are evident on electroencephalograms. These are the restful stages of sleep. A person passes through all four of these stages before returning to stage 3 and then stage 2.

2. At that point, **REM sleep** begins. This phase is characterized by rapid eye movements and is the phase in which dreams occur. REM sleep usually lasts approximately 90 minutes and a person returns to this phase of sleep several times during the night.

Processes that Regulate Sleep

There are hormonal and environmental factors that influence the mechanism of sleep.

- The hormone **melatonin** is released by the pineal gland in the brain. It regulates the natural circadian rhythm of a person to trigger sleepiness at night and wakefulness during the day. Levels tend to increase at the end of the day to promote sleep. A decrease in melatonin has been found in people suffering from depression. Melatonin secretion decreases with age, which can be a contributing factor to the poor sleep habits that many elderly people experience.
- Environmental factors that influence sleep include trying to reverse the **natural circadian rhythm** and the actual **physical environment** in which a person tries to sleep. Many people who work nights need to sleep during the day when it is light, which can be very difficult because it goes against the natural circadian rhythm instilled within us. Excessive noise, an area that feels too hot or too cold, and increased stress or anxiety can also interfere with the natural sleep process.

Sleep Disorder Risk Factors

Risk factors for a sleep disorder can be disease-related, treatment-related, or psychosocial.

- Many **cancer patients** suffer from lack of sleep. This can be due to symptoms from their illness, such as pain, nausea, and itching. Patients suffering from cancers that have effects on the respiratory system may experience shortness of breath. Electrolyte imbalances can cause muscle cramping which may prevent a person from sleeping peacefully.
- **Treatment-related risk factors** include the side effects that a person may experience from chemotherapeutic agents or radiation. These include pain, pruritus, and nausea. If a patient has undergone cancer surgery, pain or constipation may also be issues. Any extended hospital stay can interfere with a normal sleep cycle because of being in an unfamiliar environment, away from those things that are relaxing and comforting.
- **Psychosocial issues** affecting a patient's sleep pattern include anxiety, family stressors, stress from fear of the unknown and what course the illness will follow.

History and Physical Exam Findings in Patients with a Sleep Disorder

When obtaining a **history** from a patient with a sleep disorder, clarify any type of night time routine the person may have. Establish whether there is a regular set of activities that are performed each night before bed, such as reading, listening to soft music, drinking milk, or a personal care routine. Ask the patient if they having trouble falling asleep or staying asleep. Inquire about the environment in which they sleep; is there a spouse or partner who likes to read or watch TV in bed when they are trying to sleep? Ask about any smoking or drinking habits that may interfere with sleep, as well as what prescription or over-the-counter medications they have tried in the past.

On **physical exam**, some of the same findings in the patient with fatigue will also be present in the patient with a sleep disorder. Sleep deprivation can interfere with mental functioning and concentration. A patient may exhibit slurred speech, difficulty carrying on a conversation, or difficulty with decision making.

Sleep Disorder Pharmacologic Treatments

The best treatment for a sleep disorder is to treat the **cause**, whether that is due to symptoms of an illness or environmental changes that need to be made. When these conservative measures do not work, medications may need to be prescribed. The two main types of drugs which are prescribed are sedative/hypnotics and antidepressants with sedative-like qualities.

- **Sedative/hypnotics** include Ambien, Lunesta, and benzodiazepines. All of these medications can cause a physical tolerance and dependence. Many patients complain of feeling groggy several hours after taking these medications and elderly patients may have a problem with an accumulation of the drug in their system which results in more intense side effects.
- **Antidepressants** used to treat sleep disorders include Remeron and trazodone (Desyrel). These can have the same side effect of residual grogginess the morning after taking the medication. A person can also become very tolerant to these medications and need to wean off them slowly rather than stop "cold turkey."

Sleep Disorder Nonpharmacologic Treatments

Establishing a regular **night time routine** can aid in more restful sleep. A person should go to bed at the same time every night and wake up at the same time each morning. This includes weekends when the temptation is to sleep in later. A person should avoid naps during the day, unless absolutely necessary. **Smoking** cigarettes within 2 hours of bedtime can interfere with sleep, as can consuming **alcoholic beverages**. It is important to have some form of exercise during the day, but avoid this within 2 hours of bedtime. A person should avoid tossing and turning in bed if they cannot sleep. They should get up and try reading for a few minutes until they are tired again. **Relaxing exercises** such as imaging can be helpful. Flexing and relaxing alternate muscle groups can help with relaxation. Arrange to sleep in an environment where there is no noise or light distractions. Unplugging the telephone and turning off the TV and lights can provide a more relaxing environment.

Immobility

Immobility is the result of a decrease in activity. It results in the impairment of movement of all or a part of the body.

- Physical illness and fatigue can result in *excessive bed rest* in cancer patients, which can affect the ability to have full range of motion of the limbs. Weakness and muscle atrophy can occur with limited use.
- *Poor nutritional status* due to nausea and vomiting or if a patient develops cachexia can lead to immobility. These states cause the muscles to not receive the nutrients necessary to maintain adequate muscle strength.
- Effects on the *nervous system* due to cancer can cause a decrease in the ability to function physically, which can lead to immobility. This can be seen by tumors, which affect the central nervous system in the brain or spinal cord.
- Cancer tumors that directly affect other parts of the body, for example the bones, can make it impossible for patients to be mobile because of pain or decrease the ability to move as they normally would.

<u>Risk Factors</u>

Risk factors for immobility include:

- Cancers that affect the nervous system or skeletal system.
- Compression on the spinal cord or on peripheral nerves can lead to the inability to move.
- Effects on the vascular system can also lead to immobility due to pain and a decrease in nutrients being delivered to the muscle tissues.
- Effects on the cardiac or respiratory systems may also affect mobility. These include a decreased tolerance for exercise because of decreased cardiac function or respiratory compromise.
- Cancer treatments can also lead to immobility. Chemotherapy can cause incapacitating nausea, vomiting, and weakness which decreases the ability to be physically active. Cancer surgery can cause physical changes and pain that impair physical mobility.
- Patients with severe depression or anxiety because of their illness may also have a decrease in mobility if they do not have the energy to perform activities. This may be a result of anhedonia or perceived somatic complaints related to depression.

<u>History and Physical Exam in Patients with an Alteration in Mobility</u>

When taking the **history** of a patient with a risk for altered mobility, assess them for any of the risk factors for this condition. This would include any physical symptoms that prevent them from being physically mobile. Also examine which treatments the patient is currently receiving that could prevent them from being physically active, either directly or because of side effects that occur as a result of these treatments. Assess for any pain that may impede movement as well as other symptoms that impair mobility, such as shortness of breath, impaired cardiac function, or cancerous tumors that cause neurologic effects that impair mobility.

On **exam**, assess for any motor or sensory deficits and for any reproducible pain with range of motion exercises. Assess cardiovascular and respiratory function through vital signs and auscultation. Assess the skin for any vascular changes and the musculoskeletal system for any obvious deformities, loss of muscle mass, and changes in gait.

Oncologic Emergencies

Type I and II Hypersensitivity Reactions

Type I: IgE-mediated response (anaphylaxis) is an antibody-antigen reaction against an allergen, such as milk, peanuts, latex, penicillin, chemotherapeutic agents, or fish. An antigen triggers release of substances, such as histamine and prostaglandins, which affect the skin, cardiopulmonary, and GI systems. Histamine causes initial erythema and edema by inducing vasodilation. Each time the person has contact with the antigen, more antibodies form in response, so allergic reactions worsen with each contact. Initial reactions may be mild, but subsequent contact can cause severe life-threatening response.

Type II: Cytotoxic response occurs when the body produces antibodies to body constituents, such as the basement membrane of cells or the surface of red blood cells. The response is mediated by IgM and IgG. The complement cascade is implemented and produces biochemicals that destroy the antigen-bearing cells. This type of hypersensitivity reaction occurs within minutes or hours and is associated with a number of different disorders, such as myasthenia gravis (antibodies against nerve tissue), ITP, and Goodpasture syndrome (antibodies against lung and kidney tissue). Type II hypersensitivity reactions include blood transfusion incompatibility reactions. Patients may experience hemolytic anemia, pulmonary failure, and/or renal failure.

Type III and IV Hypersensitivity Reactions

Type III: Immune complex response, mediated by IgM and IgG, involves formation of immune complexes as a result of antigen-antibody binding. The allergic response occurs within 3 to 10 hours after formation of immune complexes. The complexes may be removed by phagocytic action or may deposit in the blood vessels or other tissues, especially those of the joints and kidneys. Vasoactive amines in the complexes cause increased vascular permeability and result in damage to tissues. This type of hypersensitivity reaction is common to autoimmune disorders such as systemic lupus erythematosus and rheumatoid arthritis and may occur as a result of a drug reaction.

Type IV: Delayed response does not involve immunoglobulins (antibodies) but is mediated by T cells and macrophages. The allergic response develops one to three days (and sometimes weeks) after exposure to allergen. Contact dermatitis, which may result from skin contact with antiseptics or topical medications, is an example of a type IV reaction. A positive tuberculin test also results from a type IV response.

Proper Treatment Measures of Hypersensitivity: Type I (Anaphylaxis)

Anaphylaxis syndrome may present with a few symptoms or a wide range that encompasses cardiopulmonary, dermatological, and gastrointestinal responses. This is the most common type of severe reaction to chemotherapeutic agents.

Symptoms	Treatments
Symptoms may recur after the initial treatment (biphasic anaphylaxis), so careful monitoring is essential: Sudden onset of weakness, dizziness, confusion. Severe generalized edema and angioedema. Lips and tongue may swell. Urticaria. Increased permeability of vascular system and loss of vascular tone. Severe hypotension leading to shock. Laryngospasm/bronchospasm with obstruction of airway causing dyspnea and wheezing. Nausea, vomiting, and diarrhea. Seizures, coma and death.	Establish patent airway and intubate if necessary for ventilation. Provide oxygen at 100% high flow. Monitor VS. Administer epinephrine (Epi-pen® or solution). Albuterol per nebulizer for bronchospasm. Intravenous fluids to provide bolus of fluids for hypotension. Diphenhydramine if shock persists. Methylprednisolone if no response to other drugs.

Proper Treatment Measures of Hypersensitivity: Type II, III, and IV

Hypersensitivity infusion reactions to chemotherapeutic drugs may include type II, III, and IV responses. The patient may have an allergic response to the chemotherapeutic agent itself, metabolites, or the carrier vehicles. The patient's reaction may be mild, such as mild itching, or more severe, such as rash and severe pruritus with dyspnea. With type I reactions, the only option is to stop the chemotherapeutic agent, but with other types of reactions, a mild reaction may be controlled with different approaches, as the reaction must be balanced against the patient's need. Drugs to which patients frequently develop allergic responses include alkylating agents (cisplatin, carboplatin), monoclonal antibodies (rituximab, trastuzumab), mitotic inhibitors (etoposide, teniposide), asparaginase, and procarbazine. Approaches to managing these reactions include:

- Administering antihistamines (diphenhydramine) and/or steroids before administration of the chemotherapeutic agent, such as paclitaxel.
- Administering the chemotherapeutic drugs (such as mitotic inhibitors) more slowly over 60 minutes.
- Utilizing desensitization methods.

Disseminated Intravascular Coagulation (DIC)

Disseminated intravascular coagulation (DIC) is a condition in which clotting occurs within the body when it should not. DIC is frequently fatal.

Normal **clotting** occurs after tissue injury. Steps are followed through the clotting system to cause coagulation factors and other proteins to be released and a clot is formed. If a clot is present that is not needed, other factors are released to cause fibrinolysis, or the absorption of a clot. This system usually functions appropriately within the body to maintain a normal environment of clotting and fibrinolysis.

With DIC, the clotting system is triggered in response to infection, cancer, or some other disturbance within the body. There is **no control** over the clotting system with DIC and clotting continues to occur, which can lead to organ failure. The fibrinolysis system is activated, but cannot function adequately against the amount of clotting taking place. Because of this imbalance in the hemostasis system, bleeding also occurs which causes the patient to suffer from concurrent clotting and bleeding.

History and Physical Exam Findings in Patients with DIC

When taking a **history** from patients with suspected DIC, the patient may complain of sudden appearance of small bruises, called petechiae or of pain at a site where clotting or bleeding is occurring. The patient may begin to feel dizzy with loss of blood and may complain of shortness of breath if clots are forming within the lungs.

On **physical exam**, symptoms will occur very quickly and can include a change in the patient's mental status with confusion and lethargy. There may be petechiae present as well as some discoloration of the skin over areas of bleeding. Breath sounds can be decreased and weak, heart sounds may become irregular, and blood pressure may decrease. There may be obvious bleeding from a specific site or all orifices.

Laboratory findings with DIC include an increase in the D-dimer assay and FDP titers. Decreases in platelets, fibrinogen, antithrombin III, and plasminogen levels can also be seen.

Treatments

Stabilizing the patient is the priority when treating DIC. Bleeding must be controlled to prevent hypovolemic shock. The underlying **cause** of the DIC should be identified and treated, if possible.

If the patient is suffering significant blood loss, IV fluids should be given along with any blood products that are ordered. Blood expanders can be given in an emergency situation until blood products are available. Oxygen should also be given to supplement and help meet the needs of the body tissues. With bleeding, coagulation factors may also need to be replaced to assist with hemostasis.

Clotting can be prevented with the administration of Heparin. Bleeding needs to be carefully monitored to ensure hemorrhage does not occur. PTT lab test needs to be monitored to ensure the Heparin is functioning appropriately to prevent clots and not causing additional bleeding. Antithrombin can also be given to prevent clot formation, but Heparin is usually the first line medication given for clotting in DIC.

Syndrome of Inappropriate Antidiuretic Hormone Secretion (SIADH)

SIADH is a condition in which antidiuretic hormone (ADH) is secreted in frequency and amounts that are not necessary. ADH is normally secreted from the posterior pituitary gland, but it can also come from tissue elsewhere in the body. ADH functions to cause water to be reabsorbed instead of excreted through the kidneys. The body normally regulates the amount of water reabsorbed by the renal tubules based on fluid concentrations within the body.

SIADH causes **excess ADH** to be secreted, resulting in an increased amount of water to be held by the body and not excreted. This can lead to decreased sodium levels due to decreased concentration, intracellular edema, edema within the brain, and concentrated urine. With excess water being retained, there is a strain on the kidneys and fluid volume overload can also be present within the kidneys. SIADH is rare in cancer patients, but can be fatal.

- 160 -

History and Physical Exam Findings in Patients with SIADH

When taking a **history** from the patient with suspected SIADH, ask questions about any comorbidities that may be present and what treatments the patient has received for these illnesses. SIADH is most commonly seen in association with lung cancer, so be sure to identify which type of cancer the patient has and how the cancer has been treated. Question the patient about his dietary habits including the amount of liquids drank per day and normal sodium intake. Ask about any recent infections and any recent symptoms that were unusual, such as nausea, vomiting, and headache.

On **physical exam**, the patient may show signs of confusion or even be belligerent. Weight should be regularly monitored to assess for any additional fluid retention and resultant weight gain. Check the patient frequently for changes in mental status including delirium. The patient may need to be closely observed for any seizure activity if sodium levels are diluted to very low levels.

SIADH Treatments

Treatment should be focused on the *cause* of SIADH. *Hyponatremia* can be severe with SIADH and fluid restrictions should be started to help correct this imbalance. The hyponatremia should be corrected slowly, though, because permanent changes in brain tissue can occur if the levels are raised to a normal value too rapidly.

Medications can be given that disrupt the action of ADH. These medications will either block the effects of ADH on the renal tubules or promote diuresis. Severe SIADH can be treated with IV fluids high in concentrated sodium. This can be given along with diuretics to help correct fluid volume overload. There are other treatments available, but they are still in the experimental phase.

Symptoms of hyponatremia should be monitored. Provide frequent orientation to the patient if he is confused or lethargic. Maintain seizure precautions if the patient has significantly lowered sodium levels. Closely monitor cardiac function to assess for any dysrhythmias caused by hyponatremia.

Sepsis

Sepsis is an infection that is spread throughout the body. It is usually caused by a bacterial infection, but it can also be caused by viruses and other types of organisms. More than one-half of patients who develop sepsis die from the disease.

Sepsis usually causes a **fever** >100.4° F, **pulse** >90 beats/minute, **respirations** >20 breaths/min., or a **white blood cell count** >12,000. Some patients may have all of these symptoms while others may only have two of these symptoms.

Sepsis can go through several **phases** from the initial infection to multi-organ failure. An organism or other causative agent enters the blood stream. This stimulates activation of the immune system. There are times, however, when the infection becomes too overpowering and the immune system is just not able to defeat the infection. Identification of the disease and causative organism are paramount in providing prompt treatment and avoiding possible life-threatening consequences.

History and Physical Exam Findings in Patients with Sepsis

When taking a **history** on the patient with suspected sepsis, questions should be asked regarding current medical conditions, type of cancer, and what treatments have been received. Also question the patient about past infections that have been treated. If the patient has changes in mental status due to septic shock, family members or trusted friends should be questioned. Ask when symptoms started, how high fevers have been at home, and if there has been any pain or associated symptoms with the infection.

On **physical exam**, vital signs should be monitored for any elevations in body temperature and changes in heart rate or respiratory rate. Do a thorough skin exam to check for a possible source of infection from an IV line or other break in the skin. Listen to the heart and lungs to assess for any changes. Listen to and palpate the abdomen for pain or changes. Assess the patient for any changes in mental status, though these are usually present later in the infection.

Treatments

Infections should be **prevented** at all times if at all possible. Measures should be taken to do this through properly washing hands before and after contact with patients, using aseptic technique for any sterile procedures, and performing good basic hygiene. Cancer patients who are immunosuppressed due to chemotherapy or radiation are especially susceptible to infection and extra precautions should be taken when dealing with these patients.

Once it is suspected that the patient is developing sepsis, **blood cultures** should be done to identify the causative organism. **Medical treatment** with antibiotics or other antimicrobials can be based upon results of the culture and susceptibility.

Patients should receive adequate IV fluids to maintain hydration, especially if a high fever is present. Blood products should be given if the patient is anemic. Oxygen supplementation may be necessary for the patient. Other supportive measures should be provided to keep the patient as comfortable as possible.

Septic Shock

Septic shock is a systemic response to overwhelming infection with primarily the patient's body's own endogenous flora. Endotoxin is released with the patient experiencing release of histamine, bradykinin, increased capillary permeability, and a decrease in circulating blood volume with a decrease in tissue perfusion. There are two phases to septic shock, the warm phase and the cold phase.

- The **warm phase** is the initial phase. It is when the release of endotoxin causes the dilation of the arteries and veins. There is mental confusion, chills and fever, malaise, tachycardia, tachypnea, warm dry skin, and initially normal BP.
- This state gets progressively worse with the **cold shock phase**. More endotoxin is released with the patient experiencing release of histamine, bradykinin, increased capillary permeability, a decrease in circulating blood volume with a decrease in tissue perfusion, cool skin, tachycardia, decreasing BP, hyperventilation, oliguria and a weak thready pulse.

Third Space Syndrome

Third Space Syndrome (TSS) is the shift in fluid from the vascular to the interstitial space due to lowered plasma proteins, increased capillary permeability, or lymphatic blockage from trauma, inflammation or disease. Typically, TSS is seen in patients who have undergone major surgical procedures or who are in septic shock. TSS is divided into two phases: the loss phase and the reabsorption phase.

- The **loss phase** is characterized by hypotension, oliguria, tachycardia and increased urine specific gravity.
- The **reabsorption phase** is characterized by hypertension, increased urine output, lung rales, tachycardia, jugular venous distension, elevated central venous pressure, and dyspnea.

Tumor Lysis Syndrome

Tumor lysis syndrome occurs when tumor cells are killed, as intended, by some form of cancer treatment. When the tumor cell is lysed, its **intracellular contents** are released into the body. This can cause potentially fatal abnormalities in electrolyte levels.

Disorders That May Occur Along with Tumor Lysis Syndrome

The **metabolic abnormalities** that may be present with tumor lysis syndrome include hyperkalemia, hyperphosphatemia, hyperuricemia, and hypocalcemia. These disorders can result in irregularities of the heart rate and potential renal damage. If severe, multiple organs can be involved and permanent damage can result, leading to chronic illness or even death.

Other effects that can be seen with tumor lysis syndrome include those that you would expect to see with the respective **electrolyte abnormalities**. Nervous system affects from muscle twitches to seizures, muscle cramping, diarrhea, and EKG changes can all be present. Though the goal of therapy is to destroy tumor cells, the results can be deadly if tumor lysis syndrome occurs.

History and Physical Exam Findings in Patients with Tumor Lysis Syndrome

When taking a **history** on the patient with suspected tumor lysis syndrome, review the medical history and identify what type of cancer the patient has and what treatments have been administered in the past. Ask whether the patient has been treated recently and if there were any complications from the treatment. Also question the patient about any co-morbidity(s) that may be present.

On **physical exam**, the severity of symptoms will depend upon how severe the electrolyte imbalances have become. EKG changes can be seen with elevated potassium and decreased calcium and will usually appear as ventricular dysrhythmias. If severe, the patient may go into cardiac arrest. Muscle weakness or paralysis may develop from hyperkalemia, while muscle cramping with twitching and possibly seizures can develop with hypocalcemia and hyperuricemia. Renal damage and a decrease in urine output are evident with hyperphosphatemia and the patient may experience blood in the urine with hyperuricemia. All of the electrolyte imbalances present with tumor lysis syndrome have the potential to cause changes in mental status.

Treatments

Treatment is directed at correcting the **electrolyte abnormalities** that occur with tumor lysis syndrome. The patient should be well hydrated with IV fluids to promote normal renal function.

- If **urine output** is decreased, diuretics may be given to further promote diuresis.
- If increased **uric acid** is a problem, medications such as allopurinol can be given to slow down the production of uric acid.

- If **hyperkalemia** is present, a retention enema with Kayexalate may be given. Calcium can be given IV to treat hyperkalemia that is severe. Diuretics and sodium bicarbonate may also be helpful in reducing potassium levels.
- If **renal function** is greatly impaired, the patient may need to start dialysis. This can be done via hemodialysis or peritoneal dialysis. Dialysis treatments may only be temporary if renal damage is not permanent.

Measures can be taken to try to prevent electrolyte abnormalities, such as avoiding potassium supplements and avoid foods high in potassium and phosphorous.

Anaphylaxis

Anaphylaxis is a severe allergic reaction to a foreign substance (food, medication, or other substances) that can be fatal.

When the body is exposed to a foreign substance, the immune system normally recognizes the substance and there is no allergic-type reaction. But if the immune system does not recognize a new substance, such as a new medication, it may react by forming **antigens** which will be sensitive to the medication the next time it is introduced. There may be a very mild reaction at that time or no reaction at all. The next time a medication is given, the body's immune system reacts by causing a massive release of substances that are normally present with mild allergic reactions. The large quantity of these substances can cause swelling of the smooth muscle of the airway and severe vasodilation. If not promptly treated, anaphylaxis can cause complete **respiratory arrest** because of blockage of the airway.

History and Physical Exam Findings in Patients with Anaphylaxis

The **history** in a patient with an anaphylactic reaction may be limited because of the urgency of treating the patient without delay. Information may be gathered from the family or friends or after the patient is stabilized. When taking a history from this patient, all information should be gathered regarding any medication, food, or environmental allergies that are known to that patient. Also ask about any previous reactions the patient has had from medications and how they were treated.

On **physical exam**, the patient that is beginning to have an anaphylactic reaction may begin to have complaints of difficulty breathing and wheezing may be heard. The patient may begin to develop a "wheal and flare" reaction on their skin, similar to hives, with edema and itching. The patient may complain of pressure in the chest and a decrease in blood pressure may be present. When severe, the reaction includes loss of consciousness with severe compromise in respirations, leading to respiratory arrest.

Treatments

The biggest risk with anaphylactic shock is occlusion of the airway. Maintaining patency of the airway is the first priority when a patient begins to show signs of an anaphylactic reaction. If a medication is the cause of the anaphylaxis, **stop** it immediately. The massive release of histamine during anaphylaxis causes vasodilation which may permit leakage of fluid from the capillaries. **IV fluid replacement** is necessary to maintain fluid balance.

If airway swelling is an issue, **epinephrine** is usually given to reverse the reaction. This can also be helpful for the decrease in blood pressure that frequently accompanies anaphylaxis. **Steroids** can also be given to decrease the immune response.

If a patient has a known allergy or if they are receiving medications that are more likely to cause an allergic response, **prophylactic treatment** for anaphylaxis is often given. This includes using histamine blockers (H_1 and H_2) such as Benadryl and Tagamet. Medication may also be given prophylactically to prevent a rise in body temperature (Tylenol or Motrin).

Hypercalcemia

Hypercalcemia is the most common oncologic emergency with a potentially fatal outcome, occurring in 10 to 20% of patients. It is a rise in **serum calcium levels,** due to the production of a parathyroid hormone related peptide (PTHrP), normally undetectable. This peptide results in increased calcium levels increasing bone resorption. In a second category, malignant-associated hypercalcemia accounting for approximately 20% of the cases resulted from metastatic bone sites.

Cardiac Tamponade

Pathophysiology

Cardiac tamponade is a condition in which fluid builds up around the heart and inhibits the ability of the heart to function properly. The heart is surrounded by two membranes that make up the pericardial sac. There is normally a small amount of fluid between the two membranes to provide lubrication when the heart is pumping. With cardiac tamponade, the space between the two membranes fills with more fluid than normal causing **compression** on the heart and decreasing its ability to **pump** effectively.

Cardiac tamponade can be caused by cancer that affects the pericardium. Cancer treatment with radiation can cause scarring and damage to the pericardium and restrict its movement. When cardiac tamponade occurs, there is increased pressure applied to the outside of the heart which impairs its ability to pump effectively. Blood return to the heart can be affected, also, because of decreased expansion of the chambers, which will also decrease cardiac output. These factors result in the body's tissues not receiving oxygen and nutrients necessary to function appropriately.

History and Physical Exam Findings in Patients with Cardiac Tamponade

When taking a **history** from the patient with cardiac tamponade, ask about the onset of pain and any positional changes that alter the pain. Frequently, patients will state that the pain is relieved when they lean forward and increased when lying down. Ask the patient to rate their level of pain and describe any associated symptoms they may have such as shortness of breath or cough. Question the patient whether he has a pre-existing heart condition that could exacerbate the situation.

On **physical exam**, the patient may be sitting in a forward-leaning position to relieve some of the pressure within the chest. There may be noticeable shortness of breath. Assess vital signs for any changes. Listen to heart sounds, which may be muffled or faint. The hallmark signs of cardiac tamponade are referred to as Beck's triad; these include distant heart sounds, an increase in central venous pressure, and decreased blood pressure. The disease process may be advanced, though, by the time all three of these symptoms are present.

Treatments

Invasive procedures are frequently used to treat cardiac tamponade. A **pericardiocentesis** can be done, in which a needle is inserted through the chest wall into the pericardial space and the excess fluid is withdrawn. This relieves the pressure on the heart and may remedy the situation. If there is recurrence, a **pericardial window** may be created in the pericardium to provide a space through which the pericardial fluid can drain. If cardiac tamponade is permanent and not amenable to less invasive treatment, the pericardium may be completely **removed**.

Tumors of the pericardium are treated with radiation and may help to decrease the size of the tumors and the constrictive effect they have on the heart. If the patient has received radiation to the pericardium in the past, repeat radiation treatments are not performed.

A catheter can be inserted into the pericardium and **medications** can be injected into the area to cause scarring of the pericardium. In cases that are not severe, **steroids** may be used to decrease inflammation.

Spinal Cord Compression

Pathophysiology

Spinal cord compression is a condition in which **tumors** of the cord or tumors affecting intervertebral disks cause pressure to be placed on the spinal cord. This can be an emergent situation if there is sudden neurologic dysfunction or progressive neurologic dysfunction.

The spinal cord is protected by the vertebrae and it extends from the brain stem to the level of the 1st or 2nd lumbar vertebra. Tumors can occur within the cord (intramedullary), within the lining of the cords (meningioma), within the intervertebral disk space and extending into the spinal canal, or bone metastasis causing destruction of the bone and compression on the cord.

When the spinal cord is compressed, there is **interference** in the signals transmitted from the brain to the portion of the body controlled by the nerve roots at the level of the tumor. This can result in uncontrolled movements, flaccidity, or complete paralysis. It will affect that level and all levels below because of the blockage in the cord preventing signals from being transmitted past that point.

History and Physical Exam Findings in Patients with Spinal Cord Compression

When taking a **history** from a patient with suspected spinal cord compression, assess when the symptoms started and if they have progressed since they were first noticed. Ask the patient whether he has noticed changes in motor (movement) and sensory (feeling) function. Any previous cancer treatments should be reviewed as well as any co-morbidity(s) that may be present. Also ask the patient about any pain they may be feeling from the neck to the lower back and have them rate the pain on a scale from 0 to 10. Question the patient about any problems with incontinence or sexual function.

On **physical exam**, assess whether there is any gross deformity of the spine through observation. Observe the way the patient is moving and walking to assess for any spasticity which can be a sign of spinal cord irritation. Check the patient's strength against resistance in all four extremities. Assess their sensation using a monofilament, normal touch, and pin prick. Document any changes in this sensation over time.

Treatments

Acute spinal cord compression with rapid progression of neurologic deficits requires urgent **surgery**. It is thought that the sooner surgery is performed the more likely the patient will be to return to baseline or near baseline function. If surgical intervention is delayed, progression of the neurologic deterioration will be halted, but the neurologic damage may be permanent.

- If a tumor too large to be resected, radiation treatments may be done. **Radiation** will help to shrink the tumor and relieve compression on the cord.
- **Chemotherapy** can be used, but it is usually only used when radiation has failed and surgery is not an option. Children tend to respond better to chemotherapy treatments than adults.

For medical treatment, **steroids** can be given. These will help to decrease the inflammation in the area and, hopefully, reduce some of the pressure that is being applied to the spinal cord.

Superior Vena Cava Syndrome

Pathophysiology

Superior vena cava syndrome occurs when pressure is applied to the superior vena cava resulting in decreased blood drainage from the upper body. This compression can be due to a tumor or blood clot forming in the area.

The **superior vena cava** is located off the right atrium and it is responsible for draining blood from the arms, upper chest, neck, and head into the right atrium. When a tumor occurs in the chest or around the vessel itself, the vessel can be narrowed, which causes a decrease in blood return to the heart. This will ultimately result in decreased cardiac output and decreased oxygen and nutrients going to the body's tissues, especially in the upper body. A thrombus can form in the area and cause this same problem if it is large enough. Compression of the superior vena cava can cause platelets to clump in the narrowed area and lead to thrombus formation within the vessel.

History and Physical Exam Findings in Patients with Superior Vena Cava Syndrome

When taking a **history** from a patient with suspected superior vena cava syndrome, it is important to question the patient about what type of cancer they have and what treatments they have received in the past. Also question the patient about any side effects they have experienced from treatments in the past.

On **physical exam**, assess the patient's vital signs. Examine their appearance for facial edema and edema of the upper extremities. The patient may be visibly short of breath and their voice may be hoarse. The patient may develop nasal congestion due to the increased blood flow in the upper body. If oxygen deprivation is severe, cyanosis may be seen through the upper body. Veins may appear distended over the chest and in the neck.

If severe, the patient may begin to suffer mental status changes and confusion. The visual acuity will be affected and the patient may complain of changes in balance. In the end stages, superior vena cava syndrome may cause heart failure and even death.

Treatments

Treating the **cause** of superior vena cava syndrome is the focus of treatment. The specific type of cancer is determined in order to either remove or shrink the **tumor** to reduce the compression on the superior vena cava. This is accomplished through various diagnostic tests. Biopsy of the tumor is definitive for diagnosis.

Once the histology of the tumor is determined, a treatment plan can be formulated.

- **Radiation therapy** may be performed to shrink the tumor. This may be done for a cure or as palliative treatment to reduce symptoms. If possible, surgical excision of the tumor may be attempted.
- **Chemotherapy** may be helpful in decreasing a tumor and is used when the patient has already received radiation treatment to the area of the superior vena cava.
- If a blood clot is the cause of compression on the superior vena cava, clot buster **medications** may be administered, if not contraindicated. The patient may require anticoagulant treatment to prevent future clot formation.

Increased Intracranial Pressure

Pathophysiology

Increased intracranial pressure is a condition in which the brain, the blood supply to the brain, or the cerebrospinal fluid (CSF) that is around and in the brain occupies more room than normal. This causes an increase in **pressure** because the skull is not able to expand to accommodate this increase in volume.

A **tumor** that forms within the brain tissue will press against the structures in the brain as it grows. Eventually this will compress the brain tissue enough that the normal function of that area of the brain will be impaired. A tumor can also cause compression of the ventricles where CSF is stored. This will affect the natural flow of CSF which will increase pressure within the brain. When a tumor is growing within the skull, the blood supply in the brain will expand to accommodate the nutritional needs of this growing tissue. This can also cause an increase in pressure. Certain disease processes can cause swelling within the brain tissue and an increase in intracranial pressure.

History and Physical Exam Findings in Patients with Increased Intracranial Pressure

When taking a **history** from a patient with a suspected increase in intracranial pressure, ask the patient about any unusual symptoms they may be experiencing or any changes in overall health. The patient may complain of a headache that is recurrent and that becomes more severe with position changes (leaning or bending over). Question the patient about any patterns with the headaches and about any changes experienced with vision or mental status.

On **physical exam**, vital signs may show a decrease in blood pressure and a decreased heart rate. The patient may seem confused during the exam. An eye exam should be performed to provide an assessment of visual fields. Special care should be taken to examine the optic disk with a funduscopic exam. Papilledema, or swelling of the optic disk, is traditionally a main sign of increased intracranial pressure. The patient may be nauseous with vomiting and gait may be abnormal.

Treatments

An increase in intracranial pressure is considered a **surgical emergency**. If a tumor is causing compression on the brain tissue and increasing the pressure, then resection will be attempted. Patients will be closely monitored following surgery to assess for any recurrence of increased pressure due to bleeding or edema of the normal brain tissue. After surgery is complete, the patient may receive **radiation** treatments to attempt to destroy any existing cancer cells. If there is an obstruction in the flow of CSF, a **ventriculoperitoneal (VP) shunt** may be placed. The VP shunt diverts the CSF from the brain to the peritoneal space where it is absorbed.

For immediate decrease in intracranial pressure, the patient can undergo **forced hyperventilation**. This is performed while the patient is intubated and is effective because of the effects of hyperoxygenation on constriction of blood vessels.

Some types of chemotherapy will cross the blood-brain barrier. Other treatments include steroids, antiseizure medications, and restriction of liquids.

Extravasation

Extravasation of IV medication can cause serious and permanent injury, especially with chemotherapy drugs. Some extravasations are caused by improper positioning of the IV, but some are caused by leakage around the infusion site, due to prior venipuncture in the area or brittle veins. **Prevention** of extravasation is key so most patients receiving IV chemotherapy or other vesicants will have some type of central line placed, whether a PICC line, port, or other type of access device. If extravasation occurs, stop the infusion, aspirate as much as possible, elevate the extremity, and consider the substance to decide the next treatment. For example, Regitine 5-10 mg subcutaneously times one dose in the areas of the extravasation is sometimes given for norepinephrine extravasation (it should be given within 12 hours). Totect (dexrazoxane) is FDA approved for the treatment of anthracycline extravasation and has a 98% efficacy rate with minimal toxicities. Totect infusion should be initiated as soon as possible, within six hours of extravasation. Totect is administered as a three-day infusion and is given over 1-2 hours. It should be infused in an area other than the extravasation site. Ice should be applied prior to infusion and removed 15 minutes before the Totect infusion to allow sufficient blood flow to the area to maximize the ability of the drug to reach the extravasation site.

Prevention and Treatment

Care should be taken to **prevent** extravasations when administering intravenous (IV) chemotherapy. Injuries that may occur as a result of an extravasation include tissue sloughing, pain, nerve damage, infection, and loss of mobility. **Strategies** to prevent extravasation include ensuring the IV catheter is patent and in the vein by flushing with normal saline and verifying the presence of a good blood return. Nurses should be aware of which chemotherapeutic agents are potential vesicants. The IV site should be observed before, during, and after administration of the chemotherapy. The presence of a brisk blood return should be verified throughout the course of the administration.

If an extravasation occurs, the infusion should be **stopped** immediately. The line should not be flushed as this will further advance additional chemotherapy into the tissue. Disconnect the IV tubing from the IV device and attempt to aspirate any residual fluid from the IV device using a small syringe. The IV device can then be removed. The patient's physician should be notified and the site of the extravasation assessed and documented. If an antidote exists, an order should be obtained to administer it. Hot or cold application is recommended depending on the chemotherapeutic agent. Limb elevation is also helpful for the first 24 to 48 hours to promote reabsorption of the drug.

Bowel Obstructions

Bowel obstruction is a mechanical obstruction of the passage of intestinal contents because of constriction or occlusion of the lumen or lack of muscular contractions (paralytic ileus). Bowel obstruction may occur with hematological malignancies, such as leukemia, and intraabdominal tumors. Some patients receiving vinca alkaloids may develop severe autonomic neuropathy that can result in acute intestinal obstruction.

Small Intestine Obstruction

Obstructions of the small intestine may be caused by different types of tumors:

- *Adenocarcinomas* (33%), most commonly in the duodenum or jejunum, are usually asymptomatic until the tumor has metastasized. Crohn's disease is a risk factor, and incidence is highest in those in their 60s.
- *Lymphomas* (20%) generally occur in the distal small intestine, with most classified as non-Hodgkin's B cell, but those with celiac disease are at increased risk of T cell lymphoma.
- *Carcinoid tumors* (33%) of the ileum are most common. Carcinoid tumors metastasize early with almost all tumors greater than 2 cm metastasizing to the liver.

With obstruction, fluids cannot be reabsorbed and gastric secretions and distention increase, increasing pressure in the lumen and vessels, eventually causing swelling, necrosis, rupture, and/or perforation.

Large Intestine and Colorectal Cancers

Almost all colorectal cancers are adenocarcinomas (95%) and almost half of these occur in the descending colon or rectosigmoid area. Adenocarcinomas typically result in **bowel obstruction** because of large mass or because of constricting lesions about the lumen of the intestine. Most colorectal cancers develop from precancerous adenomatous 85%) or serrated polyps (10 to 20%) with about 5% developing because of inherited polyposis syndromes. Colorectal cancers are most common in those over age 50. Patients with ulcerative colitis and Crohn's disease have increased risk beginning about 7 to 10 years after diagnosis of the bowel disorder. Dietary factors may have a role in development of colorectal cancers, especially diets high in fats and red meat. With obstruction, the large intestine is more able to expand than the small intestine, so the symptoms may be less acute initially. As pressure builds from retained intestinal contents and gas, the contents may back flow or, if unable to do so, may result in rupture or perforation. If the blood supply is impaired, then necrosis may occur.

Clinical Manifestations

Clinical manifestations of **bowel obstruction** may include abdominal pain and distention, vomiting, dehydration because of impaired reabsorption of fluids, diminished or absent bowel sounds, severe constipation, respiratory distress, shock and sepsis. Symptoms vary according to the site of the obstruction:

- *Small intestine:* Sudden and frequent nausea and vomiting in large volumes (first partially digested food and then bile and/or fecal emesis), often immediately after intake, usually indicates a bowel obstruction in the small intestine. The abdomen may become increasingly distended with severe colicky pain as peristalsis first tries to move the stool distally and then, with complete obstruction, in reverse. Patients may expel blood and mucous rectally but no fecal material. Dehydration may be severe.
- *Large intestine:* Obstructions of the colon usually result in more delayed vomiting, with fecal emesis and increasing abdominal distention and pain. Symptoms are typically less acute than with small bowel obstruction and may develop over a period of months, often beginning with chronic constipation. Dehydration is usually less severe. The stool may become smaller in size and shape as blockage progresses. With colorectal cancer, patients may begin to pass frank blood in the stool or melena and may show signs of anemia.

<u>Treatment</u>

Treatment options for **bowel obstruction** include:

- ***Small intestine:*** Resection is the treatment of choice for adenomas even if they have metastasized to control symptoms. Decompression may be needed preoperatively. Chemotherapy is also usually administered although prognosis is poor. For lymphomas, resection or debulking of tumor is usually done. With extensive disease, chemotherapy with or without radiotherapy may also be administered. For carcinoid tumors, resection is usually done if metastasis has not occurred. With signs of metastasis, treatment with somatostatin analog is also indicated to slow hepatic spread.
- ***Large intestine/Colorectal:*** The treatment of choice is resection, which may result in the need for colostomy depending on the site and extent of the tumor. Preoperative chemotherapy and/or radiation as well as postoperative chemotherapy may be administered for rectal tumors. Stage III and stage IV colon cancers are also usually treated with systemic chemotherapy. With stage IV cancer, secondary tumors (lung, liver) may be resected to increase duration of survival.

Note: If bowel obstruction is partial or inoperable, dexamethasone may relieve some of the symptoms because it reduces inflammation and swelling as well as providing relief of nausea.

Urinary Obstruction

<u>Pathophysiology</u>

Urinary obstruction associated with cancer in adults is most often the result of prostate cancer and pelvic or retroperitoneal tumors. Obstruction may occur as the result of compression of urological structures, such as ureters or urethra because of cervical or ovarian tumors, intestinal tumors, lymphoma, and metastatic tumors from the breast, prostate, or testicles. Urothelial carcinoma may block the lumens in the urinary tract. Urinary obstruction (partial or complete) may occur in the kidneys because of various types of tumors and may result in hydronephrosis, causing the kidney to swell as urine backs up into pelvis and collecting tubules. The swelling impairs circulation and can damage renal tissue and result in kidney infection. Patients may develop radiation- or chemotherapy-associated (alkylating agents) cystitis with pain and hematuria. Over time, fibrosis may occur that can lead to increased pressure in the bladder and reduced bladder compliance and capacity so that urinary output is partially obstructed.

<u>Clinical Manifestations</u>

Clinical manifestations of **urinary obstruction** vary depending on the type of obstruction and how quickly complete obstruction occurs. If both kidneys are functioning, obstruction of one ureter may not be evident because the opposite kidney will produce adequate urinary output although signs of nephrosis, such as swelling and pain may occur. With complete rapid obstruction, the patient may experience considerable pain because of the inability to urinate, especially with renal distention. With obstruction that occurs more slowly, the patient may develop dull aching abdominal, pelvic, or retroperitoneal pain and may also experience nausea and vomiting. Pain and hematuria (red blood cells, leukocytes in urine) are common as obstruction progresses and may also result from radiation and chemotherapy-associated cystitis that can cause considerable swelling and mucosal irritation. In some cases, obstruction may result from accumulation of blood clots in the bladder. Bladder cancer, especially at the bladder neck, may obstruct urinary flow, resulting in bilateral flank pain as both kidneys distend. With prostatic cancer, obstruction usually occurs over a period of time and begins with difficulty initiating flow of urine or completely emptying the bladder.

<u>Treatment</u>

Treatment for **urinary obstruction** varies according to the site and extent of cancerous lesions, but relief of obstruction is essential. This is most often achieved by resection of tumors. For example, bladder tumors may initially require transurethral resection of the bladder tumor (TURBT) for staging purposes and may then be followed by radical cystectomy with urinary diversion for invasive tumors. Patients who are not candidates for radical mastectomy may undergo TURBT followed by radiation and chemotherapy although this protocol is less effective and radiation-associated complications may occur. Metastatic bladder cancer is often treated with surgery and adjuvant chemotherapy, MVAC protocol (methotrexate, vinblastine, doxorubicin, and cisplatin). Nephrectomy is done for renal carcinoma, but chemotherapy and radiotherapy are generally ineffective although clinical trials may be advised. For prostatic cancer, treatment usually includes radical prostatectomy. Other treatment options include radiotherapy and hormonal therapy. With partial obstruction, special urethral catheters may be utilized.

Pneumonitis

<u>Pathophysiology</u>

Pneumonitis may occur because of damage to the alveoli caused by radiotherapy directed at the chest (lung, breast cancer, lymphoma) or whole-body or chemotherapy, including such protocols as MVAC (methotrexate, vinblastine, doxorubicin, and cisplatin), CMV (cisplatin, methotrexate, and vinblastine), and PCV (procarbazine, lomustine, and vincristine). Pneumonitis involves injury to the cells and inflammation of the alveoli, which become distorted and fibrotic over time. Up to 15% of patients undergoing thoracic radiotherapy develop pneumonitis. Pneumonitis typically develops over a 1 to 6-month period after treatment although damage may be permanent, especially if the patient received both radiation and chemotherapy. Phases include:

- *Initial* (0-30 days): Pneumonocytes are destroyed and loss of surfactant production results in increased serum proteins in the alveoli and interstitial edema. Pathologic changes may begin within the first two days of radiotherapy.
- *Intermediate* (to 6 months): Proteins continue to leak into alveoli, fibrotic changes begin, and patient develops symptoms.
- *Late* (>6 months): Pulmonary fibrosis with capillary loss and continues with reduction in lung volume and vital capacity. (X-rays shows "ground glass" appearance).

<u>Clinical Manifestations</u>

Clinical manifestations of **pneumonitis** vary depending on the phase. During the initial phase (0-30 days), patients usually exhibit no outward symptoms even though pathologic changes are occurring. However, as the pneumonitis progresses over the next few months, the patient will begin to exhibit a cough (generally non-productive), shortness of breath (especially on any exertion), fever, and tachycardia. Some hemoptysis may begin to occur. As the condition worsens, the patient may begin to develop pleuritic pain, chest pain, increased hemoptysis, pleural effusions, and eventually acute respiratory distress syndrome (ARDs) with hypoxemia as pulmonary fibrosis becomes severe. With hypoxemia, the patient may begin to exhibit signs of confusion. The patient may begin to sleep with the head of the bed elevated to facilitate respirations and may complain of "tightness" in the chest and constant fatigue. ARDS increases risk of infection, sepsis, pneumothorax, and pulmonary thrombosis.

Treatment

Treatment measures for **pneumonitis** include:

- ***Oral corticosteroids:*** While various medications have been tried, including ACE inhibitors, only corticosteroids have been shown to reduce progression although preventive administration has not proved effective. Oral prednisone (1mg/kg/weight) is administered when symptoms begin to occur and is continued for several weeks, and then the dose is tapered slowly to avoid exacerbation of symptoms.
- ***Fluids and electrolytes***: May be administered as needed.
- ***Oxygen***: Supplementary oxygen may help relieve hypoxemia with advanced disease.
- ***Occupational therapy:*** Can assist patients to develop energy-saving strategies to compensate for weakness and shortness of breath in order to allow them to remain independent in ADLs as long as possible.
- ***Influenza/pneumonia immunizations:*** To prevent illness that may exacerbate symptoms.
- ***Weight control:*** Excessive weight may worsen shortness of breath.
- ***Pulmonary rehabilitation:*** May include breathing exercises, nutritional advice, and stress management strategies.
- ***Smoking cessation:*** Patients should be enrolled in smoking cessation programs if they are smokers.
- ***Lung transplantation:*** This procedure may be available to some patients with advanced pulmonary fibrosis if they meet eligibility requirements.

Intracranial Hemorrhage

Bleeding into the brain can come from two etiologies, bleeding into the **substance** of the brain and bleeding into the **epidural sac**. Bleeding can be the result of excessively high blood pressure, DIC, leukemia, sepsis, trauma or thrombocytopenia. Intracerebral bleeding can result in coma, hemiplegia, and decerebrate posture. If bleeding is from a subdural hematoma, symptoms include a positive Brudzinski's sign, diplopia, dizziness, headache, nausea and vomiting, paralysis or vertigo.

Leukostasis

Leukostasis is a syndrome of intravascular sludging in patients with **leukemia**. This is present when the leukocyte count is >100,000/mm^3. This results in capillary obstruction, tissue ischemia, and decreased tissue perfusion. It is most lethal when the CNS or lungs are involved. Symptoms include high fever, acute shortness of breath, stridor, and hemoptysis. X-ray findings include pleural effusion or diffuse pulmonary infiltrates.

Carotid Artery Rupture Mortality

Carotid artery erosion and rupture occur due to cancers of the head and neck. Most cancers of the head and neck are aggressive. Invasion of the surrounding tissue happens frequently. Mortality from rupture is about 40%. Of those that do recover, 25% will have permanent neurological deficit. Rupture can occur from three different scenarios—an **exposed artery**, **impending rupture** and **acute rupture**.

Pulmonary Toxicity

- **Pulmonary toxicity** is a lung disease that occurs due to cancer treatments. The two main types are radiation-induced pneumonitis and chemotherapy-induced pulmonary fibrosis.
- **Pneumonitis** is an inflammation of the lung tissue. It can be caused by radiation treatments to the lungs. This causes irritation and inflammation of the tissue with associated pain and shortness of breath. The amount of radiation received, the amount of lung tissue that receives treatment, and the length of time the treatments are given all contribute to the severity of the illness. Radiation pneumonitis occurs in a small number of patients who receive radiation treatments, but tends to occur more frequently and more severely in older patients.
- **Pulmonary fibrosis** due to chemotherapy is a condition in which lung tissues are damaged and replaced by scar tissue. This causes the lungs to have decreased ability to function as well as decreased elasticity. It occurs more often in elderly patients and in those who have also received radiation treatments.

History and Physical Exam Findings with Radiation-Induced and Chemotherapy-Induced Lung Disease

With **radiation-induced pulmonary toxicity**, symptoms may be very vague and mimic those of an upper respiratory infection. This includes cough, some shortness of breath, and mild fever. These symptoms usually occur 2-4 months following radiation treatment.

- On **exam**, there will be fluid within the lungs that causes a productive cough and crackles on auscultation of the lungs. Adventitious breath sounds will be heard strongest over the area of the lung tissue that received the most radiation treatment. Fluid within the lungs will be present on chest x-ray.

With **chemotherapy-induced pulmonary toxicity**, the patient will complain of shortness of breath and nonproductive cough. These symptoms generally start gradually over several weeks.

- On **exam**, this patient may have an increased respiratory rate and some crackles auscultated at the end of a respiratory cycle, but some patients may be asymptomatic. Chest x-ray may also be normal.

With both illnesses, arterial blood gases will show a decrease in oxygen levels and respiratory alkalosis. Pulmonary function tests will show a decrease in total lung volume.

Medical Treatments

Radiation-induced pneumonitis is treated by attempting to control the symptoms and inflammatory response within the lungs. **Medications** can be given that help to decrease the cough and reduce fever. **Steroids** can be given to help with lung inflammation, though only about one-half of the patients who receive steroid treatment tend to improve. Patients should be slowly weaned from steroid treatments because a recurrence of the illness may occur if steroids are stopped too quickly. Patients should also be closely monitored for side effects from steroids.

The treatment of **chemotherapy-induced pulmonary fibrosis** is also aimed at symptom control. Dosages of chemotherapy drugs that cause fibrosis can be **decreased** to help prevent progression of the disease. Inflammation of the lung tissue may be treated with steroids, though this is mainly for symptom control to decrease irritation of the lung tissue and is not always effective. Cough and fever are also treated to decrease uncomfortable symptoms.

Psychosocial Dimensions of Care

Cultural, Spiritual and Religious Factors

Spiritual Distress

Some people have a strong sense of faith and beliefs which they call upon when faced with stressors in their life. **Spiritual distress** occurs when a person is no longer comforted by their beliefs and questions these beliefs. Cancer patients may feel they face something more than they can handle and not understand why this happened. They may question if they are being punished for something they did wrong or feel they have been betrayed by their God.

A **risk factor** for spiritual distress is the disease itself. The severity of the patient's illness and poor prognosis can contribute to feelings of hopelessness and abandonment. Beliefs may be questioned when faced with treatment decisions. Some faiths do not believe in certain medical treatments, which causes a dilemma for a patient. A person may not be able to practice certain aspects of their religion because of bed rest or no accessibility to a place of worship. When receiving treatments, a spiritual advisor or mentor may not be available for spiritual support.

Helping a Patient Overcome Spiritual Distress

If possible, help the patient to establish an **environment** that is conducive to their religious practices. If prayers are done during a certain time of the day, try to minimize interruptions or treatments if at all possible. Especially if a minister or other spiritual leader is visiting, provide privacy for the patient to be able to speak in confidence. Also do this if friends or family members are present to share in prayer with the patient.

If the patient has specific **dietary guidelines** they wish to follow, arrange a consultation with a dietitian to see if this is possible if not medically contraindicated. As long as it is medically safe, allow family members to bring in certain foods that may follow specific religious dietary needs.

Communication with the patient is important when ascertaining these specific needs that are necessary to help a patient maintain a healthy belief system. It is also important to accept any beliefs that may seem unusual to you.

Culture and Its Effect on Medical Treatments

Culture entails the guidelines by which a group of individuals live including their values and way of life. It influences their day-to-day lives and how they think.

Cultural beliefs can influence everything from diagnosis to treatment of cancer. Some cultures feel that diseases occur for a reason, possibly a sign or punishment, and this can influence how the person will be treated, both medically and by their community. Some cultures believe in pursuing all medical treatments available while others believe in using folk remedies and spiritual guidance rather than modern medicine to treat cancer.

Some cultures promote involvement in their **medical care** in order to be pro-active, while others do not question authority figures or may not trust medical staff. Also, in some cultures the families are dominated by an authority figure and this may not be the person with the cancer. There may be one person who makes decisions for the entire family.

How Cancer Affects Hispanics

There are more **Hispanics** living in the United States than ever, and this population is growing more each year. Hispanics suffer from the most common forms of cancer less often than Caucasians. The types of cancers that affect Hispanics are the forms that have a higher incident rate in Central and South America. These include *digestive cancers* (stomach, liver, gallbladder) and *female reproductive organ cancers* (cervix and uterine).

Digestive cancers may be more prevalent among Hispanics because of a *lower rate of colorectal screening* or possibly from dietary factors. Female Hispanics are less likely to undergo regular screening Pap smears and have a higher incidence of human papilloma virus, which may be a contributing factor to cervical cancer.

Hispanics may also not have *access to adequate healthcare* or they may not follow healthy lifestyles. Obesity is prevalent amongst Hispanics, especially women, which may be another contributing factor to cancer.

How Cancer Affects African Americans

More **African Americans** die each year of cancer than all other races combined. *Lung cancer* kills more African American men and women each year than any other type of cancer. The second leading cause of cancer death in African American women is *breast cancer*. The second leading cause of cancer death in African American men is *prostate cancer. Colorectal cancer* is the next most common type of cancer in both African American men and women.

African Americans also have the lowest survival rate for cancer than any other race, which may be due to poor health care resources because of lack of insurance. Another influencing factor is low income which prevents these individuals from seeking medical care when faced with an illness.

How Cancer Affects Asians

Asians are the least likely to have a diagnosis of cancer out of the major races (African Americans, Caucasians, and Hispanics). They also have the lowest incidence of cancer death compared to these groups. Asians are more likely to suffer from different types of cancers compared to the other racial groups. *Thyroid cancer* is prevalent, especially amongst women, and *esophageal cancer* is prevalent among men.

The most common types of cancer also vary when compared to other racial groups. For example, *uterine cancer* is much more common in Asian women, followed by *lung and breast cancers*. Asian men more commonly suffer from *stomach and rectal cancers*, followed by *liver and rectal cancers*.

It is unclear why these types of cancers are more common in Asians, but it may be attributable to certain dietary practices or uses of more traditional medicine practices instead of modern medicine.

Personal Space

Personal space is the area surrounding our body, including the physical area outside of our immediate vicinity. Individual's interpretation of personal space and appropriateness of how close you come to a person can vary in different cultures.

- The **intimate zone** is only 1 ½ feet or less from the body. Someone enters this zone for intimacy, closeness, and caring. People often feel intimated or uncomfortable when this space is invaded during casual conversation with a casual acquaintance.
- The **personal zone** is 1 ½ to 3 feet around the body. This closeness is used when communicating with a close friend or for quiet, private conversations. There is not as much of a feeling of being uncomfortable when people stand in this zone during casual conversation.
- The **social zone** is 3 to 6 feet around the body. This is the most common zone of comfort during communication and is used in casual or business conversations. This is the most comfortable zone for most people.

Types of Health Beliefs

- The **magico-religious** health belief states that a person's state of health or disease is under the direction of an uncontrollable power. Individuals who follow this belief system feel that their illness is as a result of being punished by a higher power. They also feel that their prognosis is solely in the hands of this higher power. These individuals may use traditions, rituals, and talismans for help with the healing process.
- The **scientific or biomedical** health belief follows the belief system of modern medicine. Individuals that practice this feel that there is a sound, scientific or medical reason for their illness. These individuals also believe that there is a cure for their illness, whether it is through medical procedures, medications, or by having an operation.
- The **holistic** health view adopts the theory that illness occurs because of a disruption in the natural processes that occur in the body. This belief relies strongly on homeopathic treatments using natural ingredients and not on more traditional medical treatments.

Financial Concerns

Financial Distress and Common Fears

Cancer patients are frequently too ill to maintain employment, which can bring about a fear of losing **health insurance benefits** as well as **income**. Fears may arise about continuing cancer treatments without adequate insurance coverage and about large amounts of debt incurred by medical treatments. There are federal and state laws that make it illegal for an employee to be discriminated against because of a cancer illness. Most states also have an insurance program specifically for those with reduced income. At the federal level, Medicare is available for those under the age of 65 when they are unemployable because of illness.

With a **terminal diagnosis**, patients may also face the fear of leaving their family in a financial bind. This is especially true if the patient has been the primary bread winner. There may also be concerns that any life insurance available will not be enough to provide their loved ones with the financial resources to cover any medical debts or enough income to meet their basic needs.

Poverty and Its Effect on a Patient with Cancer

Poverty is exhibited more in **minorities** than others in this country and these individuals have a poorer prognosis when diagnosed with cancer than those who are not minorities. The most obvious reason may be because of a **lack of medical resources**. Health insurance may not be available for this group of people because they cannot afford it, or they may have low-paying jobs that do not offer insurance benefits. Lack of education and possibly distrust for the medical system can also lead to an unclear understanding of their disease and poor compliance with treatment.

Patients who are poverty-stricken may not be able to participate in **regular screening practices** to help with cancer prevention and early detection. This can be due to a lack of understanding or because of low income or no insurance.

Poor nutritional status can also contribute to a poorer prognosis with cancer in a poverty-stricken patient. Poor living conditions can contribute to a poor prognosis in these individuals.

Altered Body Image

Body Image

Body image is a person's own opinion about how their body may appear to others. This includes an awareness of physical looks, how their body works, and physical feelings they experience.

The disease process of cancer as well as cancer treatments can cause a change in body image. Many patients experience profound weight loss with loss of muscle, called cachexia, which can change the outward appearance of their body. They may experience pain which inhibits them from functioning as they once did. Physical symptoms of vomiting, loss of bowel or bladder control, and shortness of breath can all cause an **impaired body image**.

Treatments that change body image include radiation and chemotherapy, which can cause hair loss and skin changes. The loss of hair, or alopecia, can profoundly affect one's perception of their appearance. Certain medications can also cause excessive weight loss or gain. Another common side effect from cancer treatments can be excessive fatigue which may interfere with a person's ability to function as they once did.

Altered Body Image

Patients may become **depressed** or withdrawn when they experience changes in their body due to cancer or treatments. These feelings may be exhibited by a lack of interest in activities, removing themselves from social interactions, or isolating themselves from others. There may also be a withdrawal from a specific body part that is primarily affected by the cancer or treatments. For example, a person who undergoes a mastectomy for breast cancer may refuse to look at their chest in a mirror for fear of how they will appear.

A patient can also experience feelings of **grief** for the loss of their previous physical appearance or function. In some this can lead to self-medicating with drugs or alcohol to overcome their perceived loss. There can be a lack of acceptance of their changed body with denial. If special care is necessary to an area of the body that has been affected, a patient my choose to avoid this or pretend it does not exist or is not necessary.

Coping with an Altered Body Image

Encourage a patient to **express** their feelings of anger, frustration, or sorrow over the change they have experienced with their body. Help them to identify what it is about the change that affects them the most and discuss what can be done to relieve these fears or feelings they may be experiencing. In some cases, **psychological counseling or group support** may be necessary to help them explore their feelings and devise ways to cope with the problem. Group support also allows them to call on other people's experiences and ways of coping with these changes.

Professional resources should be called upon for help with specific problems. For example, companies are available to fashion wigs or hair pieces that suit the patient who has experienced hair loss, or a professional orthotist to help create a prosthetic to help a patient function.

The **ultimate goal** is for the patient to gain acceptance with their new body image and prevent any changes from profoundly impacting their level of functioning.

Alopecia

Alopecia is hair loss that occurs anywhere on the body. It can have a profound effect on a person's **body image**. Causes include:

- **Treatments** that cause damage to the hair root or hair follicle may lead to hair loss that may be temporary or permanent. High doses of radiation may cause permanent hair loss. Certain types of chemotherapy may also cause alopecia, though it is usually temporary. Treating with more than one chemotherapeutic drug may increase the chances of developing alopecia.
- In very rare cases, patients who experience **extreme anxiety** and depression due to their disease may develop a condition called trichotillomania. This is a condition in which a person compulsively pulls on their hair to the point of pulling it out. This action seems to provide some sort of calming and a sense of security to the person. It is treated with clomipramine, a tricyclic anti-depressant frequently used for obsessive-compulsive disorder.

<u>Coping with Alopecia</u>

To help patients cope with **alopecia**, consider the following:

- Early **intervention** to provide measures to improve cosmetic appearance is necessary to help to prevent anxiety and depression due to an altered body image.
- There are many community resources available to help with wigs or hairpieces that are attractive and flattering. A patient should start wearing this before he or she has lost all of their hair in order to become accustomed to it. Selecting the style of the wig before losing hair is helpful, also.
- **Educate** patients in care of the scalp to promote hair regrowth. Hair may not grow in the same color or texture as it was before. Care needs to be given to sun exposure to avoid burning or loss of body heat from the bare scalp. Also educate them that there have not been any products on the market that have been medically proven to stimulate hair regrowth.

Learning Styles and Barriers

Learning Styles

Not all people are aware of their preferred **learning style.** A range of teaching materials/methods that relates to all **3 learning preferences**—visual, auditory, kinesthetic—and **appropriate for different ages** should be available. Part of assessment for teaching involves choosing the right approach based on observation and feedback. Often presenting learners with different options gives a clue to their preferred learning style. Some people have a combined learning style:

Visual learners	Learn best by seeing and reading: Provide written directions, picture guides, or demonstrate procedures. Use charts and diagrams. Provide photos, videos.
Auditory learners	Learn best by listening and talking: Explain procedures while demonstrating and have learner repeat. Plan extra time to discuss and answer questions. Provide audiotapes.
Kinesthetic learners	Learn best by handling, doing, and practicing: Provide hands-on experience throughout teaching. Encourage handling of supplies/equipment. Allow learner to demonstrate. Minimize instructions and allow person to explore equipment and procedures.

Adult Learning Principles

Adults have a wealth of life and/or employment experiences. Their attitudes toward education may vary considerably. There are, however, some **principles of adult learning** and typical characteristics of adult learners that an instructor should consider when planning strategies for teaching parents, families, or staff:

Practical and goal-oriented	Provide overviews or summaries and examples. Use collaborative discussions with problem-solving exercises. Remain organized with the goal in mind.
Self-directed	Provide active involvement, asking for input. Allow different options toward achieving the goal. Give them responsibilities.
Knowledgeable	Show respect for their life experiences/ education. Validate their knowledge and ask for feedback. Relate new material to information with which they are familiar.
Relevancy-oriented	Explain how information will be applied. Clearly identify objectives.
Motivated	Provide certificates of professional advancement and/or continuing education credit for staff when possible.

<u>Knowles' Basic Assumptions of Adult Teaching</u>

In his study on adult learning, Knowles identified some of the basic assumptions that the educator can make regarding the **adult learner**.

1. The first assumption is that as individuals grow and mature intellectually, we are able to **direct ourselves**, instead of being dependent on the directions given to us by others.
2. The second assumption is that each individual establishes his or her own **self-identity** based on unique personal experiences. These experiences (and mistakes) help the individual to establish a learning process.
3. The third assumption is that an individual's readiness to learn is based on his or her **social role**; in other words, an individual is more willing and ready to learn things that directly apply to his or her job or role in life.
4. The fourth assumption is that adults want to be able to **apply knowledge immediately**; this is sometimes called "problem-based learning," as opposed to traditional content-based learning.

Learning Theories

Behavioral learning theory states that people learn different behaviors because they observe these behaviors and receive positive reinforcement for the behaviors.

Cognitive learning theory is the process by which information is interpreted to teach a person about a certain subject. An example would be developing an acronym to help remember a list of symptoms or findings of a disease in preparation for an exam.

Social learning theory is utilizing other people to learn through observing and mimicking them. Patients can utilize this by seeing a cancer survivor who is doing very well and picturing themselves in the same position.

Motivational learning is providing a "reward" in exchange for positive behaviors. An example of this is feeling healthier in exchange for quitting smoking.

Adult learning theory states that adults utilize their past experiences to decipher new information and learn from this based on these experiences. An example of this is developing knowledge of a certain disease state after diagnosis.

Cognitive-Behavioral Therapy

Cognitive-behavioral therapy (CBT) focuses on the impact that thoughts have on behavior and feelings and encourages the individual to use the power of rational thought to alter perceptions and behavior. This approach to counselling is usually short-term, about 12-20 sessions, with the first sessions to obtain a ***history***, middle sessions to focus on ***problems***, and last sessions to ***review and reinforce***. Individuals are assigned "homework" during the sessions to practice new ways of thinking and to develop new coping strategies. The therapist helps the individual identify goals and then find ways to achieve those goals. CBT acknowledges that all problems cannot be resolved, but one can deal differently with problems. The therapist asks many questions to determine the individual's areas of concern and encourages the individual to question his/her own motivations and needs. CBT is goal-centered so each counselling session is structured toward a particular goal, such as coping techniques. CBT centers on the concept of unlearning previous behaviors and learning new ones, questioning behaviors, and doing homework.

Bloom's Taxonomy

Bloom's taxonomy outlines behaviors that are necessary for learning, and this can apply to healthcare. The theory describes 3 types of learning:

- **Cognitive** - (Learning and gaining intellectual skills to master 6 categories of effective learning.)
  - Knowledge.
  - Comprehension,
  - Application.
  - Analysis.
  - Synthesis.
  - Evaluation.
- **Affective** - (Recognizing 5 categories of feelings and values from simple to complex. This is slower to achieve than cognitive learning.)
  - Receiving phenomena: Accepting need to learn.
  - Responding to phenomena: Taking active part in care.
  - Valuing: Understanding value of becoming independent in care.
  - Organizing values: Understanding how surgery/treatment has improved life.
  - Internalizing values: Accepting condition as part of life, being consistent and self-reliant.
- **Psychomotor** - (Mastering 6 motor skills necessary for independence. This follows a progression from simple to complex.)
  - Perception: Uses sensory information to learn tasks.
  - Set: Shows willingness to perform tasks.
  - Guided response: Follows directions.
  - Mechanism: Does specific tasks.
  - Complex overt response: Displays competence in self-care.
  - Adaptation: Modifies procedures as needed.
  - Origination: Creatively deals with problems.

Barriers to Learning

The patient/family's readiness to learn should be assessed because if they are not ready, instruction is of little value. Often readiness is indicated when the patient/family asks questions or shows an interest in procedures. There are a number of factors that can be **barriers to learning**:

- *Physical factors*: There are a number of physical factors than can affect ability. Manual dexterity may be required to complete a task, and this varies by age and condition. Hearing or vision deficits may impact ability. Complex tasks may be too difficult for some because of weakness or cognitive impairment, and modifications of the environment may be needed. Health status, age, and gender may all impact the ability to learn.
- *Experience:* People's experience with learning can vary widely and is affected by their ability to cope with changes, their personal goals, motivation to learn, and cultural background. People may have widely divergent ideas about what constitutes illness and/or treatment. Lack of English skills may make learning difficult and prevent people from asking questions.

- **Mental/emotional status**: The support system and motivation may impact readiness. Anxiety, fear, or depression about condition can make learning very difficult because the patient/family cannot focus on learning, so the oncology certified nurse must spend time to reassure the patient/family and wait until they are emotionally more receptive.
- **Knowledge base /Health literacy**: The knowledge base/health literacy of the patient/family, their cognitive ability, and their learning styles all affect their readiness to learn. The oncology certified nurse should always begin by assessing what knowledge the patient/family already has about their disease, condition, or treatment and then build form that base. People with little medical experience may lack knowledge of basic medical terminology, interfering with their ability and readiness to learn.

Alteration in Mobility as a Barrier

Alterations in mobility, although not as obvious a symptom as pain, present problems that can affect the **quality of life** of the patient and the family. This alteration of mobility can affect how the family responds to the cancer patient.

- This alteration can affect the range of motion of the patient's limbs, the skin integrity (decubitus ulcers) due to the inability to turn or unwillingness to move, and observations of neurologic deficits or changes.
- Limitation affects breathing; which leads to fluid buildup in the lungs; which may lead to pneumonia.
- With alterations in mobility, detrimental circulatory changes may occur that may lead to cardiovascular problems.
- Urinary changes can occur with urinary retention and urinary tract infections as the result.
- Constipation leading to bowel impaction can occur.

The risk factors for these changes can be pathophysiologic in origin, treatment-related in origin, situational, or environmental. Each one needs to be researched. Devices such as crutches, a sling, or cane may be required. A wheel-chair, assistance in obtaining handicapped license plates, or arrangements for a home aide may still need to be made. Hospital stays are getting shorter and ambulatory care extended. The nurse may continue to be required to provide assistance in these areas, to help the patient acquire necessary devices or permissions.

Support

Support Systems Available to Cancer Patients and Family

Patient/family support systems may vary widely and can include those that provide physical and/or emotional support:

- *Family members:* Family members (parents, spouse, siblings, children, grandparents) remain the primary support system for many patients and family, especially if they live nearby and can provide assistance although even distant communication can provide emotional support.
- *Friends:* Close friends may provide support in lieu or in addition to family members and may, in some cases, be more aware of emotional needs because of longstanding close association.
- *Co-workers:* Co-workers may donate sick time, ease workload, and provide support in various manners.
- *Organizations:* Community organizations may help in provision of meals, transportation, visitors, and other types of support.
- *Religion/Spiritual organizations:* Some religions/spiritual organizations provide not only emotional support but also nursing care and financial assistance.
- *Online support groups/message boards:* Internet support systems, such as message boards for specific types of cancer, can provide emotional support as well as useful information on treatment and coping.
- *Support groups:* Local hospitals, senior centers, and organizations often provide a variety of support groups for both patients and family/caregivers, such as support groups for those with cancer.

Community/Internet Resources Available to Cancer Patients and Family

Community/Internet resources available to support patients and their families include:

- *Association of Cancer Online Resources* (ACOR): Provides information and Internet support groups for patients and families as well as information about diseases and treatment.
- *American Cancer Society:* Provides support groups and assistance with non-medical expenses, such as durable medical equipment, transportation costs, and hair replacement wigs. The "Look Good, Feel Better" program provides assistance with techniques to minimize physical changes caused by treatment.
- *Group Loop:* Provides an online support group for teens living with cancer including discussion boards, personal blogs, and video journals.
- *National Children's Cancer Society* (NCCS): Provides financial assistance for non-medical expenses.
- *Ronald McDonald House:* Provides living accommodations for families, care mobiles, family rooms (in hospitals).
- *Sibshops*: Provides workshops for siblings.
- *Songs of Love Foundation:* Provides free personalized songs for children and teens with severe illness.
- *Starlight Foundation:* Provides personalized entertainment experiences for children with life-threatening illness.
- *13Thirty Cancer Connect:* Provides online support for teens and young adults

Psychosocial Considerations

Anxiety

Anxious Patient Assessment

When questioning a patient about their symptoms of anxiety, they may often complain of a nervousness or worried feeling, but not be able to specifically **identify** exactly what they are nervous or worried about. They may even experience these symptoms to the point of developing **physical symptoms** such as pressure in the chest, nausea/vomiting/diarrhea, sweating, or not being able to take a deep breath. Patients may also say that they are consumed with these feelings and cannot seem to voluntarily stop experiencing them. If a patient is experiencing anxiety at the time they are seen, physical signs may be evident. These include shaking, pacing, lack of concentration, and possibly flushing and shortness of breath. Blood pressure and heart rate are frequently quite elevated during a state of anxiety. When anxious, a person may become short-tempered and impatient with others, and may even raise their voice or snap at another person.

Causes of Anxiety

Many times, people do not understand the complexities of their illness and may feel that they are **out of control of their own lives** and treatment. This can lead to anxiety. A fear of the course the disease may take can also produce anxiety, along with the changes in the patient's life that will need to occur to accommodate the illness.

Certain types of tumors may produce **hormones** that can cause emotional upheaval and lead to anxiety. Treatments for certain types of tumors may also do this. If side effects of treatment cause illness, anxiety may become apparent in a patient that has no control over how their body is responding.

If a patient has a **history of anxiety,** they are more susceptible to experiencing panic attacks or anxiety-filled moments than they were before the illness. If cancer progresses or metastasizes, a patient may become very anxious and begin to feel helpless or experience feelings of hopelessness.

Anxiety Treatments

Anti-anxiety medications can be used for relief of intense anxiety when conservative measures fail. Co-morbidities will need to be considered and the patient will need to be monitored for potential side effects, such as a change in mental status or drowsiness.

Non-conservative measures should be focused on eliminating the **cause** of anxiety, if possible. This can include calmly talking to a patient and communicating with them, darkening a room and providing a quiet environment, or encouraging self-relaxation techniques.

If anxiety is a **recurrent problem**, enabling the patient to perceive when their anxiety level is about to rise can help to prevent these feelings from taking over. Help the patient to practice and utilize techniques such as imagery or "talking down" to prevent anxiety from consuming their emotional state.

If a patient is no longer under direct care in a hospital, provide them with community resources to draw on when anxiety becomes unbearable. Discussing one's feelings within a group can help to relieve some feelings of anxiety.

Loss

Loss is the situation in which a person loses a relationship. This does not have to be due to death and may not always involve a relationship with another person.

Loss takes many shapes and is a subjective emotion. Depending on the severity of illness, a patient may experience a loss of their **former life** before the diagnosis of cancer. They may have also lost **social contacts** with friends or co-workers.

If extended hospital stays are involved, patients may experience loss of **familiar surroundings**. Perhaps they will not be able to return home and must deal with losing their **home and personal belongings**. This may also involve a loss of a **pet** if they are no longer able to provide care to an animal.

Patients may become active in community cancer support groups and may experience loss from **death of other cancer patients** they have befriended. This can also cause anxiety in a patient when faced with the mortality of another person in their same situation.

Helping Patients to Cope with Loss

A patient may experience loss in such a way that it deeply affects their everyday life. They may even require psychological counseling or medications to help treat depression and anxiety. Always **assess** the depth of a patient's grief and **assist** them in obtaining the resources necessary to receive help.

Treatment of emotional loss does not need to be limited to formal psychological counseling, though. Many patients respond well to *group therapies* to talk out their feelings with other persons going through the same struggles. Becoming involved in a support group and possibly helping others by sharing their own feelings can be very therapeutic for a grief-stricken person.

Physical activity, as tolerated, can also help to relieve the stress involved with emotional loss. Physical therapy can help to teach a patient how to safely exercise within their limits to not only relieve stress, but feel better about themselves and focus on something other than the object of their grief.

Stages of Grief

1. Denial
   a. *Characteristics*: Resistive to information, stunned, immobile, detached, unable to respond appropriately.
   b. *Nursing response*: Be patient and supportive and repeat information as needed.
2. Anger
   a. *Characteristics*: Lashing out, overt hostility, blaming self or others.
   b. *Nursing response*: Do not respond in anger or take statements personally, remain calm and supportive, but be alert to risk of physical attack.
3. Bargaining
   a. *Characteristics*: If-then thinking, demanding another opinion or expert, praying.
   b. *Nursing response*: Avoid making any judgmental statements.
4. Depression
   a. *Characteristics*: Tearful, crying, withdrawn, sad, isolated.

- 187 -

b. *Nursing response*: Encourage expression of feelings, remain supportive, and assure individual that feelings are normal.

5. Acceptance
   a. Characteristics: Resolution.
   b. Nursing response: Listen patiently and remain supportive.

Risk Factors for Depression

Depression is an emotional feeling of personal distress, sorrow, despondency, and desolation. It can be severe enough that a person may even consider committing suicide. For a true medical diagnosis of depression, symptoms should be present for at least 2 weeks. A major risk factor for depression is the **diagnosis of cancer**. The severity of depression associated with cancer is often dependent on the prognosis and expected recovery rate. The chronic symptoms of **pain or nausea** can also cause depression. As can a major change in the patient's **activity level or lifestyle**. Certain medications used to treat the cancer can cause feelings of lethargy and depression in some patients.

A patient with a personal or family history of depression is more likely to suffer from depression than one with no history of the illness. Also, a patient with a history of, or current, drug or alcohol abuse is more likely to suffer from depression.

Depression Signs and Symptoms

Signs and symptoms of depression will depend upon the severity of the illness. These can range from acting sad or crying to thoughts of, or attempts at, suicide. Patients may also have **physical complaints** such as nausea, vomiting, or headaches. They may have a flat affect with very little, if any, smiling at pleasurable things.

Depression can cause an increase or decrease in **weight**. Some people eat more when depressed and others cannot eat at all because of nausea. **Sleep** can also vary with some people sleeping much more than usual and others not being able to sleep. Regardless of the amount of sleep one is getting, they will also have a feeling of being chronically tired without the motivation to perform any activities.

Anhedonia may also be present, which is a disinterest in things or activities that the person once enjoyed. There may also be a noted **decrease in self-care**, with the patient not wanting to shower or change clothes.

Pharmacologic Treatments of Depression

Many advances have been made over the years in antidepressant medications. Traditional medications, such as the **tricyclic antidepressants** (amitriptyline or imipramine) have a higher incidence of side effects than newer medications. The most common class of drugs used to treat depression is the **SSRIs** (selective serotonin reuptake inhibitors). These include paroxetine (Paxil), sertraline (Zoloft), venlafaxine (Effexor), and escitalopram (Lexapro). Each medication works on a different hormonal neurotransmitter: dopamine, serotonin, or norepinephrine. Many times, patients need to try various medications until they find the one that works for them. These medications should be started at low doses and gradually increased in dose until a desired effect is reached. It may take 4-6 weeks before true effects of the medication are noticed. If insomnia is a major issue with the patient, antidepressants such as mirtazapine (Remeron) and trazodone can induce sleep and work to treat depression. An older class of drugs, the **MAO inhibitors**, is rarely used now. These have considerable side effects and are used only in cases when all other treatments fail.

Non-Pharmacologic Treatments of Depression

Psychotherapy, whether as an individual, family, or group, can be very beneficial for patients to discover the cause of their depression and learn coping methods to help with their depressed mood. There are many different techniques used in psychotherapy, such as traditional reflection and insight, hypnosis, and primal screaming therapy.

- **Holistic methods** can be used to treat depression utilizing deep relaxation techniques and meditation. There are non-prescription herbal remedies that are often available, though these have not been tested by the Food and Drug Administration for safety or effectiveness.
- **Activity** can be used to dispel feelings of depression, though it is usually more effective in mild cases. The release of endorphins when exercising can cause an improvement in overall mood.
- **Electroconvulsive therapy** is still used for depression that is not responding to any other means. It has been found to be helpful in relieving symptoms, though it can cause some temporary memory loss.

Cancer Survivor's Psychological Effects

Depression and anxiety are very common in cancer patients and survivors. This can be due to a poor prognosis, recurrence, changes in lifestyle, or medication effects. There can also be an increased level of anxiety due to a dread of recurrence of the disease. This fear can cause patients to be very concerned about every abnormal sensation they have. This fear can also border on being obsessive and greatly impact a patient's mental wellbeing.

Cancer treatments, surgery, or the disease, depending on which type of cancer is present, can cause changes in **body image** with a result in low self-esteem. For example, a woman who has undergone a mastectomy may not feel like a whole woman again after the removal of one or both breasts. Radiation treatment can cause skin changes with redness and peeling. Alterations in self-image can also occur with hair loss due to chemotherapy, which can lead to depression.

Feelings of Helplessness and Hopelessness

Feelings of **helplessness** and **hopelessness** can lead to depression. The diagnosis of cancer leaves the patient to cope with the uncertainty of life. The stress in engenders affects all aspects of the patient's life. Helplessness and hopelessness are constant factors leading to depression. The unpredictability of the course of the disease inevitably leads to the feeling of loss of control of destiny. This uncertainty leads to sadness, depression, fatalism, giving up and very poor expectations of anything positive in the future. The nurse should try to engender a **sense of purpose** or instill a feeling that counteracts these expectations of impending doom. The nurse can foster of participation by the patient to give the patient a feeling that he/she has some control. The nurse can assist in helping to moderate feelings of anger or hostility in the patient and turn this focus of negative feelings into something positive.

Loss of Personal Control

A **loss of personal control** can occur when a patient feels completely overwhelmed with their medical condition. They may feel that they are not really a participant in the illness and that they are no longer involved in the decision-making process regarding their illness.

Risk factors for a loss of personal control include *severity of disease.* If cancer progresses to the end stages, the patient no longer has control over the disease and may feel hopeless and helpless. They may need to rely on others to perform simple ADLs for them. A healthcare surrogate may need to be assigned to take over the decision making regarding continued treatment. Or family members may voluntarily take over the decision making, leaving the patient with a sense of inability to make decisions. Other risk factors include a *prolonged hospitalization* where a patient can even lose their sense of time. A great deal of *privacy* is also relinquished while staying in the hospital.

Loss of Personal Control Treatment

If a patient is mentally competent, always include them in the **medical decision-making** regarding their illness. Even if they are only able to make the simplest of decisions, be sure to make time to discuss decisions with them. Often time patients are not fully **educated** about a specific treatment or other aspect of their disease, so make sure they fully understand the situation and the impact of any necessary decisions. If the patient has another person making their healthcare decisions for them, encourage open discussion about the situation between the two. Ensure that the healthcare surrogate is completely aware of and educated on the situation at hand. Try not to overwhelm the patient with too much information at once. Space out information and treatments, if possible, to ensure that any anxiety does not accumulate. Finally, encourage as much independence as possible. Have the patient perform their own self-care activities whenever possible.

Emotional Distress

Emotional distress is the state in which a patient may experience a change in their **emotional state** due to some aspect of their disease. This can include feelings of sadness, helplessness, hopelessness, spiritual distress, and withdrawal.

Risk factors include a severe illness with poor prognosis. A change or loss of the support system can also contribute to emotional distress. If a patient is not fully educated on their disease state, stress and anxiety can cause a state of emotional distress.

Cancer patients can often face an immense feeling of being overwhelmed when faced with not only the diagnosis of cancer, but the multiple medical decisions that need to be made. Most people are unfamiliar with the treatments available to treat cancer and educated decisions will need to be made within a timely manner. This may all be too much for a patient to comprehend at once. Any barriers to learning, such as language difficulties, can increase this state of emotional distress.

Treating and Minimizing Emotional Distress
- Encourage **communication** with the patient so they can discuss any fears or concerns that may be causing them distress. Providing psychological comfort and education can help to minimize these fears. This can be done through pharmacologic methods with anti-anxiety or anti-depression medications, or by providing contacts with community and religious resources.
- Try to minimize the patient's exposure to **stress-causing situations**. Space out medical treatments and assessments, if possible, and allow adequate quiet and rest times.
- Many patients may exhibit emotional distress through **physical complaints** such as nausea, headaches, or inability to sleep. Psychological comfort can help to minimize these symptoms.

- **Pharmacologic treatments** may need to be administered to help relieve these ailments. Anti-emetics and antinausea medications can help to relieve nausea or vomiting. Analgesics may be helpful in relieving headache or other bodily aches. Sleeping aids can be administered to help patients to relax and sleep. Potential drug-drug reactions should be considered before administering any of these medications.

Social Dysfunction

Social dysfunction is the state in which a patient can no longer function adequately within their social structure. This can include changes within their family unit or on a larger scale within their living environment.

Patients may have expectations of maintaining their **previous level of functioning** while undergoing cancer treatments. These demands may include providing for their family, continuing with all of the day-to-day chores of keeping a home and raising children, or maintaining work or community obligations.

Unfair demands may also be placed on the patient by family or friends who do not fully grasp or accept the severity of the illness. This may be a state of denial, which has been adopted as a coping mechanism for dealing with the potential illness or loss of a loved one.

Other risk factors include **treatments**, which may impair the patient's level of functioning. Many of these treatments may also involve extended hospital stays with separation of the patient from their normal environment.

Treating and Minimizing Social Dysfunction

Encourage **communication with the patient** to have them express their feelings of frustration in dealing with these conflicts that are contributing to the change in their social life. This includes establishing realistic expectations and goals the patient can use to minimize frustration and feelings of helplessness.

Communicating with family members, with the patient's permission, can help to educate them on what can be expected during treatments and throughout the course of the disease. This may help to minimize any excessive demands that may normally be placed on the patient. Though realistic goals need to be set for a patient, encouragement should also be given to have them continue their **involvement** in normal activities. They may be involved in their community or church or school events, and they should continue to do this as tolerated. This will help a patient to have a continued sense of self-worth and involvement. This can also help with maintaining mental acuity.

Sexuality

Dealing with Sexuality of Patients

The oncology nurse must:

1. Be aware of the patient's sexual concerns.
2. Have the sensitivity to how personal and private this is to the patient.
3. Demonstrate a professional attitude to the sexual concerns of the patient and his/her partner.
4. Have or be able to get the knowledge to deal with this important subject.

Johnson's Behavioral Model

The **Johnson's Behavioral Model** provides a means by which a patient's sexuality can be assessed. It approaches sexuality from a more holistic approach by looking at the whole person and determining how effects on one part of their lives can affect all other aspects. This model involves various **categories**, or subsystems, which are analyzed to detect any conflicts. It is thought that a disorder in one subsystem will cause problems in the other subsystems because, though they are different, they are all interconnected. For example, if a cancer patient has a colon resection and now has a colostomy, he or she may not feel comfortable with intimacy which affects both the eliminative component and sexual component of the model.

This model allows for each patient to be evaluated individually and take into account the **full range** of affects one aspect of their illness can have on several other aspects of their lives.

PLISSIT Tool

The **PLISSIT tool** provides a structured way in which sexuality can be discussed between the nurse and patient, with questions gradually becoming more personal. The idea is to initially broach the subject and then have the conversation progress into obtaining more personal details regarding a patient's sexual activity, both past and present.

- **Permission** is the first stage and it involves the nurse asking for permission to ask questions and discuss the patient's sex life. This helps to break down any barriers and promote comfort to talk about personal issues without feeling awkward.
- **Limited Information** is when the nurse asks questions to find out what questions the patient and partner may have about their sex life as it relates to cancer and cancer treatments. Education is targeted at this level.
- **Specific Suggestions** also involves education, but at a more personal level with specific suggestions for different problems that may arise during sexual activity.
- **Intensive Therapy** is utilized if there are deep-rooted issues surrounding a patient's sexuality with possible psychological conflicts involved.

Cancer Treatments and Pregnancy

- The difficulty of treating a **pregnant** woman with cancer starts with correctly diagnosing and staging the cancer. Many of the tests that are usually done, especially those using iodine or radiation, are contraindicated in the pregnant woman because of the risk of fetal injury. CT scans expose the mother and baby to radiation, but **MRI** does not.

- **Chemotherapy** can be the most harmful during the first trimester of pregnancy, when organ development is occurring. If the cancer is a type, which is fast growing, it is advised that the mother begin treatment immediately. It may be advisable to wait until the second trimester or later to treat cancer that is slower growing.
- **Radiation treatment** is usually avoided until the baby is born because of the great risks to the fetus from radiation exposure. If it is advised that the mother begin radiation treatments sooner, a decision may need to be made regarding termination of the pregnancy.

Fertility, Infertility and Cancer Treatments

Chemotherapy can cause *fertility issues* by impairing tissue function in males and affecting hormone levels in females. Children treated for cancer with chemotherapy can have lasting infertility problems later in life. Sometimes the infertility problems will resolve after a few years, so testing should be repeated to re-assess fertility.

Hormone treatments can cause a woman to be *more fertile* and will increase the chances of becoming pregnant. These effects can last for a couple of months after treatment, so birth control methods should be reviewed.

Radiation treatments to the pelvic area greatly increase the risk of *infertility of both males and females*. About one-fourth of patients receiving radiation below the level of the diaphragm will become sterile.

If infertility is a concern with treatment, sperm samples can be collected and frozen at a sperm bank for use in fertilization later. Experiments are being conducted in harvest of eggs to be used later.

Avoiding Pregnancy

It is important to stress to the female cancer patient how important it is to **not become pregnant** while receiving cancer treatments. Exposure to radiation can cause birth defects as can chemotherapy. Any cancer surgeries that are performed increase the risk for spontaneous abortion or pre-term delivery.

For many reasons, patients may still choose to become pregnant during cancer treatment. This may be due to personal beliefs regarding birth control, or perhaps they feel this will be their only opportunity to have a child if the cancer prognosis is poor. Others may be concerned about not being able to become pregnant after completing treatments. A patient may already be pregnant when diagnosed with cancer, in which case, treatment options and risk factors must be discussed thoroughly.

Educating on various forms of **birth control** is very important, as well as helping a patient to select the form of birth control right for her. Always assess any possible contraindications to birth control due to cancer treatments. For example, oral contraceptives should not be used if the patient has a tumor that is secreting hormones.

Sexual Dysfunction and Cancer Treatments

- **Chemotherapy** does not directly cause a male to not be able to attain an erection, but its side effects can make sexual activity difficult. **Pain** can decrease libido and other side effects such as dry mouth, hair loss, and fatigue can make sexual activity undesirable.
- **Hormone treatments** can affect erection, vaginal dryness, and feminization or masculinization. There can also be a change in sex drive with hormone treatments.

- **Radiation treatments** can cause defects to nervous and circulatory tissues and lead to permanent sexual dysfunction. Radiation focused directly on the reproductive organs in both sexes is most likely to cause inability to perform sexual activity.
- **Surgery** can also affect sexual function. Removal of organs necessary for reproduction, such as the prostate gland or testes, can affect strength of an erection and ejaculation. Removal of the bladder may cause permanent nerve damage that can affect sexual function. A hysterectomy can affect sexual pleasure and may cause scar tissue to form which can make sex painful.

Cancer's Impact on Intimacy

Cancer can impact **intimacy** between the patient and his/her partner in many ways:

- *Males*: May experience erectile dysfunction.
- *Females*: May experience vaginal dryness (which can make sexual intercourse painful) and early-onset menopause and associated symptoms.

Both male and female patients may experience decreased level of interest in sexual relations as well as changes in the intensity of orgasms. Body image alterations (such as may occur with mastectomy, colostomy, disfiguring surgeries, or excessive weight loss) may make the patient feel insecure about his/her body or embarrassed. Patients may simply be too fatigued and weak to engage in sexual relations. Worry and stress dealing with cancer and treatments may negatively impact the patient's interest in sex, and partners should be patient and supportive. In some cases, sexual dysfunction may persist for years after treatment is completed because of both physical and emotional problems. Other forms of intimacy, such as cuddling, are also important and may provide comfort.

OCN Practice Test

1. Which of the following cancers is the leading killer worldwide?
   - a. Stomach
   - b. Lung
   - c. Colon
   - d. Liver

2. Cancer incidence is:
   - a. the same as prevalence
   - b. the number or percent of people alive in the population who have had a diagnosis of cancer
   - c. the number of new cancers of a specific site/type in the population during 1 year
   - d. none of the above

3. Which of the following cancer types has decreased the most in incidence during the previous decade?
   - a. Prostate
   - b. Lung
   - c. Female breast
   - d. Melanoma

4. Which of the following races has the highest mortality due to cancer?
   - a. African American
   - b. Hispanic
   - c. Caucasian
   - d. Asian/Pacific Islanders

5. Female breast cancer:
   - a. accounts for 30% of all cancer-related deaths among women
   - b. will develop in one out of eight or nine women during her lifetime
   - c. the five-year survival rate is about 50%
   - d. all of the above

6. Among the risk factors for prostate cancer are:
   - a. family history of the disease
   - b. African American heritage
   - c. increasing age
   - d. all of the above

7. All of the following have been shown to reduce the risk of breast cancer EXCEPT:
   - a. bilateral mastectomy
   - b. tamoxifen (Nolvadex)
   - c. vitamin B12 and folic acid
   - d. raloxifene (Evista)

8. According to the recent studies, modification of lifestyle (stopping smoking, better diet, more exercise) and access to proven screening methods could save this percentage of cancer deaths annually:

    a. 25%
    b. 50%
    c. 75%
    d. no such estimate exists

9. The following is NOT a risk factor for colorectal cancer:

    a. high-fiber diet
    b. familial polyposis
    c. adenomatous polyps of the colon
    d. low selenium level

10. Human papilloma virus quadrivalent vaccine, recombinant (Gardasil):

    a. eliminates the need for Pap smears
    b. prevents cervical cancers caused by papilloma virus types 6, 11, 16, and 18
    c. should be given to all premenopausal women
    d. has no effect on genital warts

11. Which of the following is not a definite environmental risk factor for cancer?

    a. Asbestos
    b. Sun exposure
    c. Electromagnetic field exposure
    d. Radon gas

12. Which of the following viruses is most closely linked to Burkitt lymphoma?

    a. Human immunodeficiency virus (HIV)
    b. Epstein-Barr virus
    c. Hepatitis B
    d. Human papilloma virus (HPV)

13. Which of the following statements about tobacco use is NOT true?

    a. It is the single most important cause of cancer mortality in the United States
    b. Inhaled tobacco smoke but not chewing tobacco is highly carcinogenic
    c. Smokers who quit before age 50 halve their risk of dying in the next 15 years
    d. Secondary smoke has not been established as carcinogenic

14. Which of the following cancers does NOT have a well-established screening procedure?

    a. Lung
    b. Breast
    c. Cervix
    d. Colon

15. Tumor markers:

    a. include PSA, CEA, CA-125
    b. may always distinguish benign from malignant conditions
    c. are always useful for diagnosis of a specific cancer
    d. are never useful gauges of effective therapy

16. Which of the following is most recommended for early detection of colorectal cancer in normal-risk persons?

    a. Fecal occult blood test (FOBT) every five years
    b. Virtual colonoscopy every 5 years
    c. Colonoscopy every 10 years
    d. Double-contrast barium enema (DCBE) every 10 years

17. Which of the following would be the best approach to early diagnosis of prostate cancer?

    a. Prostate-specific antigen (PSA) annually starting at age 40
    b. PSA and digital rectal examination (DRE) annually in men starting at age 50 who have 10 or more years of life expectancy
    c. Prostate biopsy every 5 years
    d. None of the above

18. The term lead-time bias in cancer screening refers to:

    a. cancer is detected early but this does not affect mortality; survival appears longer but is not
    b. cancer is detected when cure is still possible but treatment does not result in a cure
    c. survival is actually shortened by early detection and too aggressive therapy
    d. hose cancers that are very slow growing compared with more aggressive ones

19. Colposcopy refers to:

    a. diagnosis of pancreatic cancer via CT examination
    b. diagnosis of ovarian cancer with laparoscopy
    c. endometrial biopsy of the uterus
    d. microscopic examination of the cervix

20. Which of the following pairs of risk factors and specific cancers is true?

    a. Alcohol consumption and cancer of the esophagus
    b. Inflammatory bowel disease and colon cancer
    c. Prior thoracic radiation and breast cancer
    d. All of the above

21. According to a current theory of carcinogenesis, which of the following are required to transform normal cells into malignant ones?

    a. A carcinogenic initiating agent
    b. A promoter
    c. Both A and B
    d. Neither A nor B

22. The ras oncogene that is found in many common human cancers, such as lung, colon, pancreas and leukemias, acts to alter cellular proliferation by which of the following mechanisms?

    a. Point mutation
    b. Amplification
    c. Translocation
    d. Overexpression

23. The tumor suppressor gene p53:

    a. is the least common mutated tumor suppressor gene found in human cancers
    b. when mutated is associated with common human tumors, such as bladder, breast, colon, or lung
    c. both A and B
    d. neither A nor B

24. Typical characteristics of malignant cells include the following EXCEPT:

    a. angiogenesis
    b. invasion of surrounding structures
    c. metastases
    d. spontaneous regression

25. Well-documented carcinogens include:

    a. ultraviolet light
    b. benzene
    c. RNA viruses
    d. all of the above

26. Sarcomas:

    a. always originate in bone
    b. originate in connective tissue
    c. originate in glandular epithelium
    d. originate in squamous epithelium

27. Which pattern of cellular growth is characteristic of cancer cells?

    a. Hyperplasia
    b. Metaplasia
    c. Dysplasia
    d. Anaplasia

28. A staging workup of a patient with non-Hodgkin lymphoma (NHL) reveals disease in the cervical lymph nodes and enlargement of the hilar lymph nodes on CT scan of the chest. No mediastinal mass is seen and the rest of the examinations are negative. This would be consistent with:

    a. stage I
    b. stage II
    c. stage III
    d. stage IV

29. B lymphocytes:

    a. dwell in lymphoid tissue
    b. are associated with cellular immunity
    c. may be subdivided into helper, cytotoxic, and natural killer cells
    d. antigens can attach directly to the cell membrane and do not require macrophage presentation

30. Which of the following would confer the worst prognosis for female breast cancer?

    a. Lobular carcinoma in situ
    b. 1.0 cm tumor in left breast
    c. Inflammatory histology
    d. Estrogen-positive receptors

31. A 60-year-old man with a 40 pack-year history of cigarette smoking presents with a chronic cough but little sputum, a 10 lb weight loss, and generalized fatigue. The chest x-ray shows a possible perihilar mass but clear peripheral lung fields. Which of the following procedures would most likely provide a definite diagnosis of lung cancer?

    a. Sputum examination with cytology
    b. CT exam of the chest
    c. Bronchoscopy with brush or needle biopsy
    d. Transthoracic fine-needle biopsy

32. According to the TNM (Tumor, Node, Metastases) staging system in widespread use, which of the following would be expected to have the highest stage and most likely the worse prognosis in a case of gastric cancer?

    a. T1N0M0
    b. T1N0M1
    c. T2N2M0
    d. T1N2M0

33. Cancer of the uterine cervix:

    a. is usually an adenocarcinoma
    b. can be diagnosed by an abnormal Pap smear alone
    c. has increased in incidence in the United States over the past 50 years
    d. is often associated with certain strains of HPV

34. Which of the following is true for colon cancer?

    a. About two-thirds of these cancers occur in the cecum and ascending colon
    b. Anemia without bowel symptoms may be a presenting sign
    c. Five-year survival for those with stage I is only 50%
    d. If the tumor perforates the bowel it is considered stage IV

35. All of the following are true for ovarian cancer EXCEPT:

    a. elevated CA-125 is diagnostic
    b. it is often diagnosed in a late stage
    c. it may be suspected by a palpable ovary in a postmenopausal women
    d. it usually requires surgical staging before treatment

36. All of the following are true for prostate cancer EXCEPT:

    a. may cause a rising PSA level
    b. is usually evaluated by grade as well as stage
    c. over half of men have this disease by age 90
    d. is one of the cancers in which the incidence is higher in Caucasians than African Americans

37. The most reliable diagnostic test for Hodgkin lymphoma is:
   a. positive test for Epstein-Barr virus
   b. presence of Reed-Sternberg cells in a lymph node biopsy
   c. presence of enlarged cervical and axillary lymph nodes on physical examination
   d. presence of a mediastinal mass on CT scan

38. Which of the following is true for implantable venous access devices?
   a. Needles are not required
   b. Removal requires surgery and general anesthesia
   c. Flushing with heparin must be done several times daily
   d. They do not require sterile technique

39. A peripherally inserted central venous catheter (PICC line) has the following advantages EXCEPT:
   a. single or multi-lumen catheters are available
   b. access may be accomplished without the use of needles
   c. removal may be done under local anesthesia
   d. there is a decreased risk of infection after insertion

40. The most common complication of central venous access devices (CVAD) is:
   a. infection
   b. occlusion
   c. malposition
   d. break in the line

41. Procedures to decrease the spread of cancer during surgery include:
   a. ligation of local blood vessels and lymphatics
   b. irrigation of wounds with cytotoxic agents
   c. both A and B
   d. neither A nor B

42. A surgical procedure may be used to prevent which of the following cancers?
   a. Breast
   b. Pancreas
   c. Lung
   d. All of the above

43. Which of the following surgical procedures would be most reasonable for a patient with stage I kidney cancer, a history of recent myocardial infarction, diabetes, and poor renal function?
   a. Radical nephrectomy
   b. Total nephrectomy
   c. Laparoscopic partial nephrectomy
   d. No surgery; radiation and/or chemotherapy only

44. Which of the following is true regarding radiation therapy?
   a. Radioisotopes used in treatment emit only beta rays
   b. Therapeutic doses are often described in grays: Gy or cGY where 1 Gy equals 1 rad
   c. Radiation sources include linear accelerator and radioactive isotopes
   d. Brachytherapy refers to radiation to the arm

45. Which of the following tissues or organs respond to radiation therapy rapidly?

    a. Bone marrow
    b. Thyroid
    c. Brain
    d. Uterus

46. For patients receiving radiation implants, protection methods for hospital personnel and visitors include:

    a. portable radiation shields
    b. remaining 2 feet from patient if possible
    c. radiation warning wristband
    d. all of the above

47. Early effects of radiation therapy may cause:

    a. alopecia
    b. skin atrophy
    c. hypothyroidism
    d. pericarditis

48. Which of the following would not be appropriate therapy for noninvasive bladder cancer?

    a. Transurethral fulguration
    b. Intravesicular chemotherapy
    c. Radical cystectomy with urinary diversion
    d. Laser therapy

49. Appropriate nursing duties in patients with testicular cancer include the following EXCEPT:

    a. teaching testicular self-examination (TSE) to the patient
    b. instruction in postorchiectomy pain management
    c. discuss the possibility of sperm banking before treatment begins
    d. reassure the patient that there is no possibility of sexual dysfunction

50. Many patients with head or neck cancers will require a temporary tracheostomy. Nursing care should include:

    a. hyperoxygenate the lungs only before suctioning
    b. instill 2 to 5 mL of normal saline into the tracheostomy to lavage and stimulate mobilization of mucus
    c. be sure tracheostomy ties are loosened to 6 cm
    d. clean external suture lines with peroxide 3% and apply ointment every other day

51. Which of the following is incorrect regarding multiple myeloma?

    a. Chemotherapy is the mainstay of treatment
    b. Radiation therapy may be useful for symptomatic bone lesions
    c. Peripheral blood stem cell or bone marrow transplantation has no therapeutic value
    d. Thalidomide has been used for treatment with some success

52. Which of the following is not considered a biologic response modifier (BRM)?
    a. Dexamethasone
    b. Rituximab
    c. Interleukin-2
    d. Interferon alpha

53. Conjugated monoclonal antibodies are:
    a. derived strictly from human sources
    b. have toxins, chemotherapeutic agents, or radioactive isotopes attached
    c. naturally toxic to malignant cells
    d. none of the above

54. Some reactions that the oncology nurse must be aware of in biological agent therapy are:
    a. weight gain is common, but weight loss is not.
    b. fever uncontrolled with acetaminophen or persistent beyond typical response
    c. severe toxicity, that is usually more severe that with traditional chemotherapy
    d. all of the above

55. Antineoplastic drugs have numerous chemical structures and different modes of action.
Doxorubicin is:
    a. an anthracycline antibiotic
    b. an alkylating agent
    c. a folic acid inhibitor
    d. a corticosteroid

56. Which of the following drugs are alkylating agents?
    a. Ifosfamide
    b. Cyclophosphamide
    c. Both A and B
    d. Neither A nor B

57. Which of the following drugs inhibits folic acid metabolism?
    a. Doxorubicin
    b. Methotrexate
    c. Dexamethasone
    d. Etoposide

58. Which of the following drugs are corticosteroids?
    a. Dexamethasone
    b. Prednisone
    c. Both A and B
    d. Neither A nor B

59. Hazardous anti-cancer drugs have the following features EXCEPT:
    a. may be carcinogenic
    b. may cause skin reactions or alopecia
    c. require specialized equipment for preparation
    d. may be safely prepared by pregnant personnel

60. Which of the following would be useful in preventing graft-versus-host disease (GVHD) in a bone marrow transplant recipient?

    a. Depletion of T cells from the marrow prior to transplant
    b. Using marrow from a donor who is a 6/6 HLA match with the recipient
    c. Use of immunosuppressive drugs such as cyclosporine or methotrexate
    d. All of the above

61. The term CAM therapy usually refers to:

    a. cytotoxic administration of Mustargen (mechlorethamine hydrochloride)
    b. cyclophosphamide, Adriamycin (doxorubicin), methotrexate protocol
    c. complementary and alternative treatments
    d. none of the above

62. Which of the following is NOT true for an autograft transplantation of bone marrow or peripheral blood stem cells?

    a. Finding a matched donor is not required
    b. Graft-versus-host disease is not a problem
    c. It may be used to treat nonmalignant disorders such as aplastic anemia
    d. May be preferable in older patients with certain solid tumors

63. Nociceptive pain differs from neuropathic pain by which of the following?

    a. It is often accompanied by numbness and tingling
    b. It arises from bone, joint, or connective tissue
    c. Is centrally mediated and often accompanied by burning and aching
    d. May be maintained by central sympathetic discharge (regional pain syndrome)

64. Which of the following is not a neurotransmitter released by tissue damage?

    a. Norepinephrine
    b. Bradykinin
    c. Substance P
    d. Prostaglandin

65. Nursing evaluation of pain in a cancer patient should include:

    a. location
    b. intensity
    c. temporality
    d. all of the above

66. A 65-year-old man with metastatic prostate cancer complains of pain in the spine and hip; he has been taking naproxen and occasionally aspirin without relief. What change in his analgesic treatment would you suggest?

    a. Switch to a different nonsteroidal anti-inflammatory drug (NSAID)
    b. Add oxycodone for the pain when required (as-needed) and continue naproxen
    c. Add oxycodone on a regular basis, continue the naproxen, and stop the aspirin
    d. Stop the drugs he is taking and begin parenteral morphine

67. Which of the following should not be used in a cancer patient with neuropathic pain?

    a. Meperidine
    b. Gabapentin
    c. Amitriptyline
    d. Ketamine

68. Addiction to opioid drugs is best defined as:

    a. a continuing need to increase the dose in order to control pain
    b. dependence on these drugs for psychic gratification and compulsive use, despite harmful effects
    c. emergence of a withdrawal syndrome characterized by unpleasant physical effects when the drug is abruptly withdrawn or an antagonist is given
    d. none of the above

69. Fatigue in cancer patients:

    a. is experienced frequently by patients using chemotherapy, but rarely by those using radiation.
    b. may be caused by endogenous cytokines secreted by the tumor
    c. is more common in breast cancer than leukemia
    d. all of the above

70. Measures to manage fatigue in anemic cancer patients include all the following EXCEPT:

    a. packed red blood cell transfusion if patient is anemic
    b. erythropoietin
    c. psychostimulants
    d. iron and/or folate therapy

71. Nursing assessment of fatigue in cancer patient receiving therapy may include:

    a. use of performance scales such as Karnofsky performance status (KPS)
    b. neurocognitive screening for orientation, recall, attention, and memory
    c. both A and B
    d. neither A nor B

72. Generalized pruritus (itching) is most commonly a symptom of:

    a. lymphomas
    b. anal or vulvar tumors
    c. young patients receiving treatment
    d. those receiving low-dose radiation therapy

73. Which of the following is true about sleep in cancer patients?

    a. Less than 10% will have a sleep disorder
    b. May be caused by symptoms such as pain, fever, itching
    c. May be aided by corticosteroid treatment
    d. All of the above

74 Which of the following is not a malignant skin cancer?

    a. Actinic keratosis
    b. Kaposi sarcoma
    c. Melanoma
    d. Squamous cell carcinoma

75. In a neurological examination of the cancer patient, the Romberg test evaluates:

    a. tendon reflexes
    b. balance
    c. visual acuity and fields
    d. joint position sense

76. Which of the following skin lesions is most likely a result of cancer treatment?

    a. Mycosis fungoides
    b. Acanthosis nigricans
    c. Erythema multiforme
    d. Dysplastic nevus syndrome

77. All of the following are nursing techniques to minimize the risk of aspiration in patients with dysphagia EXCEPT:

    a. elevate the head of the bed to 45 to 90 degrees with head slightly forward during eating and for 45 to 60 minutes after oral intake
    b. encourage ingestion of milk and milk products
    c. consult with dietitian to provide food-thickening agents
    d. assist moving food to posterior oropharynx using a long-handled spoon

78. Nausea and vomiting in patients undergoing radiation or chemotherapy is preventable or reduced by:

    a. serotonin antagonists
    b. phenothiazines
    c. cannabinoids
    d. all of the above

79. Hypercalcemia in cancer patients may be caused by:

    a. tumor secretion of parathyroid hormone (PTH)–like bone-resorbing chemicals
    b. cisplatin (Platinol) therapy
    c. osteoblastic bone metastases
    d. vitamin D deficiency

80. A cancer patient reports she has lost 15 lb over the past 3 months; her normal weight is 150 lb. About how many calories per day are needed to maintain her current weight?

    a. 2000
    b. 2400
    c. 3000
    d. 3500

81. Appropriate colostomy care should include:

    a. empty pouch when full and after chemotherapy
    b. change appliance every 5 days or sooner if there is leakage or peristomal irritation
    c. both A and B
    d. neither A nor B

82. Nursing management of bowel obstruction includes all of the following EXCEPT:

    a. keeping the patient flat to diminish pain
    b. local care of nasogastric tube
    c. auscultation for bowel sounds
    d. watch for signs of peritonitis

83. Which of the following urinary diversions after radical cystectomy for bladder cancer is most likely to lead to urinary tract infections and/or renal calculi?

    a. Orthotopic neobladder
    b. Ileal conduit
    c. Continent diversion
    d. The incidence is about equal for all of the above

84. Which of the following is most likely to result in pulmonary toxicity?

    a. Methotrexate
    b. Prednisone
    c. Radiation therapy
    d. Bleomycin

85. Which of the following treatments is appropriate for a malignant pleural effusion?

    a. Thoracentesis
    b. Pericardiocentesis
    c. Lobectomy
    d. All of the above

86. Upper limb lymphedema:

    a. occurs in 50% of women undergoing a modified radical mastectomy
    b. usually occurs 5 or more years after breast surgery
    c. is most common in those women that had an axillary node dissection and radiation greater than 4600 cGy
    d. none of the above

87. Malignant pericardial effusion has the following features EXCEPT:

    a. may be associated with primary tumors of the pericardium, mesothelioma most common
    b. symptoms may include chest pain, dyspnea, and fatigue
    c. is usually not apparent on chest x-ray or echocardiogram
    d. symptoms are determined by the speed of development of the effusion

88. Thromboembolic disease in cancer patients may be associated with normal platelet counts or:

    a. thrombocytosis
    b. thrombocytopenia
    c. both A and B
    d. neither A nor B

89. The granulocyte colony-stimulating factor (G-CSF) filgrastim (Neupogen):

    a. may be given as a single dose before chemotherapy
    b. stimulates both neutrophil and monocyte/macrophage production
    c. is not indicated for patients receiving bone marrow transplants
    d. may be given by subcutaneous injection or short intravenous (IV) infusion

90. Ondansetron is:

    a. a chemotherapy drug
    b. a steroid
    c. an antiemetic
    d. an antibiotic

91. A patient with cancer is undergoing chemotherapy and develops a fever of 103.5°F; he is found to have a neutrophil count of 300/mm3. Physical exam is not helpful in pinpointing the source of infection. Cultures are pending. Appropriate initial empiric antibiotic therapy might include the following EXCEPT:

    a. a cephalosporin
    b. an antipseudomonal penicillin
    c. vancomycin
    d. a fluoroquinolone

92. Which of the following chemotherapeutic agents is not a vesicant?

    a. Cisplatin
    b. Doxorubicin
    c. Vinblastine
    d. Carboplatin

93. One of the principles of chemotherapy developed to lessen tumor resistance and avoid toxicity to normal tissue is:

    a. use of drug combinations that act by similar mechanisms
    b. use of single agents sequentially
    c. use maximum tolerated doses of the drugs
    d. all of the above

94. Which of the following would be one indication to stop antibiotic therapy in a febrile cancer patient after 7 days?

    a. Afebrile for 1 day
    b. Negative cultures
    c. Neutrophil count more than 250/mm3
    d. None of the above

95. According to cancer patients, which of the following complementary and alternative medicine (CAM) therapies is most helpful?

    a. Self-help groups
    b. Exercise
    c. High-dose vitamins
    d. Herbal/botanical supplements

96. Acupuncture:

   a. is based on the Chinese medical theory, but is ineffective in Western medicine.
   b. is ineffective in treating nausea and vomiting caused by chemotherapy
   c. usually requires cumulative treatment with sterile needles to achieve success
   d. all of the above

97. Infection control measures for nurses caring for cancer patients include all EXCEPT:

   a. hand washing before and after contact with the patient
   b. avoid administering flu or pneumococcal vaccines
   c. aseptic technique to be used for placement or inspection of IV catheters
   d. avoid invasive procedures as much as possible

98. A cancer patient undergoing treatment complains of malaise and shivering. His temperature is 103.4°F. Ideally, which of the following should be done first?

   a. Obtain blood and other cultures
   b. Tepid sponge bath
   c. Administer acetaminophen
   d. Obtain a chest x-ray

99. Anxiety is a common reaction to the diagnosis of cancer and/or its treatment. The oncology nurse should:

   a. encourage the use of alcohol, tobacco, or marijuana to calm the anxious patient
   b. avoid providing factual information about diagnosis and treatment because this may add to the patient's anxiety
   c. consider the use of anxiolytic drugs with the physician or nurse practitioner
   d. assure the patient that all will be well

100. A 50-year-old man undergoing cancer treatment complains of sadness, poor appetite, difficulty concentrating at his job, and difficulty going to and staying asleep. He has had brief suicidal thoughts. Which of the following drugs would be most appropriate to begin therapy?

   a. Lorazepam (Ativan)
   b. Trazodone (Desyrel)
   c. Fluoxetine hydrochloride (Prozac)
   d. Paroxetine hydrochloride (Paxil)

101. Among the signs and symptoms of depression are:

   a. flat affect
   b. hypersomnia
   c. hopelessness
   d. all of the above

102. Which of the following is NOT appropriate in supporting the patient's spiritual needs?

   a. Contact the appropriate clergy or spiritual leader to meet with the patient
   b. Avoid discussion of spiritual matters with the patient's family; this may lead to conflict
   c. Provide privacy and quiet for prayer or other rituals
   d. Assure the patient that the nurse or others will be available in times of spiritual crisis

103. Which of the following would LEAST describe the patient with issues related to loss of personal control?

    a. Anger over inability to work while under treatment
    b. Refusal to comply with prescribed treatment
    c. Expressions of dependency and need for assistance in activities of daily living (ADL)
    d. Expressions of low self-esteem

104. All of the following are to be discouraged in the grieving process EXCEPT:

    a. substance abuse
    b. overuse of sedatives
    c. reliance on social, religious, or cultural customs
    d. social isolation

105. Alopecia is a common adverse effect of cancer chemotherapy and higher doses of radiation. All of the following are true EXCEPT:

    a. scalp hypothermia or tourniquets may diminish or prevent alopecia
    b. most of the time hair loss is temporary and drug dependent
    c. regrowth usually begins 6 to 8 weeks after the end of therapy
    d. color and texture of regrown hair may differ from that before treatment

106. Poverty influences cancer diagnosis and treatment in the following way:

    a. incidence is about the same in middle-class backgrounds as it is in poor
    b. cancer survival rate is about 10% to 15% lower among the poor compared to the general population
    c. ethnicity alone accounts for the lower survival rate from cancer in many social groups
    d. none of the above

107. Which of the following is true for female breast cancer in whites and African Americans?

    a. Incidence is about even among whites and African Americans
    b. Survival is about the same in both groups
    c. Incidence is higher among African Americans
    d. Mortality is higher in whites

108. Good nursing practice when dealing with ethnic minorities and different cultures include:

    a. ask the patient or family about beliefs and practices that are not understood
    b. always address the client by the last name and title, if any, until permission is given for a less formal greeting
    c. be aware the matters of space and touch may be different among various groups
    d. all of the above

109. In evaluating a cancer patient's coping skills, the oncology nurse should initially:

    a. refer the patient to a psychiatrist
    b. refer the patient to a social worker
    c. discuss fears and discomforting thoughts with the patient and suggest coping skills
    d. inform the physician and leave it to him or her

110. Disseminated intravascular coagulation is a complication of some malignancies and of sepsis. Which of the following would be the most likely laboratory finding?

    a. Decreased platelet count
    b. Decreased fibrin degradation product (FDP)
    c. Increased fibrinogen
    d. Increased plasminogen level

111. Which of the following infectious organisms would be most likely to cause septic shock in an infected cancer patient?

    a. Gram-positive bacteria
    b. Gram-negative bacteria
    c. Fungi
    d. Viruses

112. Which of the following metabolic patterns would you expect in the tumor lysis syndrome?

    a. Elevated potassium, elevated uric acid, elevated calcium
    b. Low potassium, elevated uric acid, low calcium
    c. Elevated potassium, elevated uric acid, low calcium
    d. Elevated potassium, elevated uric acid, low phosphate

113. Patients with certain cancers may develop hypercalcemia. In those with advanced breast cancer or multiple myeloma, this is most likely due to:

    a. osteolytic bone metastases
    b. secretion of a parathyroid hormone–related protein (PTH-rP)
    c. hyperparathyroidism
    d. low levels of vitamin D

114. A patient with small cell carcinoma of the lung has a seizure; MRI of the brain is negative; serum sodium is found to be extremely low at 112 mEq/L and the urine osmolality abnormally elevated at 320 mOsm/L. Appropriate emergency treatment for this patient might include:

    a. slow administration of hypertonic saline
    b. fluid restriction
    c. both A and B
    d. neither A nor B

115. Anaphylactic reactions:

    a. are associated with IgG type antibodies
    b. are caused by release of chemical mediators from mast cells
    c. are always predictable
    d. may occur 24 to 48 hours after administration of an antigen

116. Increased intracranial pressure (ICP) is a complication of brain tumors or cerebral metastases among other causes. Which of the following is the most rapid imaging technique?

    a. MRI scan
    b. CT scan
    c. PET scan
    d. Myelogram

117. The oncology nurse should be alert for the early signs of increased intracranial pressure. These include all the following EXCEPT:

    a. projectile vomiting
    b. morning headache
    c. blurred vision
    d. headache that is relieved by Valsalva maneuver or bending over

118. A 65-year-old man undergoing chemotherapy for lung cancer suddenly complains of bilateral leg weakness and some back pain. An MRI scan shows metastatic disease of the lumbar spine with vertebral collapse. Which of the following would be the most likely treatment sequence?

    a. IV corticosteroids, radiation, surgery
    b. immediate surgery, radiation, chemotherapy
    c. chemotherapy, surgery, radiation
    d. none of the above

119. Nursing interventions in a patient with lymphoma undergoing radiation treatment for superior vena cava syndrome (SVCS) should include:

    a. avoid IV fluids, venipunctures, and blood pressure measurement in the upper extremities
    b. keep the head of the bed low to decrease pressure on the heart
    c. frequent physical therapy to the upper extremities
    d. All of the above

120. Warning signs and symptoms of a cardiac tamponade are:

    a. loud heart sounds
    b. chest pain improved by lying supine
    c. chest pain made worse by lying supine
    d. increased pulse pressure

121. A patient with metastatic lung cancer, including brain metastases, develops diffuse skin ecchymoses, hematuria and epistaxis. A CBC reveals a hemoglobin of 10 g/dL, WBC count of 12,500/mm3, and platelet count of 10,000/mcL. Microangiopathic red cells and large platelets are seen on the blood smear. Prothrombin time INR is 4.0, the PTT is 3 times normal, and FDP are increased. A diagnosis of disseminated intravascular coagulation (DIC) is made. Appropriate therapy would be:

    a. packed red cell transfusion
    b. administration of platelet concentrates
    c. IV heparin
    d. oral warfarin

122. Which of the following is the most important factor putting a cancer patient at risk for sepsis?

    a. Granulocytopenia
    b. Diabetes
    c. Central venous catheter
    d. Age older than 65 years

123. A 30-year-old man is undergoing chemotherapy for acute myelocytic leukemia. The next day he complains of muscle twitching, irregular heartbeat, and decreased urination. An electrocardiogram (ECG) shows "tenting" of the T waves and frequent ventricular premature contractions. Which of the following would be appropriate treatment?

    a. Acidification of the urine
    b. IV calcium gluconate
    c. Increase the dose of his chemotherapy
    d. Withhold dietary calcium and give IV potassium

124. A 45-year-old woman with a history of hormone negative stage II breast cancer and mastectomy with radiation therapy two years before now complains of lethargy and confusion, some muscle weakness, constipation, and urinary frequency. An electrocardiogram (ECG) shows bradycardia with prolonged PR and QRS intervals. A chest x-ray is negative except for one missing breast shadow. A bone scan is pending. What is the most likely cause of this patient's symptoms?

    a. Bone metastases with hypocalcemia
    b. Brain metastases
    c. Premature coronary artery disease
    d. Bone metastases with hypercalcemia

125. A 16-year-old boy with a history of penicillin allergy is given IV asparaginase for acute lymphoblastic leukemia. Fifteen minutes later he complains of generalized pruritus, feeling faint, and difficulty breathing. The most important first medical management of this situation should be:

    a. stop the drug administration but maintain an open IV with normal saline
    b. check vital signs
    c. administer emergency medications per physician's order or institutional protocol
    d. documenting the allergy and reporting it appropriately

126. A bowel and bladder program for a patient with a cord compression syndrome of the lumbar spine might include:

    a. encourage citrus foods to alkalinize the urine
    b. placing the patient on fluid restriction less than 1000 mL per day
    c. palpate the bladder after voiding to check for urinary retention
    d. all of the above

127. The oncology nurse should:

    a. have a thorough knowledge of the anatomy and function of sexual organs
    b. avoid discussion of sexual matters with the patient entirely
    c. refer the patient to his or her physician or a sexual counselor if they have sexual questions
    d. wait for the patient to ask sexually related questions before discussing the topic

128. If a cancer patient wishes to discuss possible pregnancy during treatment, the oncology nurse should:

    a. provide condoms or birth control pills
    b. explain the rationale for delaying conception for up to one year after treatment
    c. advise women already pregnant in the first trimester to have an abortion
    d. explain that while chemotherapy may be dangerous to the fetus, radiation is safe

129. Which of the following is the safest, reliable diagnostic method for a pregnant patient suspected of having cancer?

    a. CT scan
    b. Radioactive isotopic scan
    c. Ultrasound
    d. Serum tumor marker

130. A young man with Hodgkin lymphoma is about to undergo treatment. Which of the following would be least likely to cause infertility?

    a. MOPP chemotherapy (mechlorethamine, Oncovin, procarbazine, prednisone)
    b. ABVD chemotherapy (Adriamycin, bleomycin, vinblastine, dacarbazine)
    c. Total body irradiation
    d. Bone marrow transplant

131. Pelvic radiation or chemotherapy in the female may result in:

    a. dyspareunia (painful intercourse)
    b. changes that are most often irreversible
    c. later menopause
    d. all of the above

132. Which of the following is a valid recommendation for a patient undergoing HIV-related cancer treatment?

    a. Use a latex condom with water-based lubricant for sexual intercourse
    b. Use a latex condom with petroleum-based lubricant for sexual intercourse
    c. Oral sex is permissible without a condom
    d. Refrain from all sexual activity

133. In the PLISSIT model of sexual counseling, the SS refers to:

    a. safe sex
    b. sexual sophistication
    c. specific suggestions
    d. none of the above

134. Which of the following surgical procedures for cancer patients is the least likely to affect sexuality?

    a. Radical prostatectomy
    b. Bilateral salpingo-oophorectomy (BSO) and total abdominal hysterectomy (TAH)
    c. Oophoropexy
    d. Bilateral orchiectomy

135. What are prominent fears of cancer survivors?

    a. Social discrimination and isolation
    b. Financial concerns
    c. Long-term effects of treatment
    d. All of the above

136. The cancer survivors' "bill of rights" includes all the following EXCEPT:
    a. equal job opportunities
    b. freedom from blame and/or guilt for having gotten the disease and survived it
    c. freedom from worry about disease recurrence
    d. medical privacy

137. Federal legislation protecting cancer survivors' employment opportunities includes:
    a. Social Security Disability
    b. Americans with Disabilities Act
    c. Taft-Hartley Act
    d. none of the above

138. Which of the following chemotherapy drugs is most likely to cause hepatic fibrosis or cirrhosis in long-term cancer survivors?
    a. Methotrexate
    b. Doxorubicin
    c. Bleomycin
    d. Vincristine

139. Which of the following second malignancies is a possible sequel to chest radiation?
    a. Breast cancer
    b. Soft-tissue sarcoma
    c. Both A and B
    d. Neither A nor B

140. Nursing assessment of a cancer survivor should include all of the following EXCEPT:
    a. history of chemotherapy drugs and doses
    b. review and critique of treatment with the patient
    c. risk or presence of delayed effects or symptoms
    d. identification of the stage of survival

141. Which of the following drugs may cause peripheral neuropathy and hearing loss?
    a. Vincristine
    b. Etoposide
    c. Dexamethasone
    d. Cisplatin

142. Which of the following drugs may cause azoospermia/oligospermia and ovarian failure?
    a. Cyclophosphamide
    b. Chlorambucil
    c. Both A and B
    d. Neither A nor B

- 214 -

143. Which of the following second malignancies is most likely in a male patient with Hodgkin lymphoma treated with MOPP chemotherapy (mechlorethamine, Oncovin, procarbazine, prednisone)?

    a. Leukemia
    b. Brain tumor
    c. Soft-tissue sarcoma
    d. Testicular cancer

144. Social dysfunction may be a problem in cancer survivors. The oncology nurse should be aware:

    a. that cultural practices often increase social dysfunction
    b. that social dysfunction is rare in long-term survivors
    c. of inappropriate expressions of anger and violence
    d. all of the above

145. Which of the following organisms is most likely to cause infection one year or longer after a hematopoietic stem cell transplant?

    a. *Aspergillus* species
    b. Varicella-zoster virus (VZV)
    c. Pneumocystis carinii
    d. *S. aureus*

146. During the conditioning phase prior to bone marrow transplant, many patients are treated with high-dose chemotherapy, including cyclophosphamide. The latter may cause a persistent hemorrhagic cystitis. Which of the following is useful as a preventive or ameliorating agent?

    a. Continuous bladder irrigation
    b. Administering mesna (Mesnex)
    c. Both A and B
    d. Neither A nor B

147. Which of the following nursing interventions is most appropriate for the acute stage of cancer?

    a. Introduce survivorship potential and support
    b. Develop guidelines for continuing care and follow-up
    c. Keep family informed on the patient's status and prognosis
    d. All of the above

148. Dysfunctional grief responses include all the following EXCEPT:

    a. refusal to mourn
    b. prolonged denial of loss
    c. painful dejection and crying
    d. clinical depression

149. Which of the following is not helpful in resolving the grieving process?

    a. Alcohol or sleeping pills
    b. Cultural, religious, and social customs
    c. Encourage social relationships
    d. Encourage verbal communication of thoughts and feelings

150. Palliative care in the incurable patient:
   a. should not be combined with chemotherapy or radiation
   b. should first address the most distressing symptoms
   c. should only be carried out in a hospice
   d. is not a nursing responsibility

151. Regarding management of cancer-related pain at the end of life:
   a. analgesics should always be given IV
   b. adjuvant drugs are contraindicated
   c. neurologic/neurosurgical procedures for pain relief are not helpful
   d. analgesic should be given on a regular around-the-clock basis

152. Constipation is a frequent problem for cancer patients, especially those on opiates and confined to bed rest. Which of the following would be the least effective management for a patient with no bowel movement for 72 hours?
   a. Disimpaction if required
   b. Enemas until clear
   c. Senna (Senokot-S)
   d. Magnesium citrate

153. Many dying cancer patients complain of dyspnea. All of the following are true EXCEPT:
   a. hypoxia is always present
   b. thoracic muscle weakness may be a cause
   c. destruction of lung tissue by the primary cancer may be present
   d. pleural effusion or lung metastases may also be a cause

154. Cachexia and anorexia in end-of-life cancer patients:
   a. are the same phenomenon
   b. anorexia may be reversible
   c. cachexia may be reversible
   d. should always be treated with parenteral feeding

155. Which of the following is a possible cause of nausea and vomiting in a patient with advanced cancer?
   a. Bowel obstruction
   b. Chemotherapy
   c. Increased intracranial pressure
   d. All of the above

156. Total (terminal) sedation in the dying patient:
   a. is never indicated unless refractory pain is present
   b. may be ordered without the consent of the family or patient
   c. both A and B
   d. neither A nor B

- 216 -

157. A terminal cancer patient develops signs of delirium. Delirium in this patient is often:

    a. related to opioid analgesics.
    b. related to a singular cause.
    c. irreversible even if a definite cause is found.
    d. caused in part by family members staying around the clock.

158. Standards of care for the oncology nurse are all the following EXCEPT:

    a. prescription
    b. diagnosis
    c. implementation
    d. evaluation

159. The basis for evidence-based practice (EBP):

    a. is not necessarily peer reviewed, but is cost-effective
    b. is based on the results of evidence derived from well-designed clinical trials
    c. is scientifically based, not based on significantly significant data.
    d. is based on the physician's personal experience

160. Teaching the patient and his or her family appropriate methods of care is part of the oncology nurse's responsibility. Instruction should include:

    a. management of indwelling venous access devices
    b. information on how to get a second opinion from another oncologists
    c. explaining to the patient the many types of learning styles
    d. extensive psychological counseling

161. Which of the following is the leading cause of nursing error and possible malpractice?

    a. Incomplete or absent documentation in the medical record
    b. Failure to monitor a patient in restraints
    c. Medication errors
    d. Failure to educate the patient

162. An elderly cancer patient presents with abdominal pain. He appears dehydrated with abnormal vital signs. Emergency operation for a bowel obstruction is recommended by the attending surgeon. The patient seems somewhat confused and is unable to give a rational understanding and approval of informed consent. Which of the following would be the best first course of action?

    a. Delay the surgery until the patient is more rational
    b. Contact a relative or other valid representative to obtain permission
    c. Cancel surgery and attempt medical treatment
    d. Declare this an emergency and proceed with the surgery

163. Oncology nurses must frequently participate in clinical trials of new treatments that may include any or all anti-cancer modalities (e.g., chemotherapy, radiation, surgery, hormones). An investigational new drug is scheduled for clinical trials. The appropriate human dose has been determined and major toxicities have been excluded. What phase of clinical trials would be next?

    a. Phase I
    b. Phase II
    c. Phase III
    d. Phase IV

164. Among the grounds for revocation of license by the state nursing board are all the following EXCEPT:

    a. conviction of a misdemeanor
    b. substance abuse
    c. unprofessional conduct
    d. negligence

165. Impediments to collaborative relationships with other professional staff include:

    a. perceived threats to autonomy
    b. lack of recognition of knowledge, experience, and expertise
    c. both A and B
    d. neither A nor B

Answer Key and Explanations

1. B: The three leading cancer-related deaths in the global population are due to lung (17.8%), stomach (10.4%), and liver (8.8%). The industrialized countries account for the highest rates while the lowest rates tend to be in northern Africa and southern and eastern Asia. Worldwide cancer rates are expected to increase in the near term because of aging populations and unhealthy lifestyles such as smoking and probably obesity. Tobacco use alone is responsible for 10 million deaths per year and is estimated to double by 2020. Although cancer rates (usually expressed as number per 100,000 population) in the United States have declined somewhat, there has been an increase in lung cancer among women and a general rise in liver cancer.

2. C: Cancer statistics are published annually by the American Cancer Society (ACS) and are expressed as incidence and prevalence. Incidence refers to the number of new cancers of a specific site or type in a population per year. The numbers may refer to a general population or be divided into subgroups based on age, geography, gender, ethnicity, socioeconomic group, or other distinguishing categories. Carcinomas in situ (except bladder) and basal and squamous cell skin cancers are usually excluded from the general numbers because of their frequency. The number or percent of people alive on a certain date in the population who have a diagnosis of cancer is referred to as prevalence. This includes new and existing cases. The National Cancer Institute estimate of cancer prevalence in the United States at January 1, 2000 was 9.6 million with average age for men 69 and women 64.

3. A: Overall cancer incidence has declined somewhat in men (1.5%) and has stabilized for women. Prostate cancer has declined the most in recent years; there are about 3% fewer cases per year. The incidence of liver cancer has increased the most, approximately 3.9% per year. Other cancers with reduced rates include Hodgkin lymphoma and leukemia, male lung cancer, and stomach and uterine cancers. Melanomas, kidney, and thyroid have also shown a slightly increased incidence. Do not confuse incidence with survival rates. Cancer survival rates are usually expressed as five-year survival and include persons with disease still getting treatment and those who are alive at 5 years after diagnosis with no evidence of disease (NED). Improvements in the survival rate may reflect better treatments or perhaps earlier diagnosis.

4. A: According to statistics from 1996 to 2014, African American men had the highest cancer mortality, 234.1 per 100,000 population, while women in this group recorded 157.0. Caucasians and then Hispanics were next most frequent, while mortality among Asian/Pacific Islanders was the lowest of the major races, 116.9 for men and 86.2 for women. The mortality rate among African American men is about 26% higher than that for Caucasians, while for women it is 14% higher in the African American community. Lung and prostate cancers account for much of the increased mortality among the African American population: 27% higher for lung cancer and nearly twice the mortality due to prostate cancer. Interestingly, American Indians and Alaskan natives show a mortality rate lower than that of Caucasians: 132.1 versus 193.6 for men and 89.1 versus 138.6 for women.

5. B: Breast cancer accounts for about one-third of all cancer cases in women and about 15% of cancer-related deaths. Modern statistics indicate that the disease will occur in one out of eight or nine women during her lifetime. The five-year survival among Caucasian women is about 88% for all stages but less among African American women (73%), possibly due to the later diagnosis and more advanced disease among the latter group. Recent data show a small downward trend in the incidence of this disease. Median age of diagnosis in women is 63 years. Male breast cancer is quite rare but does appear to be increasing among men younger than 40. Numerous risk factors for the

disease have been identified in women, including increasing age, estrogen treatment, early menarche or late menopause (possibly related to duration of exposure to estrogen), nulliparity, family history of breast cancer, radiation exposure, and genetic factors such as the BRCA1 and BRCA2 genes.

6. D: Prostate cancer is the second leading cause of death from cancer in American men despite the fact that only about 3% of those afflicted die of the disease. This is of great interest since about 20% of American men will be diagnosed with the disease during their lifetime. The disease appears to be indolent among older men and often they die of another disease before the prostate cancer becomes life-threatening. The disease tends to be more aggressive among younger men, possibly related to testosterone levels. African American men have a higher incidence and mortality rate than Caucasian men. This may be partially related to delay in diagnosis. Risk factors include advancing age, family history of the disease, a high-fat diet, and perhaps obesity. Genetic factors are suspected to increase risk but no definite genes have as yet been identified.

7. C: Preventive measures for those at high risk of developing cancer have been the subject of a variety of clinical studies. Bilateral mastectomy, though extreme, has been used for those women who have developed a cancer in one breast and/or have a very strong family history of the disease, usually two or more direct relatives such as mother and sister. Women with the BRCA1 and BRCA2 genes may be candidates as well. Tamoxifen, a drug that interferes with estrogen activity, has been used for 30 years to treat breast cancer and for 10 years to decrease the incidence in high-risk individuals. Raloxifene hydrochloride is a selective estrogen receptor modulator (SERM) originally developed to treat osteoporosis but has been found to be useful in breast cancer prevention, with possibly an even greater efficacy than tamoxifen. Vitamin B12 and folic acid do not prevent breast cancer.

8. B: Behavioral changes, though often difficult to maintain, may be the first line of defense in cancer prevention. Tobacco use, for example, has been associated not only with an increased risk of lung cancer but many other types of cancer as well. Recently dietary measures to avoid obesity have been the subject of several cancer prevention studies. Persuading people to go for proven screening tests such as Pap smears, colonoscopies, and PSA levels may also play a larger role in detecting precancerous lesions and lead to earlier treatment. Newer techniques, such as breath analysis for lung cancer, testing for blood tumor markers, or urinary DNA for bladder cancer, may increase the potential of this approach. According to a study conducted by Harvard University in 2016, 50% of cancer deaths could be prevented in the United States (and 20-40% of cancer cases could be prevented), if behavioral changes and better access to screening tests occur widely.

9. A: Most clinical studies of high-fiber diets have concluded that this dietary change may reduce the incidence of colon cancer and colonic adenomatous polyps, a known precursor of cancer of the large bowel. One study of 500,000 individuals in 10 countries documented a 25% decrease in the incidence of colon cancer in those individuals who ate 33 g/day of fiber versus those who ate 12 g/day. Low selenium levels have been correlated with an increased risk of colon cancer, although the mechanism is uncertain. Both calcium and nonsteroidal anti-inflammatory drugs (NSAIDs) may also have protective properties. Adenomatous polyps, especially those greater than 1 cm in size, are potential precursors of colon cancer and should be removed via colonoscopy. Those individuals with familial polyposis have a very high risk of colorectal cancer and colectomy is often required for prevention.

10. B: The new vaccine Gardasil is effective against the two types of HPV that cause 70% of cervical cancers and 90% of genital warts. Originally intended for girls prior to sexual activity, the indication has now been expanded to the 9- to 26-year-old age range. There are about 30 types of

HPV, so the vaccine may protect against those types that have not yet infected an individual. It is given in three doses over six months. Since the vaccine only protects against 70% of cervical cancers, the need for Pap smears is not eliminated. Side effects include pain or erythema at the injection site, headache, fever and occasional dizziness, vomiting, or fainting.

11. C: Numerous environmental factors increase the risk of specific cancers and cancer generally. Asbestos exposure is perhaps the most documented environmental carcinogen for mesothelioma and lung cancer and may have a synergistic effect with smoking-related lung cancer. Melanoma has been firmly linked to excessive sun exposure, especially youthful sunburn, and probably plays some role in squamous and basal cell skin cancers. Radon gas exposure, especially in miners and those workers involved with nuclear waste, most likely increases the risk of lung cancer. Whether proximity to electromagnetic fields (e.g., power lines) results in an increased cancer risk has been debated for many years and studies have mostly been observational with conflicting results. The advent of widespread cell phone use has added to the controversy but no definite statement about their cancer risk may be made at this time.

12. B: Viral etiology of cancer has been studied extensively over the past two decades and links with a variety of well-established cancers. This does not imply that the virus is always a direct cause of the cancer; it may act along with genetic or environmental entities or degrade immune surveillance. HIV has been associated with Kaposi sarcoma, especially in young homosexual males. It also may increase the risk of B-cell lymphoma. Hepatitis B and C viruses may cause or lead to hepatocellular carcinoma, which accounts for the largest majority of viral-linked cancers. Epstein-Barr virus, the cause of infectious mononucleosis, has been linked to Burkitt lymphoma, predominantly in Africans, and several other cancers, including nasopharyngeal and parotid. HPV, especially type 16, is a major cause of cervical neoplasia, and the virus has also been detected in a substantial number of squamous cell carcinomas of the oral cavity, head, and neck.

13. B: Tobacco use accounts for 30% of all cancer deaths and almost 90% of lung cancer deaths. In addition to lung, cancers of the upper airway and esophagus, bladder, pancreas, kidney, and perhaps cervix and colon have been shown to be increased in smokers. While cigarette use is far and away the most important source, cigars, chewing tobacco, snuff, and secondary smoke from others are all linked to a heightened risk of cancer. While many have quit smoking, about a quarter of the population still uses tobacco in the United States, and the number is higher in many other countries. Quitting before age 50 may halve the risk of dying in the next 15 years and those who have quit have a greatly decreased risk after age 70.

14. A: Mammography has been the cornerstone of breast cancer screening for many years. T ACS recommends starting annually for women age 40 and older; NCI allows every 1 to 2 years for women older than 40. There has been a very recent conflict over these guidelines by a federal task force that suggested age 50 as the starting point for mammograms and every two years thereafter. Pap smears to detect cervical dysplasia and carcinomas at a very early stage have been well established for many years. While previously recommended for women when they become sexually active, one professional gynecology group has now stated that biannual smears starting at age 21 may be adequate. Colonoscopy with polypectomy has revolutionized colorectal cancer screening and prevention and has most likely led to the recent decline in this cancer. Lung cancer screening remains difficult. Chest x-rays and sputum cytology are inadequate and spiral CT or other sophisticated scanning techniques (e.g., PET scans) are still under evaluation.

15. A: Along with imaging studies and biopsy-cytology, tumor markers are playing an important role in cancer diagnosis and treatment. These are products in the blood either produced directly by the tumor or reflecting the body's reaction to the tumor. Some of the well-known ones are PSA, CEA,

alpha-fetoprotein, CA-125, and CA 19-9. Unfortunately, they are often nonspecific and may be produced by benign conditions. PSA may be elevated in benign prostatic hypertrophy, as well as in prostate cancer, and this has led to quite a controversy over the value of annual PSA screening tests for men. Too often, false-positives and false-negatives confound a specific diagnosis so these markers are best used as confirmatory to other diagnostic measures. Once a definite diagnosis is made, the level of the marker may often be used as an indicator of treatment efficacy. Sometimes decisions regarding treatment (e.g., surgery) are influenced by the magnitude of the tumor marker.

16. C: For many years, annual fecal occult blood testing was the only routine method of screening for early colon cancer. Unfortunately, there are many false-positives and false-negatives with this technique, although it still has a role in the detection of bowel neoplasia with annual testing. Virtual colonoscopy using computerized tomography and bowel contrast media is still under evaluation as a screening tool but is associated with high radiation exposure and the discomfort of a contrast enema. Colonoscopy every 10 years is the currently the most favored method for both sexes starting at age 50. It has the advantages of being performed under anesthesia, routine examination of the entire colon is possible, and the immediate excision of polyps or other premalignant lesions. Double-contrast barium enema has largely been replaced by colonoscopy, but when used (e.g., those with tortuous colons that are hard to colonoscope) it should be done every five years.

17. B: The best early-detection method for prostate cancer remains controversial and different professional associations differ in their recommendations. One problem is that the PSA test may be elevated more than 4 ng/ml with benign lesions, so some authorities suggest further investigation only if the level is rising over time. Also, mortality from the disease is relatively low and older men tend to have indolent disease and often die of another cause. The ACS currently recommends PSA and DRE annually for men at age 50 who have 10 or more years of life expectancy. For higher-risk individuals, those with a family history or African American heritage, starting annual testing starting at age 45 is suggested. Men with even higher risk (first-degree relative who was diagnosed with prostate cancer at a young age), are recommended to begin screening at age 40.

18. A: The concept of lead-time bias in cancer refers to an early detection of the cancer that has no impact on true survival. For example, a five-year survival rate may appear to be improved by earlier diagnosis but actual lifespan is not prolonged. This fact must be taken into consideration when evaluating cancer treatments, especially those that include five-year survival rates as an end point. There are other potential pitfalls in analyzing the efficiency of cancer screening tests and early treatment. Length bias refers to the presence of both symptomatic, aggressive cancers in a population and those with asymptomatic, less-aggressive disease. Screening may detect both but those with less-aggressive disease will appear to have a better survival. For this reason, clinical trials usually compare new treatments versus older ones with groups of patients that are as close to identical as possible (e.g., age, sex, stage of tumor, metabolic data, and performance status).

19. D: The term for microscopic examination of the cervix is colposcopy. It is usually done after a positive Pap smear and employs a long focal length dissecting type microscope with a 10x to 16x magnification. The cervix is usually treated beforehand with 4% acetic acid solution, which allows directed biopsy of suspicious lesions. Ovarian cancer is often suspected by pelvic examination and confirmed by laparoscopic biopsy but does not employ colposcopy. Endometrial biopsy may be useful for detecting endometrial and occasionally cervical cancer at the margin but does not involve colposcopy. Diagnosis of pancreatic cancer may be made by CT examination or laparoscopy and then needle or surgical biopsy but this also does not involve colposcopy.

20. D: Excess alcohol use is thought to be related to 3% of cancer mortality and includes cancers of the esophagus, upper gastrointestinal tract and colon, liver, and possibly breast. The exact

mechanism is unknown and there is evidence for either a direct or indirect effect. It is often synergistic with tobacco. Patients with inflammatory bowel disease such as Crohn disease or ulcerative colitis have an increased risk of colon cancer and require earlier and more frequent colonoscopic screening than average risk individuals. Sometimes bowel resection is the only prophylactic treatment. Among the many risk factors for breast cancer, previous thoracic radiation, usually in treatment of lymphoma or thymoma, predisposes to breast cancer, often at an early age. Routine mammography should be started within 15 years of the radiation treatment or by age 40.

21. C: According to the three-stage theory of carcinogenesis, malignant transformation of normal cells involves three distinct mechanisms. An initiator substance, which may be a chemical, physical, or biologic carcinogen, damages DNA that affects a genetic change. The damaged DNA may then undergo repair and no initiation occurs. However, if the damage is permanent (mutation) it may be subject to further modification of the cell physiology by a promoter substance that can lead to alterations in the cell's proliferative capacity or inhibit apoptosis (genetically programmed cell death). Some substances such as asbestos, tobacco smoke, or alcohol have both initiator and promoter properties. It is believed there is a threshold dose for a promoter substance to alter cell physiology that in turn depends on the nature, dose, and duration of exposure.

22. A: Oncogenes arise from mutated proto-oncogenes that normally regulate cellular growth and repair. The ras family of proto-oncogenes may be transformed to an oncogene by a point mutation of its DNA. This may lead to unrestrained cellular proliferation. Amplification overexposure or translocation are other mechanisms of genetic alteration of growth factor receptors, signal transduction proteins (transmission of membrane information to the cell nucleus), or certain nuclear regulatory proteins that control cell division. Examples are the sis proto-oncogene transformed by overexpression and associated with astrocytomas; the N-myc utilizing an amplification mechanism and associated with neuroblastoma and small cell carcinoma of the lung; and ABL associated with chronic and acute leukemias utilizing a translocation mechanism for a non-receptor tyrosine kinase enzyme.

23. B: Tumor suppressor genes refer to that portion of the genetic DNA that regulates cell division. Mutation or loss of these genes may lead to enhanced cell growth and proliferation. Some of these also carry out DNA repair, so that loss will lead to unregulated cell division. The mutated gene p53 is the most common tumor suppressor gene found in human cancers, including many solid malignancies, brain tumors, and hematologic cancers. It may also interfere with apoptosis, the genetically programmed mechanism to rid the tissue of old or defective cells. In addition to p53, some other well-described tumor suppressor genes are the BRCA1 and BRCA2 genes that are associated with breast and ovarian cancer. These have a DNA repair function. Several other tumor suppressor genes act by other mechanisms.

24. D: Whatever the causative mechanism, malignant cells have a growth advantage over normal cells and have seemingly lost their response to growth and proliferation regulatory factors. As this unregulated growth continues, the tumor cells may compress and invade adjacent tissues or organs, sometimes by secreting enzymes that break down cellular barriers. Many tumors have the capacity to secrete substances called vascular endothelial growth factors (VEGF) that stimulate new blood vessel formation, a process called angiogenesis that allows the tumor an adequate blood supply as it grows. Several new chemotherapy agents are angiogenesis inhibitors and are directed at this process. The capacity for metastatic spread of cancer cells throughout the body, whether by direct invasion, seeding of body cavities, or lymphatic or hematogenous dissemination, is another distinguishing feature of most malignant tumors. Spontaneous regression of cancer, while described, is quite unusual.

25. D: Carcinogens include ionizing radiation from natural (cosmic rays, radon gas) or diagnostic (x-rays, radioisotopes, radiation therapy) sources. Ultraviolet light is a complete carcinogen and probably causes most skin cancers including melanoma. Benzene is one of a long list of chemical carcinogens that includes such familiar substances as alcohol, arsenic, benzopyrene, beryllium, coal and tar pitch and soot, silica, smoked and pickled foods, vinyl chloride, and many others. Some therapeutic antineoplastic (e.g., alkylating agents) and immunosuppressant drugs (e.g., cyclosporine A) are also carcinogenic. Many of the common RNA viruses such as HBV, HCV, HIV and HPV are potential carcinogens. Some of the above factors act as initiators, promoters, or both; some may act by impairing immune surveillance by which the immune system is able to recognize and eliminate or inhibit growth of cancer cells.

26. B: Tumor nomenclature is usually based on the tissue of origin. Benign tumors are often named by adding the suffix -oma to the tissue of origin (e.g., lipoma from fat, neuroma from nerve) but there are exceptions. Malignant tumors are usually divided into carcinomas, which arise from epithelial tissue, and sarcomas, which are derived from connective tissue (including smooth and skeletal muscle, cartilage, bone, and fat). Carcinomas are usually subdivided into those arising in squamous epithelium (squamous cell carcinoma) and those arising in glandular epithelium (adenocarcinoma). Lymphatic and hematologic malignancies are referred to as leukemias (arising from blood cells), lymphomas (arising from lymph node tissue), and multiple myeloma (arising from plasma cells).

27. D: Numerous cells undergo growth patterns that in some cases are normal responses to injury or irritation while in others they may be precursors to malignant changes. Hyperplasia, an increase in the number of cells in a tissue, may be a normal response in wound healing or a premalignant condition but is not a defining characteristic of cancer. Metaplasia is a potentially reversible process that involves the replacement of one type of mature cell with another not usually found it that tissue. Examples are squamous cell replacement of columnar epithelial cells in the airway of smokers, or the replacement of typical cells of the distal esophagus with intestinal epithelium in Barrett esophagus. Dysplasia refers to a loss of uniformity of particular cells with changes of size, shape, and architecture. Malignant cell growth is usually described as anaplastic, which is marked by extreme cellular disorganization, immature forms, and prominent nuclei.

28. B: Staging of NHL is usually based on criteria developed by the St. Jude staging system. This includes four stages, I to IV. The stage of the disease has major implications for both prognosis and treatment. Generally, stage I disease is limited to a single nodal or extranodal area; II reflects two nodal or non-nodal areas on the same side of the diaphragm; III indicates disease on both sides of the diaphragm or any intrathoracic tumor or extensive intraabdominal disease; IV means involvement of the central nervous system or bone marrow. Additionally, lymphoma staging may sometimes include a sub-staging of either *A* or *B*, where *A* lymphomas are generally asymptomatic, while *B* lymphomas will present with symptoms such as fever, night sweats, pruritus, or significant weight loss. This classification level, however, is utilized more often in Hodgkin's lymphoma. Regardless of staging, the total burden of disease is perhaps the most significant prognostic factor and may correlate with serum LDH and serum IL-2 receptor levels as well as stage and histologic type.

29. A: The distinction between B lymphocytes associated with humoral immunity and T lymphocytes associated with cellular-mediated immunity is important in understanding the immune system. B cells originate in bone marrow and lymphatic tissue. Antigens are usually presented to B cells for processing by macrophages that acquire antigens and unused B cells react with specificity to one type of antigen. Some B lymphocytes differentiate into plasma cells and produce circulating protein antibodies while others retain the capacity to do so, called memory

cells. T cells (originally thymus derived) are responsible for cellular immunity and may accept antigen from macrophages or via direct attachment to the cell membrane. T cells may be helper T cells that regulate cellular immunity by secretion of cytokines, or cytotoxic T cells that may kill target cells by several mechanisms. Natural killer (NK) cells are a form of T cell that attaches to and perforates target cell membranes and destroys them with granular enzymes.

30. C: Numerous factors influence the prognosis for female breast cancer, including histology and grade, tumor size, lymph node involvement, hormone-receptor status, tumor proliferative index, and several others. Lobular carcinoma is often an incidental finding that does not show up on mammography and carries an increased risk for invasive breast cancer, approximately 1% per year in either breast. Tumor size is an important marker for prognosis and tumors over 5 cm may increase the stage from II to III and worsen the prognosis. Inflammatory carcinoma of the breast often appears suddenly with skin changes but no discrete nodule and confers a poor prognosis. Tumors associated with estrogen and/or progesterone receptors tend to have a better prognosis than those that are receptor negative.

31. C: The clinical description in the question is classic for lung cancer but other possible causes such as chronic obstructive lung disease, sarcoidosis, lymphoma, metastatic cancer, and tuberculosis must be ruled out. Only a biopsy can confirm a diagnosis of lung cancer. Chest x-rays may show suspicious lesions but false positives and false negatives are common and can only suggest a diagnosis. CT scans of the chest tend to show most lung cancers well and are quite helpful in localizing the lesion(s) and assisting in staging. Both bronchoscopy with brush or needle biopsy and transthoracic fine needle biopsy may provide a definite diagnosis. The latter is most useful in peripheral or diffuse lesions of the lung while the former tends to be more useful in centralized bronchogenic carcinomas. Sputum cytology may or may not be positive but usually cannot be relied upon for staging and in planning treatment.

32. B: In the common TNM system for assessing stage. T refers to the size or degree of invasion of the primary tumor. In gastric cancer, T1 would show invasion of the lamina propria or submucosa while T2 would show invasion of the muscularis layer. N refers to nodal involvement with N0, indicating none, and N1 and N2, indicating perigastric nodal involvement with cancer: N1 within 3 cm of the primary tumor and N2 beyond 3 cm or in distant nodes. M refers to distant metastases: M0 none, M1 any metastases. Thus, answer A would be stage 1A; B stage 4 because of metastatic disease, C stage III, and D stage II. Interestingly, this cancer is very common in Japan and relatively uncommon in the United States, though the incidence has been rising here recently. Dietary factors likely play a role.

33. D: Cancer of the cervix is usually squamous in nature (85% to 90%), while adenocarcinoma tends to occur in younger women and carries a worse prognosis. Lesions may be exophytic, ulcerative and necrotic, or endophytic projecting into the cervical canal. The incidence has dramatically decreased in the United States since the advent of the Pap smear in the 1940s, though worldwide it remains a significant cause of morbidity and mortality. Pap smears may report abnormal cells but the usual diagnostic methods are cone biopsy, endocervical curettage, or colposcopy directed direct biopsy of a lesion. Recently, DNA testing for high-risk strains of HPV, considered the cause of cervical cancer, may contribute to the diagnostic arsenal.

34. B: Colon cancers are usually adenocarcinomas and some two-thirds arise in the rectosigmoid and sigmoid sections of the colon. Only about 14% arise in the cecum and ascending colon. They most often arise in adenomatous polyps. Typical symptoms are abdominal pain, bowel obstruction, or changes in stool habits; however, the cancer may present without bowel symptoms and may be detected by stool positive for occult blood. Therefore, anemia may be the only presenting sign. This

demands a bowel investigation such as barium enema or colonoscopy, especially in persons older than 40 or with a family history of bowel cancer. Five-year survival rates run from 90% to 95% for those with stage I (tumor limited to submucosal invasion with no nodal or metastatic disease) to 5% for those with stage IV (metastatic disease). Even if the tumor perforates the bowel but does not involve lymph nodes or have distant metastases it is considered stage II, which has a 75% to 80% five-year survival rate.

35. A: Ovarian cancer remains a highly lethal disease with a peak incidence in the 60- to 64-year-old age group. One of the reasons for its lethality is that it often lacks symptoms until the disease is in an advanced stage. Although the CA-125 tumor marker and transvaginal ultrasound have been used as screening tools in high-risk women (e.g., those positive for BRCA genes or with a family history), their use for this purpose remains controversial. CA-125, like many tumor markers, is not specific for ovarian cancer. Bimanual pelvic exam remains the screening method most often leading to a suspected ovarian cancer, by palpation of an ovary in postmenopausal women or of a mass or irregular ovary. Surgical staging is usually required for pathologic examination of ovaries, tubes and uterus, and pelvic lymph nodes, and possible seeding of tumor into the abdominal cavity. Surgical debulking of tumor is also carried out.

36. D: Prostate cancer tends to be more aggressive in younger men but may be present in more than 50% of men who reach the age of 90. Nearly 95% of these tumors are adenocarcinomas and most arise in the peripheral portion of the gland. Symptoms, if present, are most often referable to urinary function, although local invasion or distant metastases may give rise to other localizing symptoms, especially metastatic disease of bone. The disease is evaluated by 1) grade: Gleason score based on the sum of abnormality in two areas (primary and secondary) of biopsied specimens with higher scores indicating more aggressive disease and a poorer prognosis; and 2) stage by the usual TNM criteria. African Americans tend to have a higher incidence and poorer prognosis than Caucasian men.

37. B: The hallmark diagnostic criterion of Hodgkin lymphoma is the presence of the eponymous Reed-Sternberg cells, almost always found in a lymph node biopsy. These are giant cells with polypoid or multiple nuclei and eosinophilic nucleoli. These represent a minority, only 1% to 5% of the cell population against a background of small lymphocytes and fewer other cell types such as granulocytes and fibroblasts. Immunochemical markers that are especially positive for CD30 and CD15 are also helpful in distinguishing Hodgkin from non-Hodgkin lymphomas. There are four main histologic subtypes that are important in prognosis and treatment decisions. In addition to these, nodular lymphocyte predominant form occurs with tight-packed nodules under low-power microscopy. While enlarged cervical and axillary lymph nodes may be enlarged or a mediastinal mass present, these are not diagnostic of Hodgkin lymphoma.

38. B: Implantable venous access devices require surgical insertion with a port placed in a subcutaneous pocket in the upper chest or abdomen and the catheter threaded into the superior vena cava. They are quite useful for drawing blood and/or blood and electrolyte infusions but special needles (Huber) are required that may be left in place for up to a week. Sterile technique must be employed if withdrawing blood or administering fluids. Flushing with heparin is only required once a month and after the device is accessed. Surgery under general anesthesia is required for removal. All central venous access devices (internal and external) should be placed early in a patient's course to avoid sclerosing peripheral veins.

39. D: Peripherally inserted central venous catheters have advanced the effectiveness of blood withdrawal and administration of fluids and blood products without the need for repetitive needle sticks that are painful and may compromise the peripheral veins. They can be placed by specially

trained nurses and left in place for as long as 60 days. They are usually threaded through an arm vein to the superior vena cava. Daily dressing changes and flushing with heparin/saline using sterile technique is required. They do, however, provide a potential entry port for bacteria and must be removed if this occurs. One other disadvantage is that they may limit activities such as athletics or swimming or distort the patient's body image, resulting in shame or avoidance of socialization.

40. A: The most common problem with CVAD is infection. The incidence may range from 2% to 60% depending on the type of device, the length of time it is in place, or on the antiseptic care it receives. Infection may affect the device at its exit site, inside the tubing, or surrounding the port pocket. Some infections can be cleared without removal of the device but many cannot and the CVAD will need to be replaced. Occlusion is the second most common problem and may be caused by thrombus in the line, fibrin accumulation at the tip, or by precipitation of drugs given with incompatible fluids. Clearing of the line may sometimes be successful with fibrinolytic drugs (e.g., tissue plasminogen activator [tPA]) or ethanol or sodium bicarbonate. Malpositioning may also impair line function and, if it cannot be corrected by manipulation, will have to be replaced. Finally breaks in the line can cause bleeding or air embolus or infection.

41. C: A major principle of cancer surgery is to avoid spreading cancer cells locally or systemically. This is especially important during excision of a localized cancer with curative intent. Several techniques are employed to diminish the risk of spread. These include ligation of local blood vessels and regional lymphatics to preclude spread by interfering with typical pathways of tumor dissemination; irrigation of wounds and cleansing of surgical instruments with cytotoxic agents; changing surgical gloves frequently; and using a "no-touch" technique in handling malignant tissue. One of the objectives of postoperative chemotherapy is the destruction of microscopic tumor cells that may have spread from the main tumor.

42. A: Using a surgical procedure to prevent a cancer is often considered for high-risk individuals. Prophylactic mastectomy may be employed for those women with a very strong family history of the disease or those who are positive for one of the BCRA genes, or those who have had a malignancy in the contra- lateral breast. This is nearly always an elective procedure but the availability of cosmetic reconstruction surgery has made this a viable option for many high-risk women. This approach has also been used for cryptorchid testes with orchiopexy, colectomy in patients with familial polyposis or inflammatory bowel disease, or oophorectomy in those with a strong family history of ovarian cancer. Many premalignant lesions such as Barrett esophagus, colonic adenomatous polyps, or dysplastic skin lesions are often excised as well. The future may hold the possibility of removal of vital organs such as the pancreas or lung for replacement with natural or artificial ones.

43. C: The possible consequences of radical surgery for cure must often be weighed against the risk of possible complications or even death. Patients with metabolic disorders, such as diabetes, and poor cardiac, pulmonary, or renal function present a higher risk. In the current case, stage I kidney cancer indicates the tumor is less than 7 cm in its widest diameter and confined to the kidney. While total or even radical nephrectomy might have been considered in the past, the availability of laparoscopic surgery with subtotal nephrectomy may now be the treatment of choice for such a patient. Five-year survival rates for stage I kidney cancer approach 90% but nephron-sparing surgery should be strongly considered in this type of high-risk patient.

44. C: Radiation therapy constitutes an important treatment modality for many cancers and it is estimated that some 60% of cancer patients receive some sort of radiation therapy. This may be in the form of external beam (teletherapy) or localized from a sealed radiation source

- 227 -

(brachytherapy). The latter is often used with implants to treat prostate cancer or other localized malignancies. X-rays and gamma rays may be produced by a linear accelerator or cobalt60 while radioactive isotopes such as iodine131 or cesium137 emit both beta and gamma rays. Dose measurements are now usually expressed in grays (Gy) or centigrays (cGy) where an absorbed dose of 1 Gy equals 100 rads (the older unit of absorbed dose) and 1 cGy equals 1 rad. Radiation protective badges are usually expressed in dose equivalent units called millirem (mrem).

45. A: The purpose of radiation therapy is to kill malignant tissues while affecting the surrounding normal tissue as little as possible. All tissues respond to ionizing radiation but differ in the speed and magnitude of response. Likewise, some tumors are considered radiosensitive (e.g., lymphomas) while others are more resistant (e.g., some squamous cell tumors). Rapidly proliferating tissues such as bone marrow, gastrointestinal epithelium, or skin tend to respond acutely and account for early side effects in these sites. Skin erythema, neutropenia, and gastrointestinal disturbances are all common early side effects. Lung, liver, kidney, brain, and heart are considered intermediate responders while late effects are more often seen in such organs as the pancreas, thyroid, pituitary, cartilage, and uterus. Different body areas have certain dose limitations and shielding of tissues surrounding the tumor is an important part of radiation therapy.

46. A: Protection from radiation for hospital personnel and visitors is important to avoid contamination. Portable radiation shields are useful tools and patients are often placed in private rooms with specialized equipment for radiation protection and disposal. All body fluids and items that come in direct contact with these patients must be disposed of in specialized containers. Radiation warning signs are placed not only on the patient's wristband, but also in their chart, and on the door of the room. Most hospitals have radiation safety officers who are responsible for monitoring exposure and usually test exposure at 1 meter from the patient behind the shield and at the door of the room. Hospital personnel and visitor should remain 6 feet from the patient if possible. Sometimes it is possible to temporarily remove the radiation source from the patient receiving brachytherapy while nursing personnel or visitors are present.

47. A: Side effects of radiation therapy are usually divided into acute, which occur during or shortly after the treatment, and intermediate/late, which occur months to years afterwards. Acute changes are most often seen in rapidly proliferating tissues such as skin and hair follicles, gastrointestinal mucosa, and bone marrow. Therefore, erythema, moist or dry desquamation, and some pigmentation are acute skin reactions, while delayed ones include fibrosis, atrophy, and telangiectasia. Carcinogenesis is a general late radiation reaction that may occur at all sites. Head and neck irradiation may lead to late hypothyroidism and dental caries while chest radiation may cause delayed pulmonary fibrosis, pericarditis or myocardial infarction, and esophageal stricture. Abdominal targets may cause late bowel stricture and obstruction while pelvic radiation may lead to eventual ovarian failure and sterility in women.

48. C: The major goals of treatment for noninvasive bladder cancer are to prevent invasive disease, prevent the loss of the bladder, and improve survival. Most bladder cancers are urothelial (formerly called transitional cell carcinomas) and may be multifocal in origin. Hematuria is the most frequent sign. The treatment approach is to eradicate the noninvasive cancer by transurethral resection, often using electrical fulguration or laser treatment. Intravesicular chemotherapy, often with mitomycin C alone or in combination, has been shown to prevent recurrence of the cancer in many cases. Radical cystectomy with urinary diversion is appropriate treatment for invasive bladder cancer; preoperative chemotherapy has been found to prolong survival compared with surgery alone.

49. D: Testicular masses, often painless, are the most common presenting sign of testicular cancer. Men, especially adolescent to young adult men, should be trained in periodic testicular self-examination. This should be done even in patients that have been treated because a second tumor may arise in the intact testicle. Pain is often an issue after surgical removal of the tumor and since this is often an outpatient procedure, reviewing appropriate analgesics and intervals of ingestion with the patient should be done. Sperm banking prior to treatment is an option that should be discussed with the patient, especially if chemotherapy or radiation is the scheduled therapy. Long-term sexual dysfunction may occur post treatment in up to 25% of these patients, and the patient (and sexual partner) should be made aware of this possibility.

50. B: Postoperative tracheostomy care is important to ensure the patient has adequate oxygenation and avoid pulmonary atelectasis and mucus accumulation that may lead to obstruction or aspiration pneumonia. Suctioning is critical for airway clearance, and the patient should be hyperoxygenated before and after suctioning. Normal saline may be used to lavage the upper airway to assist in mobilization of mucus and prevent plugging. Tracheostomy ties should be comfortable for the patient, about 2 cm (one fingerbreadth) ease underneath the ties. External suture lines should be inspected for breakdown and cleaned with a half-and-half solution of normal saline and peroxide and prescribed ointment applied every 4 to 8 hours. A similar solution may be used to cleanse the inner cannula of mucus and crusts.

51. C: Multiple myeloma is a plasma cell malignancy that usually produces an elevated blood level of monoclonal immunoglobulin and lytic lesions of bone, probably by secreting an osteoclast activating factor. While solitary plasmacytomas may occur, diffuse disease is more common. Chemotherapy with such drugs as melphalan and prednisone or vincristine, doxorubicin, and dexamethasone has shown good results though cure is uncommon. Most patients die of the disease. In recent years, thalidomide has shown useful activity. Targeted radiation treatment to painful or fracture-threatening bone tumors is often added to the therapy, if required. Autologous or allogenic stem cell transplantation and bone marrow transplantation have been used as consolidation measures and have shown success in selected patients.

52. A: Biologic response modifiers are usually low molecular weight cytokines or monoclonal antibodies that bind to cell membranes and influence cellular signaling pathways, enzymatic activity, or cell growth regulators. They have the property of preferential attack on malignant cells so that side effects are generally less prominent than with traditional chemotherapeutic agents. Rituximab is a chimeric monoclonal antibody that targets certain B-cell non-Hodgkin lymphomas. It must be given as an infusion with gradually increasing doses; premedication with an antihistamine and acetaminophen is suggested. Interleukin-2 is a cytokine that stimulates natural killer and cytotoxic T cells, and is FDA approved for metastatic renal cell carcinoma and melanoma. Interferon alpha is an antiviral and antiproliferative agent that has activity in hairy cell leukemia, AIDS-related Kaposi sarcoma, chronic myelogenous leukemia, and several other malignancies and benign conditions. Dexamethasone is a steroid that is useful in lymphoid malignancies but is not a BRM.

53. B: Unconjugated monoclonal antibodies (Mab) bind to specific antigens on the cell and initiate immune activity to kill cancer cells. Examples are Herceptin, Avastin, and Erbitux. Conjugated monoclonal antibodies are able to bind to antigens on the cell surface but are not naturally toxic to cancer cells. They have a cytotoxic agent attached. This may be a chemotherapeutic agent or a radioactive isotope (e.g., radioiodine) that is cytotoxic to the malignant cell. Radioactive agents bound to Mabs may also be toxic to surrounding normal tissue. Examples of conjugated Mabs are Mylotarg, Zevalin and Bexxar. Bexxar has iodine131 bound (gamma and beta emitter) and Zevalin has yttrium90 (beta emitter). These drugs are indicated for certain non-Hodgkin lymphoma. Most

- 229 -

therapeutic monoclonal antibodies are murine (mouse-derived), chimeric (30% murine, 70% human), or humanized (5% murine, 95% human).

54. B: While usually less severe than toxicity associated with traditional chemotherapy, biologic agents have several important side effects that the nurse must be aware. Short-term fever is common with many of these agents and is usually controllable with prophylactic acetaminophen. However, persistent or very high fever despite prophylaxis is an ominous sign and must be investigated. Other common side effects are weight gain (greater than 10 lb per week or 3 lb per day) or loss (greater than 10% of body weight per month), overwhelming fatigue, dyspnea at rest with increased severity on exertion, and marked changes in urinary volume. Chest pain, irregular heartbeat, allergic reactions, and rashes are also possible.

55. A: Doxorubicin is an anthracycline antibiotic that has antineoplastic activity. It is isolated from a species of bacterium (Streptomyces peucetius var. caesius). The drug intercalates between the base pairs of the DNA helix, preventing replication and ultimately blocking protein synthesis. It also forms oxygen free radicals that contribute to its major toxicities: cardiac and cutaneous. It is used frequently in combination with other drugs in the treatment of a variety of tumors. Patients are sensitive to its cardiotoxicity and a strict cumulative dose limitation must be employed in its use. Extravasation of the drug during IV administration can result in severe skin toxicity so close monitoring of peripheral venous drug infusion is mandatory. Alopecia is prominent.

56. C: Both ifosfamide and cyclophosphamide are alkylating agents derived from nitrogen mustard. These drugs alkylate (add saturated hydrocarbons) and form DNA crosslinks, preventing DNA strand separation and replication. They also have immunosuppressive properties. Both are prodrugs that require activation by liver microsomal enzymes. Both drugs have numerous toxic effects, most prominently bone marrow depression with cytopenias, nausea and vomiting, alopecia, and occasional hemorrhagic cystitis with cyclophosphamide. Both drugs have been incorporated into multiple drug combinations for a variety of adult and pediatric tumors. Some of these are lymphomas, sarcomas, and neuroblastoma. Alkylating agents have a long-term risk of carcinogenesis due to their action on DNA.

57. B: Methotrexate is an antimetabolite and antifolate drug that is used for both cancer and noncancerous conditions (e.g., psoriasis, rheumatoid arthritis). It binds to and inhibits the dihydrofolate reductase enzyme that is critical in the folic acid metabolic pathway. This causes an inhibition of purine nucleotide formation and thymidylate synthesis, both of which are dependent on the folic acid metabolite and critical in the formation of DNA and RNA. The drug also has immunosuppressant properties. It may be given orally or intravenously and is often used in high-dose regimens in many antineoplastic protocols. Folinic acid (leucovorin) may be given to reverse a methotrexate overdose or to limit exposure to the drug's therapeutic effects.

58. C: Both dexamethasone and prednisone are synthetic adrenal corticosteroids with powerful anti-inflammatory effects. Dexamethasone is somewhat more potent and the drugs differ slightly in several pharmacologic effects. They are used in the treatment of cancer, predominantly in lymphomas and lymphoid leukemias based on their strong lympholytic properties, and in multiple myeloma and brain tumors. They tend to suppress the immune system and have numerous side effects with long-term use: increased risk of infections, elevated blood glucose and worsening of diabetes, osteoporosis, increasing tendency for ulceration of the upper gastrointestinal tract, weight gain, hypertension, Cushing syndrome, and psychological disturbances. Because of their many side effects, they are often used in a cyclic high-intensity fashion for cancer chemotherapy (e.g., two weeks on the drug followed by two weeks off).

59. D: Hazardous drugs are those that may cause potential harm to those who obtain, prepare, administer, and dispose of them. This includes many chemotherapy agents, as well as certain antivirals, immunosuppressives, and biologic agents. Exposure may be direct (e.g., skin or mucous membrane contact, ingestion, inhalation, needle stick) or indirect (e.g., excreta or body fluids of patients who have been treated with these agents). Long-term effects include liver damage, chromosomal damage, reproductive problems, and carcinogenesis. Protective equipment such as ventilation hoods, gloves and protective clothing, face shields or goggles, and surface pads should be employed by nursing personnel charged with preparation and administration of hazardous drugs. Employees who are pregnant, attempting to conceive (male and female), or breastfeeding should avoid any exposure to hazardous drugs.

60. D: GVHD is an acute or chronic disorder in bone marrow transplant patients due to immunocompetent cells from the donor marrow attacking the recipient's tissues. This may result in rashes, liver abnormalities, and gastrointestinal disturbances such as diarrhea. Reducing the number of T cells in the marrow before transplantation diminishes its immunocompetency and lowers the risk of GVHD; using 6/6 HLA matched siblings as donors also limits the incidence of GVHD. The HLA antigens of class I are termed A, B, and C, while the class II antigens are called DR, DQ, and DP. The risk of GVHD is higher among mismatched related donors (3/6 to 5/6 match) and matched unrelated donors (5/6 to 6/6 match). Immunosuppressive drugs such as cyclosporine A or methotrexate or steroids are often used to prevent and/or treat GVHD.

61. C: CAM usually refers to complementary and alternative treatments employed by patients and some professionals to fight cancer. Vitamins, often in high doses, and herbs are perhaps the most common form of CAM. Unfortunately, they carry the most potential for harm since the vitamin-herbal industry is largely unregulated and their products do not require FDA approval. In addition, such entities as mind-body medicine, chiropractic or massage, and spiritual or energy healing all have their proponents. The experience with all these methods in cancer is limited and unproven. In addition, non-Western techniques such as acupuncture and naturopathic or homeopathic medicine also have adherents. Unfortunately, there is a significant charlatan industry in cancer treatment that defrauds and steals from desperate patients and sometimes delays accepted cancer therapy.

62. C: Allografting involves the transplantation of bone marrow or peripheral blood stem cells to a genetically different individual. This usually requires a 5/6 or 6/6 match of HLA antigens from a family member or stranger. Graft-versus-host disease is frequently a problem. Autografting involves the administration of the patient's own marrow or peripheral blood stem cells (or umbilical cord blood if available) back into the patient, often after chemotherapy or radiation therapy. Graft-versus-host disease is not a problem and obviously there is no need to find a matched donor. It is often preferred in older patients with certain solid tumors since the morbidity and mortality of allografts is higher than in younger patients. There must be a functioning bone marrow to provide the autograft so the technique cannot be used for disorders such as aplastic anemia or sickle cell anemia. The technique should be used in those tumors where the bone marrow has a low risk of infiltration with malignant cells.

63. B: Pain is usually divided into two patterns: nociceptive, which usually arises in bone or soft tissues, and neuropathic, which results from compression or damage to peripheral, sympathetic, or central nervous system fibers. Neuropathic pain is often accompanied by tingling, burning, or numbness, along its innervation route. Nociceptive pain may be of somatic origin such as muscle, joint, or bone, and is usually well localized, or of thoracic or abdominal visceral origin, which is often less well localized and has an aching or cramping sensation. It is activated by pain receptors in deep or cutaneous tissues. Both types may occur in cancer patients and may be due to

progression of the tumor or of therapy. Pain is also subdivided based on duration and cause into acute (less than 3 months), chronic malignant, and chronic nonmalignant (greater than 3 months).

64. A: Nociceptive pain sensation begins with tissue damage, which causes the nociceptors to release a variety of chemical neurotransmitters. Some of these are bradykinin, substance P, prostaglandins, and histamine, depending on the tissue involved. These chemical substances lead to an influx of sodium and an efflux of potassium ions, which generates an action potential and conduction of the nerve impulse to the dorsal horn of the spinal cord. Secondary pain fibers then conduct the pain sensation to the thalamus, usually by spinothalamic tracts. The pain signal is then transmitted to higher centers of the brain to register pain perception. Fibers originating in the brainstem descend to the dorsal horn to modulate the pain signal by release of other neurochemicals such as serotonin, norepinephrine, and endogenous opioids.

65. D: Nursing evaluation of patient's complaint of pain should include five aspects of the symptom. Location may be described by the patient or drawn on a body chart by the patient or nurse. Often there may be more than one site or there is pain radiation from one anatomical site to another. Intensity of the pain may be graded as mild, moderate, or severe, or increasingly by a 0 to 10 rating scale with 0 being no pain and 10 the worst possible. It is important to know what painkillers and other drugs that may modify pain sensation the patient is taking. Sometimes the patient's description of the quality of the pain is diagnostically helpful: pricking, aching, throbbing, burning, or stabbing are all possible descriptions. Temporality, what changes the pain undergoes with time or conditions, may also be useful for diagnosis: onset, duration, exacerbating factors. In addition, how the pain affects the activities of daily living should be evaluated: sleep, work, self-care, physical activity, emotions.

66. C: Treatment for cancer pain is often suboptimal and new guidelines for appropriate analgesic therapy have been issued by the American Pain Society and the World Health Organization. Initial treatment for pain such as that described in this patient with probable metastatic lesions in bone may be an NSAID, such as ibuprofen or naproxen. If this does not control the pain, addition of an opioid, such as oxycodone, on a regular basis is indicated. Switching to a different NSAID is unlikely to be successful. It should be noted that many oral opioids (e.g., Vicodin) are marketed in a fixed-dose combination with acetaminophen or aspirin, so these drugs should not be given in addition. IV morphine is usually reserved for severe pain unresponsive to lesser treatment or for acute pain with an anticipated short duration (e.g., postoperative). It should also be noted that a variety of nonanalgesic adjuvant drugs may be useful in supplementing pain control at any intensity.

67. A: Numerous drug classes may serve as adjuvants, usually in combination with true analgesic drugs. Some anticonvulsants such as gabapentin (Neurontin), phenytoin (Dilantin), or carbamazepine (Tegretol) may have activity in neuropathic pain such as brachial or lumbosacral plexopathies or chemotherapy-induced neuropathies. Antidepressants such as amitriptyline (Elavil) or nortriptyline (Pamelor) are also commonly used adjuvants. NMDA (N-methyl-d-aspartate) antagonists such as ketamine may also show some activity in neuropathic pain. Many of these drugs are not FDA approved for pain control but since are all on the market, the physician is free to prescribe them as adjuncts for pain control. Each has its own side effects that may cause confusion in sorting out the source. Meperidine (Demerol) is a synthetic opiate but its use in cancer patients is discouraged since its metabolite normeperidine may accumulate and cause CNS toxicity.

68. B: The long-term use of opioids, even in cancer patients, has been controversial and long-term prescribing has often led to conflict between doctors and law enforcement. Clarification of the phenomena associated with the use of these drugs should be understood. All opiate drugs continuously taken will lead to a state in which the dose must be increased to achieve a good

clinical result; this is referred to as tolerance and should not be confused with addiction. Drug dependence is also common in patients on long-term opioid therapy; it is characterized by a physical withdrawal syndrome on immediate cessation of the drug or the administration of an antagonist. Rapid withdrawal may lead to exacerbation of pain, shivering, nausea and vomiting, muscle spasms, and a host of unpleasant physical effects. True addiction implies the repetitive use of opioids to satisfy a psychic craving, a drug-centered lifestyle, and continued use despite physical and socioeconomic harm.

69. B: Fatigue is the most common symptom in cancer patients and may be related to the tumor itself or to treatment. Anemia is often the cause, especially in those malignancies that infiltrate the bone marrow (e.g., leukemia, metastatic small cell carcinoma) or cause bleeding (e.g., gastric or colon cancer). Many tumors secrete chemical substances that act on muscle or even the brain to engender a sense of fatigue and exhaustion. Complications of cancer such as cachexia, depression, or infection may contribute to the fatigue. Electrolyte imbalance may also be a cause. Fatigue is also the most common side effect of chemotherapy, especially a few days after administration. This may be due to destruction of tumor cells and release of fatigue-inducing chemicals. Nearly all radiation therapy patients experience a cumulative fatigue between the second and sixth week of treatment.

70. C: Anemia is a common finding in cancer patients. It may be due to bleeding with resulting iron deficiency, poor absorption of iron or folic acid due to the tumor or gastrointestinal side effects of treatment, infiltration of the bone marrow with tumor, or anemia of chronic disease where the tumor most likely secretes a chemical substance that depresses red cell production. Packed red cell transfusion may be indicated if the hemoglobin level is less than 8 to 9 g/dL and the patient is symptomatic. Erythropoietin has been used to stimulate erythropoiesis in cancer patients so that transfusion may be avoided. However, this hormone has recently been shown to be associated with an increased incidence of strokes so caution in its use is emphasized, avoiding hemoglobin levels above 11 to 12 g/dL. Psychostimulants such as amphetamines or high-dose caffeine are sometimes helpful for fatigue but may complicate anemic patients by causing cardiac arrhythmias.

71. C: The oncology nurse may employ numerous methods to assess the level of cancer patient fatigue and advise coping mechanisms. There are several scales based on daily activity and required assistance that are helpful in determining the effect of the cancer and/or treatment. One of these is the Karnofsky performance scale (KPS) that is widely used in oncology. The scale is based on activities of daily living and ranges from 10 (moribund) to 100 (normal, no evidence of disease). It is useful for both prognosis and following the course of the disease. Many cancer treatment trials include a minimum KPS number for admission to the study. Neurocognitive factors may also be evaluated by simple tests for orientation (name, place, and date), recall and memory (usually words given in groups), and attention (counting or reciting the alphabet backwards). Review of laboratory findings, such as hemoglobin level, oxygen saturation, and electrolyte and glucose values, should also be done.

72. A: Itching is a common symptom in cancer patients, including those receiving treatment. It is similar in physiology to pain in that a variety of chemical mediators stimulate C pain fibers that are perceived as pruritus. Some of these are histamine, prostaglandins, and substance P. Drugs commonly given to cancer patients may have a side effect profile that includes pruritus: opioids, phenothiazines, or certain hormones.

Lymphomas, especially Hodgkin lymphoma, frequently cause generalized pruritus, although it is no longer used as a symptomatic classification for the disease stage (B symptom). Anal and vulvar tumors usually cause localized itching or irritation. Pruritus is more common in elderly patients (older than 70 years) and those receiving radiation therapies greater than 20 Gy.

73. B: Nearly 30% to 50% of cancer patients will have some interruption of a normal sleeping pattern: either inability to fall asleep or frequent nocturnal awakening. Certain symptoms such as pain, itching, dyspnea, or restless legs are obvious causes. Steroids tend to exacerbate restful sleep, whether they are given as therapy or are secreted in some paraneoplastic syndromes. Increased age, female gender, and depressive thoughts all tend to interfere with restful sleep. Often, hospitalizations with IV lines, frequent interruptions for assessment of vital signs, or excessive time in bed are contributors. There are numerous nonpharmacological methods to assist falling and staying asleep. Hypnotics include benzodiazepines (flurazepam, triazolam), nonbenzodiazepines such as zolpidem (Ambien) or zaleplon (Sonata), and sedating antidepressants such as amitriptyline or doxepin. All must be used judiciously to avoid side effects, especially in elderly patients.

74. A: Actinic keratoses are precursor lesions to squamous cell carcinomas of the skin and require biopsy to exclude progression to squamous cell carcinoma. They are often found in the same areas as skin cancers: those with high sun exposure such as the head, neck, dorsal hands and arms. Multiple lesions are common. Malignant melanoma is the deadliest form of skin cancer. The lifetime risk is still increasing in the United States, especially among white men. Sun exposure, especially sunburns at a young age, is a major risk factor. Squamous cell carcinoma is another primary skin cancer. Early lesions are usually asymptomatic and appear as firm red papules or plaques, which may go on to ulcerate. Kaposi sarcoma was a rare disease of elderly Mediterranean and Eastern European men. Now it is a common malignancy among HIV-infected patients, although the newer antiviral therapies have decreased the incidence dramatically. Lesions are usually flat, purple plaques that arise on skin or mucous membranes and may progress to nodules.

75. B: Cancer patients are subject to numerous neurological abnormalities, both as a function of their disease and of its treatment. The oncology nurse should be aware of the common signs and symptoms of these patients and consider the source. The Romberg test has the patient stand with arms and feet together with the eyes closed. A slight sway is normal but marked shifting or obvious loss of balance may suggest cerebellar disease or impaired proprioception. Diminished visual acuity or impaired visual fields may be observed in ocular or brain tumors but is usually confirmed by ophthalmologic methods. Testing of joint position sense and deep tendon reflexes may reveal impairment of peripheral nerves, not uncommon in a variety of tumors that compress or infiltrate nerves. It also may be a manifestation of neurotoxic chemotherapy with drugs such as vincristine or platinum compounds.

76. C: Cancer may involve the skin in several ways: primary skin cancers such as melanoma or basal cell carcinoma; cutaneous infiltration or metastases from other sites; or paraneoplastic syndromes such as acanthosis nigricans or Paget disease. Mycosis fungoides is a slow-growing cutaneous T-cell lymphoma that often masquerades as other skin diseases. Acanthosis nigricans is a dark, thick, and sometimes velvety change that accumulates in skin folds, such as armpits or groin. It is sometimes associated with certain cancers but may also be a manifestation of benign disease or inherited. The dysplastic nevus syndrome is an inherited disorder in which dysplastic skin nevi have a high risk of transformation to melanoma. Erythema multiforme appears as scattered, cutaneous vesicles and is usually associated with multiple drug therapy.

77. B: Dysphagia is common in cancer patients whether from tumor involvement of the swallowing mechanism or of the upper gastrointestinal tract. Therapy-induced nausea and vomiting may also contribute. Complete obstruction of the upper airway with food is a medical emergency. Attempts to avoid aspiration of food or esophageal-gastric contents should be carried out. Certain mechanical methods may enhance swallowing comfort and effectiveness. Elevation of the head of the bed with the patient's head tilted slightly forward lessens regurgitation. Avoiding milk and milk products,

alternating liquids and solids, and thorough chewing enhance effective swallowing. Thickening of foods may also minimize aspiration. Placement of food in the posterior pharynx with a long-handled spoon or syringe also is effective.

78. D: Nausea and vomiting are among the most unpleasant side effects of cancer treatment and often lead the patient to delay or terminate therapy. Pretreatment or concurrent treatment with a variety of pharmaceutical agents has been successful in diminishing vomiting during and after treatment. Serotonin antagonists (e.g., ondansetron) alone or in combination with corticosteroids have been successful even for highly emetogenic drugs such as platinum-containing compounds. Phenothiazines (e.g., prochlorperazine) have been used traditionally as antiemetics, although their potency alone may not be as effective as some of the other drug classes. Cannabinoids, either via synthetic tetrahydrocannabinol (THC)–containing drugs such as dronabinol (Marinol) or smoking marijuana, have been found to be effective in preventing emesis in many patients. Corticosteroids or benzodiazepines in combination with other antiemetic drugs may be synergistic.

79. A: Hypercalcemia is often present with such tumors as lung, breast, and multiple myeloma. It may be due to the secretion of substance(s) that have a PTH-like effect on bone or by other osteoclast-activating chemicals that promote bone reabsorption. In some cases, lytic bone lesions such as those found in myeloma may be responsible for elevated serum calcium. Platinum-containing drugs may cause hypocalcemia; low calcium is often found in those patients with low magnesium levels as well. Osteoblastic bone metastases tend to reduce serum calcium level. Vitamin D is necessary for proper calcium absorption and deficiency is common in cancer patients, leading to lower calcium levels.

80. B: Anorexia, weight loss, and cachexia are common symptoms of cancer. Weight loss of 10% of usual or greater over three months is considered significant. Causes may be disease-related, treatment-related, or a combination of both. Provision of adequate calories is critical to maintaining weight. These may be provided by oral consumption of increased calories for the underweight patient. If this is not feasible, enteral (nasogastric or gastroenterostomy tube) or parenteral (IV) feeding must be considered. A simple estimate of daily caloric requirements to maintain current weight may be derived from multiplication of the current weight by 18 for underweight, 16 for normal weight, and 13 for overweight patients; for the above described patient: 18 x 135 = 2430 or about 2400 calories.

81. B: Colostomy care is frequently required in cancer patients who have undergone abdominal surgery for obstructing lesions of the bowel or resection of rectosigmoid or anal cancer. The stoma may be temporary or permanent and of the end, loop, or double-barrel type, depending on the nature of the neoplasm and the required surgery. Most colostomies become functional three to five days after placement. The pouch should be emptied when it is one-third to one-half full and before chemotherapy. The appliance should be changed every five days or sooner if there is leakage or peristomal skin discomfort. Skin protective paste may be useful in preventing peristomal irritation. Type of appliance is selected on the basis of location and type of effluent, abdominal contour, cost, and ease of use for the patient.

82. A: Mechanical obstruction most often affects the small intestine and accounts for 90% of bowel obstructions. This may be caused by extrinsic or intrinsic lesions or blocking of the intestinal lumen with impacted stool or foreign bodies. Appropriate nursing care should ensure that the patient's bed is raised to 45 degrees to avoid aspiration and promote respiration. Most of these patients will have a nasogastric (or longer) tube that requires frequent local care with lubricant and saline irrigation. Auscultation for bowel sounds is important in distinguishing mechanical obstruction (loud, tympanitic sounds) from paralytic ileus (diminished to absent bowel sounds) due to

abdominal surgery or electrolyte imbalance. Signs of peritonitis include fever, board-like rigidity of the abdomen, and increased pain on movement.

83. B: Urinary diversions are performed when the cancerous bladder is removed by radical cystectomy. The surgery usually includes prostatectomy and removal of the pelvic lymph nodes in men and removal of the ovaries, tubes, and uterus in women. Urinary diversion may be employed by an ileal conduit in which the ureters are implanted into a segment of small bowel with the distal end brought out to the abdominal wall via a stoma. This is a freely refluxing system and urinary infections and subsequent stone formation may occur with some frequency. Other diversions include a continent diversion in which a urine reservoir is created from bowel tissue and continence is maintained by construction of a one-way flap valve; or an orthotopic neobladder in which an artificial bladder is constructed from stomach or intestinal tissue and attached to the urethra. These tend to preserve continence and decrease the likelihood of urinary infection and calculi.

84. D: Pulmonary toxicity due to radiation therapy or chemotherapeutic agents is common and must be looked for in patients undergoing treatment with either and especially when these modalities are combined. Radiation therapy to the chest leads to some evidence of pulmonary toxicity in 5% to 15% of patients. Elderly patients tend to be more susceptible perhaps because of preexisting lung disease or history of smoking. Radiation dose, volume of lung irradiated, and fractionation schedule all influence the extent of lung damage. Many chemotherapy drugs cause pulmonary damage. Most notorious is bleomycin, which has both direct and hypersensitivity properties leading to pulmonary fibrosis and should be dose-limited to less than 400 units. Methotrexate may cause a hypersensitivity pneumonitis in some patients but is rarely a cause of severe pulmonary toxicity by itself. Prednisone is a corticosteroid and is often used to treat drug- or radiation-induced pulmonary toxicity.

85. A: Pleural effusion is a frequent finding in cancer patients, especially those with lung, breast, or lymphatic tumors. Diagnosis is usually made by diminished breath sounds at the lung base and a chest x-ray showing a blunted costophrenic angle. Thoracentesis is frequently used to exclude benign causes, look for malignant cells, and provide temporary relief of dyspnea. Longer-term drainage may be provided by a chest tube inserted into the pleural space and connected to continuous underwater seal suction. This promotes adherence of the pleural surfaces by removal of fluid. Longer-term therapy for recurrent effusions may include sclerotherapy: an intrapleural injection of a sclerosing agent (tetracyclines, nitrogen mustard, bleomycin, or talc). Newer, relatively noninvasive surgical techniques (e.g., videothoracoscopic pleurectomy) are replacing open pleurectomy. Treatment of the underlying cancer if sensitive to radiation or chemotherapy may also bring relief.

86. C: Lymphedema is caused by damage or obstruction of the lymph vessels draining a particular anatomical area. Damage to the venous side of capillary blood flow may also contribute. While tumor infiltration or obstruction may be the underlying cause, the most common form of upper limb lymphedema in breast cancer patient's results from modified radical surgery of the breast followed by radiation therapy, as many as 5% to 10% of these patients will develop the condition. Axillary lymph node dissection for staging the tumor may result in lymphedema, usually occurring within one year of the surgery. It is less common in those whose lymphatic dissection is confined to the sentinel node. Avoiding injections or blood drawing or carrying heavy objects in the affected extremity are two of many preventive measures.

87. C: Pericardial effusion is usually caused by impaired lymphatic and venous drainage of the heart with accumulation of fluid in the pericardial sac; this leads to impaired ventricular filling and

- 236 -

diminished cardiac output. Symptoms include chest pain, usually nonpositional, dyspnea at rest, nonproductive cough, and fatigue, and are usually related to the speed at which the effusion accumulates. Rapid accumulation may be a medical emergency and require transthoracic needle aspiration of the pericardial fluid. It is usually associated with primary tumors of the pericardium such as mesothelioma but may also arise from direct invasion from lung, breast, and esophageal tumors or thymomas and lymphomas. High doses of radiation to the heart or chemotherapy with cyclophosphamide or cytosine arabinoside may also increase the risk. The effusion may be seen on chest x-ray as a widened mediastinum or water bottle–shaped cardiac silhouette. Ultrasonography is a more definitive test and most often is the diagnostic method of choice.

88. C: Thrombotic disease with or without embolization is common in cancer patients. Some cancers predispose to this by release of procoagulants or by obstruction of blood vessels; obesity, prolonged immobilization, or therapy with estrogenic hormones may also be contributing factors. Thrombocytosis, seen in myeloproliferative disorders, predisposes to clot formation, especially at counts greater than 400,000/mm3. Thrombocytopenia may be a manifestation of disseminated intravascular coagulation (DIC) or thrombotic thrombocytopenic purpura (TTP) in which the platelet count will be low. Deep vein thrombosis (DVT) or pulmonary embolus (PE) is a presenting sign in 5% to 10% of cancer patients and many authorities still suggest cancer screening for those, especially older patients, who present with idiopathic DVT/PE.

89. D: Filgrastim (Neupogen) is a granulocyte colony-stimulating factor that raises the absolute circulating granulocyte count by stimulating a committed marrow precursor. It has been very useful in avoiding severe neutropenia (absolute count less than 500/mm3) and subsequent fever and infection in cancer or some leukemia patients receiving cytotoxic chemotherapy. It is also indicated for bone marrow transplant recipients and for recruiting neutrophil precursor cells into the blood for harvesting by leukapheresis. It does not stimulate monocyte/macrophage production. It is given in multiple doses daily by subcutaneous or IV administration and should not be started earlier than 24 hours after the administration of cytotoxic chemotherapy. A pegylated (covalently bound to polyethylene glycol) form named pegfilgrastim (Neulasta) is longer acting and may be given as a single dose. Bone pain is a side effect of both forms.

90. C: Ondansetron (Zofran) is an antiemetic drug used to prevent or treat nausea and vomiting during or after chemotherapy. It may also be used to control postoperative and postradiation therapy nausea and vomiting and perhaps for gastrointestinal disease induced as well. It is thought to reduce the activity of the vagus nerve that connects to and activates the vomiting center in the brainstem as well as block serotonin in the chemoreceptor trigger zone. Interestingly, it has little effect on vomiting caused by motion sickness. It may be given orally and is sometimes combined with dexamethasone to enhance the antiemetic effect. The drug is usually well tolerated with constipation, headache, and dizziness the most common side effects. It has no significant drug interactions.

91. C: Choosing the correct empiric antibiotic therapy for cancer patients with fever and neutropenia is a complex matter and to some extent depends on a high degree of suspicion as to the source and nature of the infection. It also requires some knowledge of the bacterial profile within a particular institution. For high-risk patients, an IV infusion of an antipseudomonal cephalosporin or penicillin (e.g., ceftazidime or piperacillin-tazobactam) or a carbapenem may be used. Use of vancomycin is controversial unless there is a strong suspicion of methicillin-resistant Staphylococcus aureus (MRSA). This is because frequent or prolonged use of vancomycin has led to the development of resistant organisms, especially enterococcus. Fluoroquinolones such as ciprofloxacin or levofloxacin may be used but should not be used alone.

92. D: Numerous cytotoxic drugs are vesicants that cause tissue damage if infiltration from the IV line occurs. Others are considered irritants if they cause a local inflammatory reaction but not true tissue necrosis. Anthracyclines, some platinum compounds, and vinca alkaloids all may cause significant tissue damage and are considered vesicants. Carboplatin, however, may cause burning and inflammation at the injection site but is considered an irritant. Basic principles of treatment include stopping the infusion quickly and administering a cold compress (for many drugs) or warm compress for vinblastine or etoposide. This should be followed by administration of an antidote if one is available (e.g., sodium thiosulfate for cisplatin). Many drugs can be irritating even without extravasation. Often a cold compress and slowing the infusion rate will help. The toxic effects of many drugs when administered peripherally have been bypassed by the development of indwelling devices to facilitate central venous administration.

93. C: The concept of using drug combinations in cancer treatment evolved in the 1960s. Use of single agents sometimes resulted in remissions but these were usually short-lived. The experience with drug combinations such as MOPP (mechlorethamine, Oncovin, procarbazine, and prednisone) for Hodgkin lymphoma showed dramatic improvement in remission rates and survival. Drugs were and still are chosen on the basis of single drug tumoricidal activity. Multiple short, intense treatment periods with maximum tolerated doses followed by a rest period (called the cycle of chemotherapy) proved quite effective. Often it is beneficial to include both cell cycle specific drugs (plant alkaloids, antimetabolites) and cell cycle nonspecific agents (alkylating agents, antitumor antibiotics, hormones) in the combination to reduce the development of drug resistance.

94. B: Infection is probably the most common complication of cancer patients undergoing treatment and is often the cause of death. Sometimes the source of infection is uncertain so that after appropriate cultures are obtained from the febrile patient, antibiotic therapy, usually in combinations to cover a variety of possible bacteria, is started immediately. Choice of empiric antibiotics is a complex task but a broad spectrum to cover the likely organisms from that institution is often given. If cultures are negative and the patient is afebrile for three days and the absolute neutrophil count is greater than $500/mm^3$, antibiotics may be stopped and the patient observed for physical findings and/or recurrent fever. Prolonged use of multiple antibiotics without a definite source of infection may lead to untoward side effects and bacterial resistance.

95. A: There are numerous alternative and supplemental nonpharmacologic therapies for cancer patient. Few have been subject to rigorous clinical trials for effectiveness, although some are beginning to be looked at in a more scientific way than before. This area is subject to quackery and outright criminal activity; so many desperate patients get no benefit and lose considerable amounts of money. According to a 2000 study of patients undergoing clinical trials, self-help groups were the most popular form of complementary treatment, followed by spiritual, massage, and exercise. Imagery, relaxation techniques, and lifestyle changes were considered of moderate benefit while high-dose vitamins and herbal/botanical dietary supplements were last on the list.

96. C: Traditional Chinese medicine is based on the theory that a deficiency or stagnation of vital energy or life force (qi) is the cause of most disease. This qi runs along specific body meridians that determine the treatment location. Thin sterile needles are placed at the strategic site(s) and left in place for a minimum of 20 minutes. Cumulative treatments are thought to be required for most conditions. This technique has been used extensively for pain control and is thought by many experts to be effective in reducing chemotherapy-induced nausea and vomiting. Many believe that it is also beneficial for dental pain, musculoskeletal disorders, headache, and gastrointestinal or urinary symptoms, possibly by relieving stress and body tension.

97. B: Infection in cancer patients, especially those that are neutropenic from treatment, is a major problem. Every effort should be made to avoid external contamination. This requires hand washing or use of sterilization gels before and after all patient contact. Use of sterile gloves is also advised. Indwelling catheters (e.g., Foley or IV) are a frequent source of infection so sterile technique should be used for placement and inspection, and frequent changes according to protocol must be carried out. Avoid invasive procedures such as rectal temperatures, enemas, bladder catheterization, or venipunctures if at all possible. Ventilators and tracheal suctioning are a frequent source of bacterial or fungal invasion. While in many cancer patients the immune system is impaired, this does not generally rule out immunization with influenza or pneumococcal vaccines. The manufacturer's contraindications for use and possible side effects should be checked before administration and knowledge of common hospital pathogens and their route of entry are also helpful.

98. A: Fever and chills are quite common in cancer patients, especially those hospitalized and undergoing cytotoxic therapy. Ideally, blood and other cultures would be obtained initially, then acetaminophen and a tepid sponge bath would be given, and finally a chest x-ray would be obtained. However, hospital logistics often preclude the above sequence of tests and treatments. If one must wait for the lab technician to come to do blood cultures and other blood tests, symptomatic treatment with a sponge bath and acetaminophen should be given while waiting. If one must wait for the drug to come from the pharmacy, this is another source of delay. Similarly, the patient should be subjected to a brief physical examination, including vital signs. If hypotension or other signs of sepsis are present, a portable chest x-ray should be ordered. While it is less precise than regular PA and lateral films, it may be dangerous to allow the patient to leave the unit and be away from direct nursing supervision.

99. C: Anxiety is perhaps the most common psychological reaction to a diagnosis of cancer. It may range from vague uneasiness and apprehension to panic attacks. Self-medication or use of alcohol, tobacco, or illegal drugs is not a recommended course of action. Usually, the facts of the diagnosis, even if discouraging, should be discussed frankly with the patient in a calm, sympathetic, and soothing manner. However, do not tell the patient that "all will be well" if it is not true. For more extreme anxiety states and panic attacks, anxiolytic medications may relieve psychological and somatic symptoms. This should be discussed with other responsible members of the health care team. Psychiatric consultation is appropriate in extreme cases.

100. B: Cancer patients often experience symptoms of depression and require support. This may include psychiatric or psychological referral and/or pharmacologic intervention. There are many antianxiety and antidepressive drugs from which to choose. Some are more dangerous than others and suicide risk must be considered. Side effect profile is also important as some drugs have prominent anticholinergic, CNS, and cardiovascular side effects. Benzodiazepine antianxiety drugs, such as lorazepam, are not true antidepressants and may lead to daytime confusion or dizziness. Trazodone has prominent sedative effects, a low anticholinergic side effect profile, and only a moderate orthostatic hypotension risk. It is probably the best drug to begin with for this patient. Selective serotonin reuptake inhibitors (SSRIs), such as fluoxetine and paroxetine, have low side effect profiles and are effective antidepressants but do not have much sedative activity. Traditional sleeping pills may pose a risk because of suicidal thoughts.

101. D: Clinical depression is very common in cancer patients and the oncology nurse should be aware of the major signs and symptoms. In general, the symptoms should persist for longer than two weeks. Sleep disturbances, either insomnia or hypersomnia, are frequent and should be asked about in the patient's history. Crying, depressed mood, and feelings of hopelessness and guilt are fairly obvious indicators, as are fatigue and weight loss or gain without other explanation.

Observation of the patient may offer clues: flat affect, lack of spontaneity, changes in eye contact, inactivity, or excessive agitation may all signal an underlying depression. The nurse should inquire about past episodes and treatments for depression and mental illness in general. Inquiry about current and past use of psychotropic drugs is also indicated.

102. B: Assisting a cancer patient's spiritual needs is sometimes difficult, especially if the nurse does not share them. This subject requires delicacy and discretion and should be discussed with a spouse or other family members. The appropriate member of the clergy should be contacted if the patient so desires. It should be noted that there is a wide variety of beliefs and practices even among members of the same or similar faith. This must be taken into account in supporting a patient's religious practice. It is important that the nurse listens to the patient carefully and with empathy. The nurse should assure the patient that he or she will be available to support spiritual or cultural needs.

103. C: A sense of loss of personal control is common in cancer patients and many patients who are chronically ill. The inability to carry out ADL or continue an established work schedule is particularly burdensome to these individuals. These feelings may be expressed with anger or aggressive behavior, or failure or refusal to cooperate with medical staff or comply with prescribed treatments. Anxiety and symptoms of depression may be prominent. In many patients used to being in charge or who have major work or family responsibilities, the loss of personal control that arises in a clinical situation is a particularly difficult coping problem. Refusal to participate in decision making and to express emotion are clues to this problem; there are often complaints about medical personnel or other staff members responsible for the patient care without much basis in fact.

104. C: While people deal with loss and grief, especially of a loved one, there are some common responses that should be watched for and discouraged, if possible. Substance abuse with either illegal or legal drugs, especially sleeping pills, tranquilizers, and narcotics, should be limited and excess use reported to appropriate individuals, family or professional. Withdrawal to social isolation is all too frequent in those who have lost someone close or in those who have received a diagnosis of cancer. Participation in support groups and individual counseling is often helpful for patients as well as close relatives. Most cancer centers and oncology units have lists of outside support groups for referrals. The patient or grieving relative should be encouraged to seek social, religious, or cultural support in dealing with the emotional trauma.

105. A: Alopecia is one of the frequent side effects of many cancer drugs (e.g., alkylating agents, anthracyclines, antimetabolites) and combination chemotherapy usually enhances hair loss. This is among the common distortions of body image sustained by cancer patients and is quite visible to the outside world. Patients should be reassured that most of the time hair loss is temporary and will regrow after the treatment is completed. However, the hair may regrow in a somewhat different color or thickness than previously present. Caps and wigs are often used to minimize social embarrassment. Head covering to prevent heat loss and sun exposure should be recommended. There is no good evidence that scalp hypothermia or tourniquets during drug administration will prevent alopecia but may actually be detrimental by diminishing the amount of drug reaching the scalp vessels.

106. B: Poverty has a deleterious effect on cancer patients: delay in diagnosis, irregular or inadequate treatment, and inability to afford regular medical care are all factors. Cancer incidence is higher in the poor population, probably because of harmful social and environmental causes, such as smoking, excess use of alcohol, obesity or chronic malnutrition, and exposure to toxic materials in poor neighborhoods and in the workplace. Survival rates are about 10% to 15% lower among the poor. Poverty should be distinguished from ethnicity in evaluating cancer rates and

survival. There may be confusion and overlapping of statistics since many ethnic minorities in the United States tend to be poorer than the general population.

107. A: New breast cancer cases have equalized among white women and African American women (approximately 126 per 100,000) based on 1999 to 2014 statistics. Mortality from breast cancer, however, is higher in the African American population (approximately 28 per 100,000) than in white (approximately 20 per 100,000). These statistics have changed since 2000, when incidence among white women was 140.8 per 100,000 and African American women was 121.7 per 100,000. The mortality rate among African American women has been consistently higher from 2000 to 2014.

108. D: Dealing with minority ethnic and cultural groups may be difficult, especially for inexperienced nurses. Usually a language barrier is the biggest problem, followed by ignorance of cultural beliefs. These should be ascertained through a family member who speaks English or via a competent translator. Do not make assumptions about cultural beliefs and traditions based on skin color because there are many subgroups based on religion, country of origin, or degree of "Americanization." Personal habits and exposure of private parts are frequently a source of embarrassment and should be handled in a sensitive but matter-of-fact manner. The patient's attitude toward intimate touching in the course of examination and nursing care should be taken into account. Initially addressing the patient by the last name and title (e.g., Mrs. Lopez, Dr. Washington) shows respect and indicates professionalism. The patient will usually state if he or she wishes a less formal appellation

109. C: Evaluation of the patient's emotional distress and instructing him or her in coping skills is an important nursing function for cancer patients. Based on history and symptoms, a decision should be made as to whether the patient has a psychiatric disorder or is merely undergoing the natural fear and anxiety of a cancer diagnosis and treatment. Often, allowing the patient to verbalize anxiety and emotions is therapeutic. Teaching the patient about the disease and treatment and what to expect may alleviate considerable anxiety. Referral to support groups is often a good idea so that the cancer patient may be reassured by others who have been through it. Referral to a psychiatrist or social worker may be indicated but the nurse should initially evaluate the patient and attempt simple remedial measures. The nurse's frequent contact with the patient may make his or her intervention more supportive than that of the physician.

110. A: In certain cases of malignancies, infection, or trauma, the intrinsic or extrinsic blood clotting cascade is activated. This may be due to injury to vascular endothelium or procoagulants released by the tumor. Diffuse microthrombosis occurs. Clotting factors are consumed at a rapid pace and normal replacement is inadequate. The platelet count and fibrinogen are decreased and diffuse bleeding often occurs. Fibrinolysis is activated by the increased thrombosis and there is an increase in the fibrin degradation products, but these are only slowly removed from the circulation so that the level increases. Plasminogen is activated and converted to plasmin; thus the plasminogen level is decreased. Plasmin activates the kinin and complement systems and this leads to hypotension and increased vascular permeability. Treatment of the underlying disease and replacement of critical coagulation factors and platelets (if count less than 20,000) are the mainstays of treatment. Heparin, widely used in the past, is now rarely indicated because of the risk of worsening bleeding.

111. B: Septic shock is a dreaded complication of infected patients, usually caused by endotoxins released into the blood by invading organisms. It is characterized by fever, chills, tachycardia, tachypnea, hypotension, and hypoperfusion. It is usually preceded by bacteremia. About 40% of the time this is due to gram-negative bacteria (e.g., E. coli, Klebsiella or Pseudomonas); about 5% to 10% of cases are due to gram-positive bacteria such as Staphylococcus aureus or Streptococcus

pneumoniae. Most infections arise from endogenous flora but the use of invasive techniques (catheters, vascular access devices, endotracheal intubation) and cytotoxic drugs that injure mucosal surfaces has caused an increase in recent years. Other less common causative organisms are fungi, viruses, anaerobic bacteria, and protozoa.

112. C: Rapid killing of tumor cells by cytotoxic therapy, especially in leukemia and lymphomas, can lead to an accelerated release of intracellular potassium, phosphate, and nucleic acid into the circulation. Phosphate binds to calcium, resulting in hypocalcemia, and the nucleic acids are converted to uric acid, resulting in hyperuricemia. This pattern may lead to cardiac arrhythmias and renal and/or multiorgan dysfunction. Prevention with hypouricemic drugs (e.g., allopurinol) and IV hydration to maintain a urine flow of 150 to 200 mL per hour prior to treatment is recommended. Alkalization of the urine with bicarbonate is also helpful. External sources of potassium should be discontinued and measures to lower serum potassium (e.g., Kayexalate, glucose and insulin, loop diuretics) should be undertaken if the serum potassium level is more than 6.5 mEq/L and/or if ECG changes are present. Dialysis is occasionally required.

113. A: Hypercalcemia is common in cancer patients, in as many as 10% to 20%, usually as a late complication. Tumors of the breast, lung, head, and neck, and multiple myeloma are most frequently associated with elevated calcium levels. Hypercalcemia is defined as a serum level greater than 11 mg/dL but this may require correction based on the level of serum albumin. Normal calcium homeostasis is largely controlled by parathyroid hormone (PTH), which stimulates calcium release from bone, enhances renal resorption of calcium, and promotes vitamin D–dependent calcium absorption from the gastrointestinal tract. Malignant tumors may raise the calcium level by secreting a PTH-rP, called humoral hypercalcemia of malignancy (HHM); or by metastatic invasion of bone with osteolytic bone lesions, called local osteolytic hypercalcemia (LOH). Advanced breast cancer and myeloma are associated with malignant osteolytic bone lesions. Low levels of vitamin D tend to impair calcium absorption, and hyperparathyroidism is most often associated with adenomas of the parathyroid gland.

114. C: This patient has the syndrome of inappropriate antidiuretic hormone (SIADH). ADH (arginine vasopressin) is synthesized in the hypothalamus and secreted by the posterior pituitary gland. It controls plasma osmolality and volume via its action on the renal tubules. SIADH may be found in a variety of tumors, especially small cell carcinoma of the lung. It may also be caused by drugs, including several antineoplastics (e.g., cyclophosphamide, vincristine, cisplatin), infections, hemorrhagic or traumatic disorders of the brain, pulmonary infections, or in postoperative patients. The serum sodium level is characteristically low and the urine concentrated with an elevated osmolality. Milder cases may be treated with fluid restriction and oral agents, such as demeclocycline, urea, or lithium. A serum sodium below 110 to 115 mEq/L and/or seizures and other CNS symptoms constitutes a medical emergency and requires use of hypertonic saline.

115. B: Anaphylaxis is an immediate, unpredictable, and sometimes overwhelming reaction to an administered antigen, often a drug, which may result in bronchospasm, smooth muscle spasm, increased capillary leak with hypotension, cardiovascular collapse, respiratory failure, and possibly death. It is considered a medical emergency. It may be provoked by some cytotoxic drugs, such as asparaginase, taxanes, or platinum compounds. The antigen-specific antibody of the IgE class is produced by B-lymphocytes and combines with a previously sensitized mast cell. This leads to degranulation of the mast cell and release of a variety of vasoactive and other chemical substances (e.g., histamine, serotonin, leukotrienes) that cause the syndrome.

116. B: Increased intracranial pressure may result from an increase in volume of brain tissue, vascular tissue, or cerebrospinal fluid (CSF) within the intracranial cavity. Since this is a closed

space, there will be a corresponding rise in pressure. Abnormalities resulting in ICP include tumor expansion, brain edema, and obstruction of CSF flow or angiogenesis associated with tumor growth. The CT scan of the brain is the most rapid imaging technique since it requires little patient preparation with or without contrast media and is available in practically all hospitals and larger clinics. MRI usually presents a superior image but takes longer and some machines are still claustrophobic to the patient. PET (positron emission tomography) scans are precise and may distinguish between tumor recurrence and radiation necrosis in treated patients. PET scan machines are quite expensive and not available in many medical facilities. Myelography is an invasive technique that is best used for searching for dropped metastases.

117. D: Early signs of increased intracranial pressure may be cranial (headaches), neurologic, and/or gastrointestinal. Early morning headache is a classical sign that may be bilateral or diffuse. It may be described as discomfort in the head. It is usually exacerbated by Valsalva maneuver, bending over, or cough. It is usually progressive and may or may not respond to simple analgesics. A variety of neurologic signs and symptoms may be present: blurred vision, diplopia, lethargy and confusion, and diminished consciousness are a few common ones. These tend to progress without treatment. Gastrointestinal function may be an early sign with loss of appetite, nausea, and projectile vomiting most characteristic. Cardiovascular and respiratory symptoms and signs appear as the pressure increases.

118. A: This patient has a spinal cord compression that must be addressed immediately. It is most common in tumors that invade the spine, leading to vertebral collapse and compression of the cord. It may also occur with invasion of the spinal canal or with primary tumors of the spinal cord. Most patients complain of back pain and there are usually neurologic findings consistent with the level of the cord that is compromised. Most likely treatment sequence is administration of corticosteroids to reduce inflammation and edema (and may be oncolytic for some tumors such as lymphomas) followed by radiation therapy to a dose of 3000 to 4000 cGy given over several weeks if the tumor is radiation sensitive. Otherwise, surgery is an option and may take precedence is there are profound neurologic changes present and a surgical decompression is possible. Chemotherapy is less effective, especially in a patient already receiving it, except in some childhood tumors.

119. A: The superior vena cava syndrome refers to obstruction of this thin-walled vessel of the mediastinum that collects blood from the head, neck, upper extremities, and thorax, and conducts it to the right atrium. The obstruction may be caused by tumor invasion or external compression, enlarged lymph nodes, or internal thrombus formation. Lung cancer and lymphomas are perhaps the most common tumors that may compress the SVC and lead to this syndrome. Symptoms and physical findings include dyspnea, swelling of the face and neck, visible collateral vessels on the chest wall, and many others related to impaired venous return. Radiation therapy is the primary treatment modality for cancer-induced SVCS. Removal of a central venous catheter and anticoagulation is indicated for an obstructing thrombus. Avoiding upper extremity manipulations, semi-Fowler positioning of the patient, and observation for respiratory compromise are all appropriate nursing responsibilities for these patients.

120. C: Patients with primary cardiac tumors or metastatic invasion of the pericardium are most at risk for this emergency. Mesothelioma and Kaposi sarcoma (in HIV/AIDS patients) are also possible causes. Radiation greater than 4000 cGy to a field that includes the heart may also be causative. Chest pain is a prominent symptom and is typically made worse by lying supine and improved by sitting up and leaning forward. Heart sounds are usually muffled because of pericardial fluid accumulation and there is tachycardia, tachypnea, and a diminished pulse pressure due to reduced systolic and increased diastolic pressures. Echocardiography is a precise diagnostic test and treatment may be surgical (pericardial window or total pericardectomy) or radiation therapy for

- 243 -

those who have not received prior chest radiation. In an extreme emergency situation, transthoracic needle pericardiocentesis is indicated.

121. B: In patients with DIC, treatment of the underlying disease is always primary but in the patient described it may be delayed or impossible. Supportive therapy is therefore required. This patient has relatively minor bleeding so that an immediate packed RBC transfusion is not necessary. Hemoglobin (Hb) and hematocrit (Hct) should be followed aggressively and transfusion given if the Hb falls below 8 g/dL or brisk bleeding ensues. Administration of platelet concentrates is indicated for active bleeding or counts below 20,000. Heparin, which might be antithrombotic, is dangerous in a situation with brain metastases and possible intracranial bleeding. Warfarin (Coumadin) is a vitamin K–dependent anticoagulant and is contraindicated.

122. A: Cancer patients undergoing treatment are at higher than average risk for infectious complications and possible sepsis. The single most important factor that places the patient at high risk for sepsis is granulocytopenia. The granulocyte count nadir usually occurs 7 to 10 days after chemotherapy, although this may be modified somewhat with the use of granulocyte colony-stimulating factor. Hospitalization, especially in an ICU setting, tends to expose the patient to more virulent organisms. Underlying diseases such as diabetes or organ-related disorders also increase the risk. Cellular and/or humoral immunity is diminished in many cancers, especially where the bone marrow is compromised as in leukemia. Invasive appliances such as indwelling PICC lines or urinary catheters or endotracheal intubation with respiratory therapy also increase the risk, patients older than 65 are also at higher risk of sepsis.

123. B: This patient is a prime candidate for tumor lysis: a highly proliferative tumor treated with chemotherapy and without apparent preventive measures. Rapid destruction of malignant cells results in hyperkalemia, hyperphosphatemia, hypocalcemia, and elevated uric acid. In this patient with the ECG changes as described, potassium levels greater than 6.5 mEq/L are likely and steps to reduce this should be taken immediately as a life-threatening arrhythmia may occur. IV calcium gluconate or glucose and insulin and exchange resin (Kayexalate) orally or by enema are possible treatments. Oliguria or anuria may occur so that brisk diuresis should be induced with IV hydration, loop diuretics, or mannitol. Alkalinization of the urine with bicarbonate may preclude uric acid nephropathy and aid potassium lowering. Additional chemotherapy or withholding calcium and giving potassium are obviously contraindicated.

124. D: This woman with a history of stage II premenopausal, hormone-negative breast cancer is at an increased risk of recurrent disease. While brain metastases may occur, spread of the cancer to bone with osteolytic lesions is more likely. Her symptoms are strongly suggestive of hypercalcemia: confusion, muscle weakness, constipation, and polyuria are typical symptoms of an elevated serum calcium. Her ECG findings are also typical for hypocalcemia. There is no suggestion by symptomatology or ECG of premature coronary disease. Most likely, the bone scan will be positive for osseous lesions. It should be noted that hormone-positive breast cancer patients may be taking tamoxifen (Nolvadex), which has been reported to be an occasional cause or trigger for hypercalcemia. This drug should be inquired about and temporarily discontinued until the full clinical situation is known.

125. A: A history of allergies and immediate hypersensitivity reactions experienced by the patient must be obtained and noted prominently on the chart and perhaps the wrist identification bracelet in hospitalized patients, but this is not emergent in this situation. Several chemotherapy agents, especially a bacterial product such as asparaginase, may cause immediate hypersensitivity reactions and result in anaphylaxis. Skin testing and premedication with antihistamines (types H1 and H2), acetaminophen, and possibly a corticosteroid is usually indicated for a high-risk individual

and even for those without an allergic history. In the event of a suspected drug reaction, the drug should be discontinued immediately and the IV line maintained with normal saline at a rapid rate. Vital signs must be checked quickly. If wheezing or stridor is present, the possibility of laryngospasm must be considered. Epinephrine 1:1000 solution should be administered, oxygen given, and arrangements for emergency intubation made. If significant hypotension is present, dopamine or other pressor is indicated.

126. C: Spinal cord compression is a common complication of metastatic cancer and may range from mild impairment of motor, sensory, and autonomic nerve function to complete paralysis of the extremities. Primary tumors of the spinal cord such as ependymoma, astrocytoma or glioma may also cause this syndrome. Lumbosacral involvement often leads to bowel and/or bladder dysfunction that is quite disconcerting for the patient. Some of the bladder function may be enhanced by encouraging foods to keep the urine pH under 7. Instruction in self-catheterization if needed, limiting fluid intake after 7 PM, and palpation of the bladder after voiding are additional measures to assist bladder function. Many of these patients become constipated, so adequate fluid intake, stool softeners and laxatives, and checking for fecal impaction are all appropriate measures.

127. A: Sexuality is an important part of life and is affected by many different cancers and/or their treatment. It is imperative for the oncology nurse to be aware of both the physical and psychological manifestations that the diagnosis and therapy cause. The anatomy and normal functioning of the sexual organs and the common causes of impairment in cancer patients are basic. Too often nurses and other professional staff will not initiate discussion of these matters with patients for fear of embarrassment or engendering patient hostility. Discussions of intimate matters should not be feared and avoided. If there are complex problems that require expert knowledge, appropriate consultation from a sex counselor, gynecologist, or urologist is in order.

128. B: Conception and pregnancy during cancer diagnostic testing and treatment often raise thorny issues. In general, it is best avoided at least until one-year post treatment. While different birth control methods may be suggested, caution is advised since hormonal methods may enhance growth of some tumors. Prescription of birth control methods should be by a physician or nurse practitioner; it is inappropriate to provide birth control appliances or drugs to the patient. Women already pregnant, especially in the first trimester when the fetus is most sensitive, present a difficult problem if radiation therapy or chemotherapy is scheduled. In some cases, treatment of slow-growing tumors may be deferred until later in the pregnancy and radiation shielding of the pelvis and use of drugs that do not cross the placenta may be employed. While an abortion is a consideration, it is such a controversial matter and subject to so many social, religious, and cultural factors that a firm recommendation is best avoided. In non-pregnant patients, it is best to advise delay of conception.

129. C: Pregnant patient undergoing diagnostic imaging studies present a problem. Plain x-rays may not be adequate and present a radiation risk to the fetus. However, bilateral mammography exposes the fetus to less than 500 cGy radiation and perhaps adequate shielding may reduce this even further. CT scans emit high-dose radiation and though reliable diagnostically, many oncologists would order MRI scanning for a pregnant patient. Radioactive isotopic scans (e.g., bone, thyroid, and lung) expose the fetus to radiation and should be avoided if possible. Serum tumor markers are safe but may not be reliable in a pregnant patient where nonspecific elevation and false-positive results are possible. Ultrasound is safe in that it does not emit ionizing radiation and is usually accurate. It may be wise to obtain a pregnancy test on all females of childbearing age before decisions regarding diagnosis and therapy are made.

130. B: Nearly all combination chemotherapy results in some degree of infertility in males. For this reason, pretreatment sperm collection and banking is advised. Of the listed treatment regimens, ABVD is the least toxic to spermatogenesis; about 35% of men receiving this combination will have fertility affected and it usually recovers. MOPP will cause infertility in about 80% of patients. Radiation to the pelvis will also cause oligospermia and sterility, permanent if the dose is greater than 5 cGy. High-dose cytotoxic conditioning treatment before bone marrow transplantation will usually cause permanent sterility. Therefore, in males, sperm banking, gonadal shielding, and careful selection of chemotherapy drugs is standard treatment.

131. A: Decreased vaginal lubrication from nerve or vascular damage by pelvic radiation is common. A premature menopause may result that may have considerable consequence for sexual function. Painful intercourse (dyspareunia) and resulting loss of sexual desire are not uncommon sequelae. Diminution of vascular supply makes the area more susceptible to infection and loss of sexual pleasure. Chemotherapy with certain drugs may also result in similar anatomic changes and physiologic dysfunction. In these patients, hormone therapy and sexual counseling may be appropriate. There are certain products that enhance libido and clitoral blood flow that may improve sexual experience. Pelvic floor exercises and even vaginal reconstruction in women may improve sexual functioning and pleasure.

132. A: Several cancers are associated with HIV/AIDS, including Kaposi sarcoma and primary lymphomas of the brain, as well as more typical non-Hodgkin lymphomas. In addition, there appears to be an increased incidence of squamous cell carcinoma of the cervix and perhaps Hodgkin lymphoma in HIV-positive patients, but no clear causation has been established. Since the advent of highly active antiretroviral therapy (HAART), the incidence of malignancies, especially Kaposi sarcoma, is declining. The virus may be transmitted to an uninfected partner by vaginal, rectal, or oral routes, so a condom should be used for all sexual activity that involves penetration or external manipulation of these structures. Water-based lubricant is preferred since petroleum or cream-based lubricants are more likely to weaken the condom; breakage may occur and permit viral transmission. Abstention from sex, though effective in avoiding transmission of HIV, is usually not a practical solution.

133. C: A variety of excuses interferes with sexual counseling by nurses, such as: the patient is not interested, someone else will do it, I don't have the time, or I don't know enough about it. The PLISSIT system is a model for sexual counseling based on a nurse's knowledge and comfort in discussing sexual matters with a patient. P stands for permission; all nurses should be able to inquire about sexual concerns and discuss effects of treatment without guilt or embarrassment; LI indicates limited information, the next step which most nurses can incorporate into their comfort zone and knowledge base; and SS refers to specific suggestions such as proposing the use of topical hormone vaginal creams for women or possible use of erectile dysfunction treatments for men. IT refers to intensive therapy that requires an expert sexual counselor or mental health practitioner, often based on long-standing sexual and psychological problems.

134. C: Surgical procedures, both curative and palliative, may have profound effects on sexuality in cancer patients. Some are direct and obvious, such as bilateral orchiectomy in which both testes are removed (castration). Others are indirect, such as nerve injury during prostatectomy that may lead to impotence and incontinence. BSO and TAH in women may have direct and indirect effects (vaginal dryness, diminished libido). Some procedures, far removed from the genitalia, will also have effects on a patient's sexuality. For example, mastectomy or facial surgery may lead to psychological problems and a sense of altered body image and loss of sexual attractiveness for both patient and partner. Ostomy surgery falls into a similar category. Oophoropexy is used to move the

ovaries out of the field for pelvic or lower abdominal radiation. It has about a 50% chance of preserving fertility and usually does not affect sexuality.

135. D: Return of the cancer is the most obvious fear. Financial concerns are also a great source of anxiety among cancer patients, including loss of wages and job position; adequate insurance coverage and ability to obtain coverage after cancer treatment; and ability to pay for high cost of hospital and drug expenses. Employment problems and job benefits should be discussed with a labor and employment attorney; there are several federal and state laws governing discrimination against cancer survivors and those with disabilities. People, even family members, often treat cancer survivors differently or avoid them, leading to social or personal isolation, sometimes accompanied by feelings of guilt for having survived. Many long-term side effects and disabilities are associated with cancer treatment, including surgical, chemotherapy, or radiation. Consider referral to a support or self-help group for cancer survivors.

136. C: The American Cancer Society has developed a four-point cancer survivors' "bill of rights" to enhance the quality of life for cancer survivors and educate the public and health care professionals. The major categories are: 1) the right to lifelong medical care, as needed; 2) the right to the pursuit of happiness; 3) equal job opportunities including privacy of their medical history and advancement based on ability; 4) ensure adequate health insurance coverage. Even if survivorship has been prolonged, patient complaints should not be dismissed by health care professionals. Although fear of recurrence diminishes with time, complete freedom from worry is probably an impossible goal. Health insurance coverage may be a difficult problem for cancer survivors as they often are consigned to the "preexisting condition" exclusion or subject to astronomical premiums.

137. B: Several acts of Congress have precluded cancer survivors and others with disabilities from workplace discrimination. Cancer survivors often face numerous employment-related problems, such as demotion or lack of promotion, job loss, and inability to change jobs because of fear of loss of insurance benefits, and possible avoidance or special treatment by coworkers. Several pieces of federal legislation have assisted those with disabilities or those perceived as having disabilities by prospective employers. These include the Federal Rehabilitation Act of 1973 and the Americans with Disabilities Act of 1990. Social security disability is intended for those who are disabled and unable to work for longer than six months. The Taft-Hartley Act involves labor law and collective bargaining but does not specifically address employment discrimination against those with a history of cancer.

138. A: Nearly all chemotherapeutic drugs have acute and long-term side effects. While many of the acute effects are short-lived or reversible, some of the long-term effects are not. Factors that may influence chronic toxicity are cumulative dose of the drug, the nature of the tumor, combination with other drugs or radiation, and the presence of underlying disease prior to the cancer treatment. Methotrexate and actinomycin D may cause hepatic fibrosis or cirrhosis. Liver biopsy is sometimes indicated in patients who have received these drugs and develop abnormal liver function tests. Cardiotoxicity is the chief long-term side effect of doxorubicin, which is subject to cumulative dose and any underlying heart disease. Pulmonary fibrosis is the main consequence of bleomycin and peripheral neuropathy of vincristine. Long-term follow-up is indicated for any cancer survivor who has received chemotherapy.

139. C: Development of a second malignancy as a long-term consequence of cancer chemotherapy and/or radiation is among the major fears of cancer survivors. Intelligent choice of chemotherapy regimens and radiation shielding and dose-fractionation schedules may diminish but not eliminate the likelihood of a second cancer unrelated to the one treated. Breast cancer and soft-tissue

- 247 -

sarcomas may arise after chest irradiation. The overall risk of second malignancies is relatively low and should not preclude optimal treatment of the initial cancer. In addition to solid tumors, acute and occasionally chronic leukemias may arise, especially in those patients receiving alkylating agents. Although the incidence is low, cancer survivors must be warned of this possibility so that symptoms are not be ignored and long-term medical follow-up is indicated.

140. B: Oncology nursing assessment of a cancer survivor should include identification of the stage of survival: acute (still undergoing treatment); extended (treatment completed or on maintenance therapy); or permanent (long-term survival, "cured"). History of treatment including surgery, chemotherapy, radiation, and biotherapy should be noted and recorded. Attention should be paid to the risk of recurrent disease, chronic signs or symptoms, and delayed onset of symptoms that may be related to original treatment. The impulse to criticize the treatment the patient has undergone should be suppressed because this may lead to conflict with other members of the health care team and even lawsuits (e.g., telling a prostate cancer patient complaining of impotence and incontinence that he should have had radioactive implants rather than a prostatectomy).

141. D: Vincristine, etoposide (VP-16), and cisplatin can all cause a peripheral neuropathy, and in the case of vincristine this side effect is the dose-limiting toxicity. The usual manifestations are tingling, numbness, and loss of reflexes in the extremities. Nerve conduction studies performed before and after treatment may document the presence and severity of the nerve damage. Ototoxicity (hearing loss) may be caused by cisplatin and other platinum-containing drugs. It may be severe and there is no current treatment that is reliable. Audiometry before and during treatment may be indicated. Aminoglycoside antibiotics also may cause ototoxicity and are best avoided while a patient is undergoing treatment with cisplatin. It is thought that both drugs may bind to melanin in the small vessels of the cochlea or generate reactive oxygen species (free radicals). Dexamethasone is a corticosteroid and does not cause neuropathy or hearing loss.

142. C: Both cyclophosphamide (Cytoxan) and chlorambucil (Leukeran) may interfere with oogenesis and spermatogenesis, leading to sterility in both sexes, which is sometimes irreversible. Dose and duration of therapy are determining factors as is the state of gonadal function prior to treatment. Cyclophosphamide may cause amenorrhea with decreased estrogen and increased gonadotropin levels in women but normal menses is usually restored several months after therapy is completed. The drug may be teratogenic so that pregnancy should be discouraged during treatment and birth control recommended. Chlorambucil may cause chromosome damage and both reversible and permanent sterility in both sexes has been reported. This drug may also cause amenorrhea. Autopsy studies of ovaries in women receiving this drug have shown fibrosis, vasculitis, and depletion of primary follicles.

143. A: Second malignancies are not uncommon in patients with Hodgkin lymphoma who have received combination chemotherapy containing alkylating agents or combined with radiation therapy. The most frequent solid malignant neoplasm (SMN) reported were those of the lung, gastrointestinal tract, and female breast. According to one study, the overall 25-year follow-up data of 1111 patients of all age groups showed an SMN rate of nearly 20%. There was a decrease in the risk after 25 years of survival. The overall leukemia risk at 15 years post treatment, according to a second study, was 4.2% with two peaks: 3 and 8 years after treatment. Those who had extended-field radiation therapy or combination chemotherapy with alkylating agents had the highest risk. Those who received involved field radiation only had a lower risk. No leukemias were found in those who received combination chemotherapy with ABVD (Adriamycin, bleomycin, vinblastine, and dacarbazine).

144. C: Suicidal behavior, substance abuse, social withdrawal, and anger and/or violent outbursts may all be manifestations of social dysfunction in cancer patients, even in long-term survivors. Support groups or individual counseling should be suggested to the patient. Family should be made to understand the stress the patient is undergoing and remedial suggestions are appropriate. Professional evaluation and pharmacologic treatment may be needed and should be discussed with the patient's physician. The patient should be made aware of his or her strengths in coping with a difficult time and perhaps a depressive outlook on the future. Activities or work that the patient previously enjoyed should be encouraged. Spiritual and cultural practices should also be encouraged in order to bring the survivor back into social integration.

145. B: Bone marrow transplant (BMT) patients are susceptible to numerous infectious agents, ordinary and opportunistic. The risk of various infections may be divided into those that are most likely to occur acutely (first month after transplant), then 1 to 4 months and 4 to 12 months after transplant. Long-term survivors (more than 1 year) are still at risk of certain organisms. VZV and cytomegalovirus (CMV) are two viruses that may attack at this late stage. The former causes a typical zoster rash (shingles) while the latter may invade pulmonary or hepatic sites. *Aspergillus* is a fungus that may infect sinuses and lungs, skin, and central nervous system but usually during the initial year after BMT. Pneumocystis carinii is a protozoan opportunist that may cause pneumonia during the first year after BMT but is less likely in long-term survivors. *S. aureus* infections may occur at any time, especially on skin or in sinopulmonary sites, but is less common in survivors after one year.

146. C: Hemorrhagic cystitis is common after high-dose cyclophosphamide or ifosfamide chemotherapy and may be persistent after the cessation of treatment. It is usually accompanied by pain in the bladder area and hematuria and sometimes dysuria. Preventive measures include high volume fluids with frequent voiding before and during chemotherapy or continuous bladder irrigation. A chemoprotective agent such as mesna may also be given intravenously or as a pill before or during the chemotherapy. The drug leaves a bad taste, so addition of strong-flavored liquids to the oral preparation is recommended. There are few other side effects. Antispasmodics and analgesics may also be given to the patient to diminish discomfort.

147. A: Oncology nursing interventions are critical to good patient care and the patient's resumption of as "normal" a life as possible. Guidelines for different phases of the illness and survivorship have been developed to assist oncology nurses' participation in patient care. For acute stage patients, informing the patient and family about survivorship potential and referral to support groups, within the hospital setting or in the community, may ease the burden of the diagnosis on the patient and family. Developing guidelines for continuing care and relating this to patient and family is an important step during the extended stage of treatment. Keeping the family informed and enlisting their support is also an appropriate measure during this second phase. For long-term permanent stage survivors, encouragement to resume previous personal and public activities and social interactions is valuable for many patients.

148. C: Grief is the emotional response to loss. In cancer patients, this loss may include the diagnosis, poor prognosis, questionable results, and possible recurrence. These are all possible reasons for grief among the patient's friends and loved ones, with prolonged disability and death as obvious bases for the grieving process. Crying, painful dejection, outbursts of anger, and changes in eating, sleeping, or sexual habits are typical grief responses and are considered normal. Persistence of these for long periods is considered abnormal and dysfunctional. Depression, which shares some of the same symptoms, should not be confused with normal dejection. Some symptoms of the dysfunctional grieving process are refusal to mourn, prolonged denial of the loss, and somatic complaints (e.g., headaches, gastrointestinal disturbances, muscular tension).

149. A: The nurse should attempt to assist the patient and/or family members with the grieving process. Interventions should be respectful and supportive but obvious deleterious thoughts and behavior should be discouraged. Prolonged dependence on alcohol or sleeping pills or suicidal thoughts must be discouraged and referral for professional counseling strongly considered. On the other hand, encouragement of social relationships and support group participation is often valuable. Cultural, religious, or ethnic customs in dealing with death and dying may assist many individuals with the grieving process and avoid development of dysfunctional attitudes or behavior. Verbal expressions of thoughts about the dying or departed are often useful in relieving sadness and guilt, and may be expressed to lay persons or professional individuals (counselors, psychologists, and clergy).

150. B: Palliative care for the dying patient or one with an incurable disease is an important responsibility of an oncology nurse. The decision to stop aggressive treatment and continue only that which provides symptomatic relief is often difficult and subject to ambivalence on the part of the patient and/or family. Both physician and nurse should counsel them and present options, but the decision should not be dictated. Hospice care is an excellent option where expertise in palliative care is available, along with medical and psychological support. However, palliative care may be offered in a hospital or home setting. Most disabling symptoms should be addressed initially (e.g., dyspnea, pain, altered consciousness). It should be noted that palliative care does not necessarily require the cessation of disease-directed treatment with chemotherapy drugs or radiation because these may provide some symptomatic relief.

151. D: Management of cancer pain at the end of life is a complex and frequently contentious issue. Many physicians are not well schooled in pain management and there is often a tendency to overmedicate or undermedicate the patient. Basic principles include oral analgesia followed by IV if the former is not successful; use of adjuvant drugs such as steroids, antidepressives, or anticonvulsants; prescribing analgesia on a regular, around-the-clock schedule with provision for managing "breakthrough" pain. While most pain in terminal cancer patients is related to the cancer itself (75%), some may be due to treatment-related causes (e.g., mucositis, radiation dermatitis). Neurologic procedures for pain relief may be considered if anatomically possible: intraspinal or epidural infusion of painkillers or direct procedures on nerves such as chemical blockade.

152. C: A stepwise approach to managing constipation should be used in cancer patients receiving opioid analgesics or other drugs that tend to impair normal bowel function. Some other cancer-related problems also provoke a reduction in peristalsis such as dehydration, hypercalcemia, low-fiber diet, or spinal cord damage. Senna is most useful as a prophylactic agent to be given to those patients in whom a constipation problem is anticipated. The laxative may be switched to bisacodyl (Dulcolax) if there is no bowel movement within 48 hours. If there is no bowel movement in any 72-hour period, one should check for impaction; if it is present, disimpaction followed by enemas until clear is a reasonable treatment. If impaction is not present, one or more of several laxatives may be tried: magnesium citrate, magnesium with mineral oil, lactulose, or phosphate enemas. Efforts to correct other contributors should also be undertaken: hydration, high-fiber diet, or correction of metabolic abnormalities.

153. A: Many dying cancer patients complain of shortness of breath or difficulty breathing. This may be more distressing to some than pain. Blood gases should be checked and if hypoxia is present, then oxygen therapy is indicated. Some patients are not hypoxic and the sensation of dyspnea may have other causes (e.g., anemia, elevated carbon dioxide). Replacement of lung tissue by a primary lung cancer is a common cause as is metastatic disease to the lung, with or without pleural effusion or pneumothorax. The latter may be treated with intrapleural chest tube placement and suction. Sometimes patients are so weak that chest or even diaphragmatic muscle is unable to sustain a full

respiratory excursion. In all cases, oral or more likely IV opioids should be considered because this will usually provide some symptomatic relief. Ventilator therapy may be considered but may be excessive treatment in a terminal patient.

154. B: Both anorexia and cachexia may occur in terminal cancer patients but are distinct in nature and probably cause. Anorexia is a loss of appetite and a reluctance to eat that leads to weight loss but may be reversible with careful food preparation and/or drugs that stimulate the appetite. Cachexia is a metabolic syndrome, sometimes referred to as wasting, in which there is a loss of muscle and body fat and bone mineral content. It is generally irreversible. Enteral feeding may be helpful but one must consider the discomfort to the patient and the prognosis. This treatment has been the source of controversy in end-of-life care, often leading to conflict among family members. Parenteral feeding is sometimes tried but is usually inappropriate in the end-stage cancer patient.

155. D: Nausea and/or vomiting are very common in terminal cancer patients and every effort should be made to offer relief from this discomforting symptom. There are many causes. Gastrointestinal irritation, obstruction, and hepatobiliary disease are all possible, and treatment may require a change of diet, oral antacids, or bowel decompression. Chemotherapy and radiation are notorious causes and may be ameliorated with a variety of antiemetic drugs. Other drugs such as opioids, antibiotics, or anticonvulsants may also be emetogenic. Increased intracranial pressure from a brain primary or metastatic tumor and cerebral edema may also lead to nausea and vomiting. Fluid and electrolyte imbalances and hypercalcemia may be at fault and require correction if possible. Finally psychogenic factors such as fear and anxiety may be responsible and should be addressed with appropriate medication.

156. D: The subject of terminal or total sedation of the dying patient is controversial and has been the basis of lawsuits against the ordering physician or hospital and nursing staff. While refractory pain, dyspnea, agitation, and restlessness are all possible indications, dose is critical if accusations of euthanasia are to be avoided. Consent of the patient, if possible, or family is imperative. One should attempt all reasonable palliative measures before deciding on this course. Still, it is widely used and not always well documented in the medical record and permission is not always obtained. While there may be an empathic desire to relieve the patient by "turning up the morphine," this impulse should be resisted unless permission is obtained and the order well documented.

157. A: Cancer patients often display signs and symptoms of delirium at the end of life. This may take the form of hallucinations, meaningless verbal communication, altered consciousness, and possibly progress to coma. It may fluctuate so that at one time during the day the patient is quite rational while at another he or she is not. Preterminal restlessness and agitation may accompany the pattern. The causes are numerous and include steroids or opioid analgesics, tumor directly affecting the central nervous system, toxic or metabolic abnormalities that affect the brain, or local and remote effects of infection. If a definite cause is found, specific measures may be taken to reverse the delirium, if available. Delirium is often very upsetting to family who may wish to converse with the patient before death.

158. A: There are six categories in the standards of care for the oncology nurse: 1) assessment in which the nurse collects health data from the patient; diagnosis in which the assessment data is analyzed and a 2) nursing diagnosis made; 3) expected outcome; 4) planning in which the nurse develops an individual and holistic plan of care to achieve the desired outcome; 5) implementation in which the plan of care is carried out; and 6) evaluation in which the result of the interventions are evaluated and modified if required. Prescription is not usually assigned to nursing care since it remains the responsibility of the physician. However, suggestions for therapy are always in order

and a collegial relationship with other members of the health care team is usually beneficial to the patient.

159. B: Evidence-based practice is the use of valid clinical evidence, usually derived from well-designed trials, which should offer the cancer patient the best possible and most cost-effective outcome. All too often, decisions regarding patient care are made on the basis of the nurse or physician's personal experience and may not be supported in the medical literature. Anecdotal evidence is often used but should not take precedence over scientifically based and statistically significant data. Peer review is an essential part of developing new or alternative therapies and should be mandatory when evaluating new treatments. The nurse is expected to be familiar with current knowledge and treatment protocols for cancer therapy. Attending lectures and discussions and reading of professional journals are strongly recommended.

160. A: The oncology nurse is the individual largely responsible for patient education in self-care and in signs and symptoms of disease recurrence, oncologic emergencies, and side effects of treatment. Most hospital oncology units and outpatient clinics have written detailed instructions covering these matters and what to do in case they occur. However, it is the nurse's responsibility to go over the list with the patient and/or family to be sure there is an understanding of all aspects of at-home care. Some examples include management of indwelling venous access devices such as a central venous catheter, what to do in case of fever, treatment of mucositis caused by chemotherapy, diet and hydration measures, and what to do in case of emergency. Information on getting a second opinion is a very fragile subject and should not be routinely included. The patient doesn't need to be taught that there are many types of learning styles, the nurse only needs to figure out the patient's learning style and teach him this way. Extensive psychological counseling should be referred to a professional.

161. C: The most common cause of error by nurses (including oncology nurses) is that of dispensing medication: failure to give the prescribed drug, administration of the wrong drug, or a dosing mistake. In the late 1990s, the Institute of Medicine issued a study that claimed 98,000 hospital deaths annually were caused by medication errors; a recent follow-up showed not much has changed. Certainty in administering medications is particularly important for oncology nurses who deal with chemotherapy drugs that have a high morbidity and mortality if the wrong drug or dose is given. Computerized orders and pharmacy preparation of dangerous drugs may alleviate this situation somewhat, but if there is doubt, double-checking is always in order. Incomplete or absent documentation in the medical record is another possible source of negligence that may lead to patient injury. Failure to educate the patient or monitor the patient in restraints are both deviations from the standard of care but are less common.

162. B: This is an admittedly difficult situation but one that comes up often. If the patient is disoriented and judged unable to give permission for informed consent, much depends on how emergent the situation is and how promptly must treatment be given. If the patient has signed a power of attorney for health care and appointed someone specific as his medical representative, that person (usually a family member or occasionally a lawyer) should be contacted. If not, a close family member may be adequate. If no one is reachable and the situation is grave, then an emergency may be declared and the surgery begun without informed consent. This should be well documented in the medical record, preferably by two staff members. If the situation is such that medical treatment may be employed temporarily, an appropriate representative may be contacted or the patient's mental state may improve enough to sign an informed consent document.

163. B: A phase I trial, often using a limited number of subjects, is intended to establish the appropriate dose and schedule for humans and to exclude major toxicities. Phase II, usually using

more study subjects, is designed to test the drug's efficacy against a particular form of cancer and if side effects are associated with it. Therefore, the drug described in the question would be ready for a phase II trial. If the drug has significant activity and manageable side effects, then a phase III study comparing it with the best available treatment for the cancer is next. This trial usually involves a greater number of randomized patients and strict clinical guidelines established as to which patients may enter the study. Phase IV refers to a long-term study that will determine delayed side effects and efficacy of the drug over time. This type study is less common and most new drugs will enter the market prior to completion of long-term analysis.

164. A: There have been many recent news accounts of sanctions against nurses from state boards. The greatest publicity has been for those accused and/or convicted of felonies, including kidnapping, murder of patients, euthanasia, and stealing controlled drugs for personal use or sale. All of these are grounds for criminal action and revocation of a nursing license. Although state boards vary in their policies, misdemeanors may result in sanctions but rarely complete loss of license. Substance abuse, negligence, and unprofessional conduct are also adequate reasons for loss of license. Some of these unprofessional activities may be handled at the institutional level without reporting to the state board but different states and medical institutions have varying policies. Acts of omission and commission may be subject to termination of employment alone.

165. C: Collaborative relationships with other members of the health care team or an administrator is an ideal that is often not obtained. The great tendency in medical facilities for individuals to stake out a particular area based on specialty knowledge or administrative methods may interfere with optimal patient care or simply work against a pleasant employment environment. A perceived threat to autonomy is especially common among physicians but may also be a problem with nurses or any staff member with supervisory or specialty responsibilities. Often, communication between members of the health care team or administrators is fraught with difficulty because neither party will recognize the other's knowledge or experience. Disputes may arise in front of patients, leading to a lack of confidence or trust in one or more members of the professional staff. This should obviously be avoided.

How to Overcome Test Anxiety

Just the thought of taking a test is enough to make most people a little nervous. A test is an important event that can have a long-term impact on your future, so it's important to take it seriously and it's natural to feel anxious about performing well. But just because anxiety is normal, that doesn't mean that it's helpful in test taking, or that you should simply accept it as part of your life. Anxiety can have a variety of effects. These effects can be mild, like making you feel slightly nervous, or severe, like blocking your ability to focus or remember even a simple detail.

If you experience test anxiety—whether severe or mild—it's important to know how to beat it. To discover this, first you need to understand what causes test anxiety.

Causes of Test Anxiety

While we often think of anxiety as an uncontrollable emotional state, it can actually be caused by simple, practical things. One of the most common causes of test anxiety is that a person does not feel adequately prepared for their test. This feeling can be the result of many different issues such as poor study habits or lack of organization, but the most common culprit is time management. Starting to study too late, failing to organize your study time to cover all of the material, or being distracted while you study will mean that you're not well prepared for the test. This may lead to cramming the night before, which will cause you to be physically and mentally exhausted for the test. Poor time management also contributes to feelings of stress, fear, and hopelessness as you realize you are not well prepared but don't know what to do about it.

Other times, test anxiety is not related to your preparation for the test but comes from unresolved fear. This may be a past failure on a test, or poor performance on tests in general. It may come from comparing yourself to others who seem to be performing better or from the stress of living up to expectations. Anxiety may be driven by fears of the future—how failure on this test would affect your educational and career goals. These fears are often completely irrational, but they can still negatively impact your test performance.

> **Review Video:** 3 Reasons You Have Test Anxiety
> Visit mometrix.com/academy and enter code: 428468

Elements of Test Anxiety

As mentioned earlier, test anxiety is considered to be an emotional state, but it has physical and mental components as well. Sometimes you may not even realize that you are suffering from test anxiety until you notice the physical symptoms. These can include trembling hands, rapid heartbeat, sweating, nausea, and tense muscles. Extreme anxiety may lead to fainting or vomiting. Obviously, any of these symptoms can have a negative impact on testing. It is important to recognize them as soon as they begin to occur so that you can address the problem before it damages your performance.

> **Review Video:** 3 Ways to Tell You Have Test Anxiety
> Visit mometrix.com/academy and enter code: 927847

The mental components of test anxiety include trouble focusing and inability to remember learned information. During a test, your mind is on high alert, which can help you recall information and stay focused for an extended period of time. However, anxiety interferes with your mind's natural processes, causing you to blank out, even on the questions you know well. The strain of testing during anxiety makes it difficult to stay focused, especially on a test that may take several hours. Extreme anxiety can take a huge mental toll, making it difficult not only to recall test information but even to understand the test questions or pull your thoughts together.

> **Review Video:** How Test Anxiety Affects Memory
> Visit mometrix.com/academy and enter code: 609003

Effects of Test Anxiety

Test anxiety is like a disease—if left untreated, it will get progressively worse. Anxiety leads to poor performance, and this reinforces the feelings of fear and failure, which in turn lead to poor performances on subsequent tests. It can grow from a mild nervousness to a crippling condition. If allowed to progress, test anxiety can have a big impact on your schooling, and consequently on your future.

Test anxiety can spread to other parts of your life. Anxiety on tests can become anxiety in any stressful situation, and blanking on a test can turn into panicking in a job situation. But fortunately, you don't have to let anxiety rule your testing and determine your grades. There are a number of relatively simple steps you can take to move past anxiety and function normally on a test and in the rest of life.

> **Review Video:** How Test Anxiety Impacts Your Grades
> Visit mometrix.com/academy and enter code: 939819

Physical Steps for Beating Test Anxiety

While test anxiety is a serious problem, the good news is that it can be overcome. It doesn't have to control your ability to think and remember information. While it may take time, you can begin taking steps today to beat anxiety.

Just as your first hint that you may be struggling with anxiety comes from the physical symptoms, the first step to treating it is also physical. Rest is crucial for having a clear, strong mind. If you are tired, it is much easier to give in to anxiety. But if you establish good sleep habits, your body and mind will be ready to perform optimally, without the strain of exhaustion. Additionally, sleeping well helps you to retain information better, so you're more likely to recall the answers when you see the test questions.

Getting good sleep means more than going to bed on time. It's important to allow your brain time to relax. Take study breaks from time to time so it doesn't get overworked, and don't study right before bed. Take time to rest your mind before trying to rest your body, or you may find it difficult to fall asleep.

> **Review Video. The Importance of Sleep for Your Brain**
> Visit mometrix.com/academy and enter code: 319338

Along with sleep, other aspects of physical health are important in preparing for a test. Good nutrition is vital for good brain function. Sugary foods and drinks may give a burst of energy but this burst is followed by a crash, both physically and emotionally. Instead, fuel your body with protein and vitamin-rich foods.

Also, drink plenty of water. Dehydration can lead to headaches and exhaustion, especially if your brain is already under stress from the rigors of the test. Particularly if your test is a long one, drink water during the breaks. And if possible, take an energy-boosting snack to eat between sections.

> **Review Video: How Diet Can Affect your Mood**
> Visit mometrix.com/academy and enter code: 624317

Along with sleep and diet, a third important part of physical health is exercise. Maintaining a steady workout schedule is helpful, but even taking 5-minute study breaks to walk can help get your blood pumping faster and clear your head. Exercise also releases endorphins, which contribute to a positive feeling and can help combat test anxiety.

When you nurture your physical health, you are also contributing to your mental health. If your body is healthy, your mind is much more likely to be healthy as well. So take time to rest, nourish your body with healthy food and water, and get moving as much as possible. Taking these physical steps will make you stronger and more able to take the mental steps necessary to overcome test anxiety.

> **Review Video: How to Stay Healthy and Prevent Test Anxiety**
> Visit mometrix.com/academy and enter code: 877894

Mental Steps for Beating Test Anxiety

Working on the mental side of test anxiety can be more challenging, but as with the physical side, there are clear steps you can take to overcome it. As mentioned earlier, test anxiety often stems from lack of preparation, so the obvious solution is to prepare for the test. Effective studying may be the most important weapon you have for beating test anxiety, but you can and should employ several other mental tools to combat fear.

First, boost your confidence by reminding yourself of past success—tests or projects that you aced. If you're putting as much effort into preparing for this test as you did for those, there's no reason you should expect to fail here. Work hard to prepare; then trust your preparation.

Second, surround yourself with encouraging people. It can be helpful to find a study group, but be sure that the people you're around will encourage a positive attitude. If you spend time with others who are anxious or cynical, this will only contribute to your own anxiety. Look for others who are motivated to study hard from a desire to succeed, not from a fear of failure.

Third, reward yourself. A test is physically and mentally tiring, even without anxiety, and it can be helpful to have something to look forward to. Plan an activity following the test, regardless of the outcome, such as going to a movie or getting ice cream.

When you are taking the test, if you find yourself beginning to feel anxious, remind yourself that you know the material. Visualize successfully completing the test. Then take a few deep, relaxing breaths and return to it. Work through the questions carefully but with confidence, knowing that you are capable of succeeding.

Developing a healthy mental approach to test taking will also aid in other areas of life. Test anxiety affects more than just the actual test—it can be damaging to your mental health and even contribute to depression. It's important to beat test anxiety before it becomes a problem for more than testing.

> **Review Video: Test Anxiety and Depression**
> Visit mometrix.com/academy and enter code: 904704

Study Strategy

Being prepared for the test is necessary to combat anxiety, but what does being prepared look like? You may study for hours on end and still not feel prepared. What you need is a strategy for test prep. The next few pages outline our recommended steps to help you plan out and conquer the challenge of preparation.

Step 1: Scope Out the Test

Learn everything you can about the format (multiple choice, essay, etc.) and what will be on the test. Gather any study materials, course outlines, or sample exams that may be available. Not only will this help you to prepare, but knowing what to expect can help to alleviate test anxiety.

Step 2: Map Out the Material

Look through the textbook or study guide and make note of how many chapters or sections it has. Then divide these over the time you have. For example, if a book has 15 chapters and you have five days to study, you need to cover three chapters each day. Even better, if you have the time, leave an extra day at the end for overall review after you have gone through the material in depth.

If time is limited, you may need to prioritize the material. Look through it and make note of which sections you think you already have a good grasp on, and which need review. While you are studying, skim quickly through the familiar sections and take more time on the challenging parts. Write out your plan so you don't get lost as you go. Having a written plan also helps you feel more in control of the study, so anxiety is less likely to arise from feeling overwhelmed at the amount to cover. A sample plan may look like this:

- Day 1: Skim chapters 1–4, study chapter 5 (especially pages 31–33)
- Day 2: Study chapters 6–7, skim chapters 8–9
- Day 3: Skim chapter 10, study chapters 11–12 (especially pages 87–90)
- Day 4: Study chapters 13–15
- Day 5: Overall review (focus most on chapters 5, 6, and 12), take practice test

Step 3: Gather Your Tools

Decide what study method works best for you. Do you prefer to highlight in the book as you study and then go back over the highlighted portions? Or do you type out notes of the important information? Or is it helpful to make flashcards that you can carry with you? Assemble the pens, index cards, highlighters, post-it notes, and any other materials you may need so you won't be distracted by getting up to find things while you study.

If you're having a hard time retaining the information or organizing your notes, experiment with different methods. For example, try color-coding by subject with colored pens, highlighters, or post-it notes. If you learn better by hearing, try recording yourself reading your notes so you can listen while in the car, working out, or simply sitting at your desk. Ask a friend to quiz you from your flashcards, or try teaching someone the material to solidify it in your mind.

Step 4: Create Your Environment

It's important to avoid distractions while you study. This includes both the obvious distractions like visitors and the subtle distractions like an uncomfortable chair (or a too-comfortable couch that makes you want to fall asleep). Set up the best study environment possible: good lighting and a comfortable work area. If background music helps you focus, you may want to turn it on, but otherwise keep the room quiet. If you are using a computer to take notes, be sure you don't have any other windows open, especially applications like social media, games, or anything else that could distract you. Silence your phone and turn off notifications. Be sure to keep water close by so you stay hydrated while you study (but avoid unhealthy drinks and snacks).

Also, take into account the best time of day to study. Are you freshest first thing in the morning? Try to set aside some time then to work through the material. Is your mind clearer in the afternoon or evening? Schedule your study session then. Another method is to study at the same time of day that you will take the test, so that your brain gets used to working on the material at that time and will be ready to focus at test time.

Step 5: Study!

Once you have done all the study preparation, it's time to settle into the actual studying. Sit down, take a few moments to settle your mind so you can focus, and begin to follow your study plan. Don't give in to distractions or let yourself procrastinate. This is your time to prepare so you'll be ready to fearlessly approach the test. Make the most of the time and stay focused.

Of course, you don't want to burn out. If you study too long you may find that you're not retaining the information very well. Take regular study breaks. For example, taking five minutes out of every hour to walk briskly, breathing deeply and swinging your arms, can help your mind stay fresh.

As you get to the end of each chapter or section, it's a good idea to do a quick review. Remind yourself of what you learned and work on any difficult parts. When you feel that you've mastered the material, move on to the next part. At the end of your study session, briefly skim through your notes again.

But while review is helpful, cramming last minute is NOT. If at all possible, work ahead so that you won't need to fit all your study into the last day. Cramming overloads your brain with more information than it can process and retain, and your tired mind may struggle to recall even previously learned information when it is overwhelmed with last-minute study. Also, the urgent nature of cramming and the stress placed on your brain contribute to anxiety. You'll be more likely to go to the test feeling unprepared and having trouble thinking clearly.

So don't cram, and don't stay up late before the test, even just to review your notes at a leisurely pace. Your brain needs rest more than it needs to go over the information again. In fact, plan to finish your studies by noon or early afternoon the day before the test. Give your brain the rest of the day to relax or focus on other things, and get a good night's sleep. Then you will be fresh for the test and better able to recall what you've studied.

Step 6: Take a practice test

Many courses offer sample tests, either online or in the study materials. This is an excellent resource to check whether you have mastered the material, as well as to prepare for the test format and environment.

Check the test format ahead of time: the number of questions, the type (multiple choice, free response, etc.), and the time limit. Then create a plan for working through them. For example, if you have 30 minutes to take a 60-question test, your limit is 30 seconds per question. Spend less time on the questions you know well so that you can take more time on the difficult ones.

If you have time to take several practice tests, take the first one open book, with no time limit. Work through the questions at your own pace and make sure you fully understand them. Gradually work up to taking a test under test conditions: sit at a desk with all study materials put away and set a timer. Pace yourself to make sure you finish the test with time to spare and go back to check your answers if you have time.

After each test, check your answers. On the questions you missed, be sure you understand why you missed them. Did you misread the question (tests can use tricky wording)? Did you forget the information? Or was it something you hadn't learned? Go back and study any shaky areas that the practice tests reveal.

Taking these tests not only helps with your grade, but also aids in combating test anxiety. If you're already used to the test conditions, you're less likely to worry about it, and working through tests until you're scoring well gives you a confidence boost. Go through the practice tests until you feel comfortable, and then you can go into the test knowing that you're ready for it.

Test Tips

On test day, you should be confident, knowing that you've prepared well and are ready to answer the questions. But aside from preparation, there are several test day strategies you can employ to maximize your performance.

First, as stated before, get a good night's sleep the night before the test (and for several nights before that, if possible). Go into the test with a fresh, alert mind rather than staying up late to study.

Try not to change too much about your normal routine on the day of the test. It's important to eat a nutritious breakfast, but if you normally don't eat breakfast at all, consider eating just a protein bar. If you're a coffee drinker, go ahead and have your normal coffee. Just make sure you time it so that the caffeine doesn't wear off right in the middle of your test. Avoid sugary beverages, and drink enough water to stay hydrated but not so much that you need a restroom break 10 minutes into the test. If your test isn't first thing in the morning, consider going for a walk or doing a light workout before the test to get your blood flowing.

Allow yourself enough time to get ready, and leave for the test with plenty of time to spare so you won't have the anxiety of scrambling to arrive in time. Another reason to be early is to select a good seat. It's helpful to sit away from doors and windows, which can be distracting. Find a good seat, get out your supplies, and settle your mind before the test begins.

When the test begins, start by going over the instructions carefully, even if you already know what to expect. Make sure you avoid any careless mistakes by following the directions.

Then begin working through the questions, pacing yourself as you've practiced. If you're not sure on an answer, don't spend too much time on it, and don't let it shake your confidence. Either skip it and come back later, or eliminate as many wrong answers as possible and guess among the remaining ones. Don't dwell on these questions as you continue—put them out of your mind and focus on what lies ahead.

Be sure to read all of the answer choices, even if you're sure the first one is the right answer. Sometimes you'll find a better one if you keep reading. But don't second-guess yourself if you do immediately know the answer. Your gut instinct is usually right. Don't let test anxiety rob you of the information you know.

If you have time at the end of the test (and if the test format allows), go back and review your answers. Be cautious about changing any, since your first instinct tends to be correct, but make sure you didn't misread any of the questions or accidentally mark the wrong answer choice. Look over any you skipped and make an educated guess.

At the end, leave the test feeling confident. You've done your best, so don't waste time worrying about your performance or wishing you could change anything. Instead, celebrate the successful completion of this test. And finally, use this test to learn how to deal with anxiety even better next time.

> **Review Video:** 5 Tips to Beat Test Anxiety
> Visit mometrix.com/academy and enter code: 570656

Important Qualification

Not all anxiety is created equal. If your test anxiety is causing major issues in your life beyond the classroom or testing center, or if you are experiencing troubling physical symptoms related to your anxiety, it may be a sign of a serious physiological or psychological condition. If this sounds like your situation, we strongly encourage you to seek professional help.

Thank You

We at Mometrix would like to extend our heartfelt thanks to you, our friend and patron, for allowing us to play a part in your journey. It is a privilege to serve people from all walks of life who are unified in their commitment to building the best future they can for themselves.

The preparation you devote to these important testing milestones may be the most valuable educational opportunity you have for making a real difference in your life. We encourage you to put your heart into it—that feeling of succeeding, overcoming, and yes, conquering will be well worth the hours you've invested.

We want to hear your story, your struggles and your successes, and if you see any opportunities for us to improve our materials so we can help others even more effectively in the future, please share that with us as well. **The team at Mometrix would be absolutely thrilled to hear from you!** So please, send us an email (support@mometrix.com) and let's stay in touch.

If you'd like some additional help, check out these other resources we offer for your exam:

http://MometrixFlashcards.com/ONCC

Additional Bonus Material

Due to our efforts to try to keep this book to a manageable length, we've created a link that will give you access to all of your additional bonus material.

Please visit **https://www.mometrix.com/bonus948/ocn** to access the information.